AF248630

Complete in All Its Parts

Complete in All Its Parts:

Nursing Education

at

the University of Iowa, 1898-1998

Lee Anderson   *Kathy Penningroth*

Introduction by Dean Melanie Dreher

Ann Arbor

THE UNIVERSITY OF MICHIGAN PRESS

Acknowledgments

The authors brought to this case study in nursing education an un-settling lack of knowledge of nurses and nursing. So, at least, it surely seemed to our collaborators in the University of Iowa College of Nursing. For that reason, we owe a generous debt of gratitude to those who guided us through a maze of contemporary nursing issues and lent insight as well into nursing's past. Their remarkable forbearance made this book possible.

Particularly deserving of mention are Geraldene Felton, dean of the college from 1981 to 1997 and currently Kelting Professor of Nursing, who gave generously of her time to push this project forward; Myrtle Kitchell Aydelotte, the college's first dean and an unstinting champion of nursing education, who a gave us the benefit of a professional lifetime spent at the center of American nursing; Laura Corbin Dustan, dean of the college from 1964 to 1972, whose enthusiasm made her own history and that of the college come alive; Etta Rasmussen, longtime professor in the college, who kindly shared her reminiscences and who, over the years, has diverted a storehouse of college documents to the University of Iowa Archives; and Eva Erickson, who provided background on the much-embattled program in nursing service administration. In addition, Professors Kathleen Buckwalter, Joanne Comi-McCloskey, Toni Tripp-Reimer, and Joann Eland each helped us to understand not only her own area of interest but also the internal workings of the college. Finally, University Archivist Earl Rogers and his staff were, as always, invaluable resources, as were the staff of the dean's office in the College of Nursing.

Special thanks go to the reviewers whose comments and suggestions made this book, whatever its faults, far better than it would otherwise have been; to Dr. Samuel Levey of the University of Iowa Program in Hospital and Health Administration, who gave the authors much of his time and counsel; and to Rebecca McDermott of the University of Michigan Press whose support and interest carried the project to a happy conclusion.

Contents

Foreword

This history of nursing education at the University of Iowa was written by persons educated as historians. Such attention to accuracy and historical details is logically consistent with the need to understand academic nursing and the nurse's role—what it has been, and what it might become.

The nationally recognized excellence of the University of Iowa College of Nursing reflects a long and illustrious history of innovation in nursing education. What eventually became known as the College of Nursing had its beginnings in 1898 as a hospital diploma program for the preparation of nurses under the auspices of the University Hospital of the State University of Iowa. Established as the Training School for Nurses, it became the School of Nursing in 1928.

In 1919 a five-year curriculum combining Liberal Arts and Nursing and leading to a Bachelor of Science degree was adopted alongside the existing graduate nurse certificate program. This plan continued until 1949 when the first students were admitted into the Bachelor of Science in Nursing degree program in the College of Nursing, which became the tenth autonomous college of the University of Iowa authorized by the State Board of Regents. In December 1971, all activities of the College of Nursing were consolidated in the new College of Nursing Building.

No single element of the history of the College of Nursing at Iowa is unique. Yet an aggregate of elements creates a distinctive environment: its work culture, its combination of baccalaureate and graduate programs, its location within a health sciences center that includes one of the largest university-owned teaching hospitals in the world, its critical mass of faculty involved in nursing research, and its collaborative relationships within and without the college. Our faculty play important roles in this state and elsewhere. All this makes the College a visible focus and rallying point for better nursing education, responding to the demands of sophisticated technology, the changing needs of patients, and the fact that health care policies have grown progressively more complex as change has become a force in its own right.

The College of Nursing has long recognized that legislators are not interested in supporting the nursing profession for nursing's sake. The orientation of legislators is that nursing is a means to an end—the overall improvement of the nation's health—not an end in itself. The real driving force behind funding nursing education, nursing practice models, and nursing research is access to care and the need to ensure that such care is high-quality and cost-effective. This means we cannot afford to think of nursing alone when we communicate with constituents outside the profession. We must be able to discuss nursing within the much broader context of health care.

One reason I was persuaded to come to Iowa was a fascination with the history of this school. The College is attentive to new challenges and has a sense of its mission, an ability to focus on goals, an orientation about consensus as strength, and a faith in itself and its destiny. Also, the faculty and staff communicate that they will be there for each other, showing love, respect, and support as friends and adversaries and as people.

It is an exciting prospect that the College is reaffirming the nature of nursing: reevaluating the viability of its historical rituals and practices and discovering nursing science and learning how to document and communicate nursing knowledge to other health care practitioners.

I have been chosen the new academic leader of this College. Leadership, however, is a complex concept, among other things a way of thinking about institutional heirs and about stewardship in terms of relationships of assets and legacy, of momentum and effectiveness, and of civility and values. Leadership is also about continuity, about institutional culture, about missions and values that guide decisions, strategies, and actions, about directions that emerge from the history and traditions of the College and from the synthesis of positions, suggestions, and ideas elicited from multiple sources throughout the College, the University, and beyond.

This manuscript sets out the traditions and the heritage, the beliefs, values, attitudes, and behaviors that have evolved over the life of this College and that have guided professional life and re-

sponsibility within its confines. In illuminating years of history
and memory and culture, it is eloquent and persuasive about change
and the College's capability to respond to new demands.

—Dean Melanie C. Dreher, January 1997

Introduction

Nurses and Nursing History

This is a case study of nursing education at a single institution, known originally as the University of Iowa Training School for Nurses, later the University of Iowa School of Nursing, and, since 1949, the University of Iowa College of Nursing.[1] It is not a general history of American nursing, although developments in nursing at large inevitably play a major part in the narrative. Nor does it purport to be a general history of nursing education in America, although this study does, to the extent practicable, view local developments within a national context. Likewise, this is not a case study of nursing education at a prestigious eastern institution, either hospital or university, but at a public university in Iowa City, Iowa, deep in the American heartland well beyond the Hudson River and the Appalachians.

Alone among the older health care professions, nursing in America has, from its origins in the late nineteenth century, always been women's work. In contrast, medicine was a fiercely defended male preserve until the 1970s, and women's gains over the past quarter century—first among the ranks of undergraduate medical students, later in graduate medical education and in medical practice, and, most recently, in academic medicine—have been hard fought and in some important respects limited. Pharmacy, too, was an overwhelmingly male profession prior to 1970, but, as pharmacy practice shifted from the pharmacist-owned corner drug store to large retail outlets and to institutional settings, women made striking advances in the profession, comprising fifty percent of the undergraduate pharmacy student population by 1980 and some forty percent of pharmacy practitioners by the mid-1990s. Notwithstanding quite recent changes in medicine, pharmacy, and some other health care professions, nursing still stands apart by virtue of its overwhelming domination by women. For such reasons, the history of nursing, more than that of any other health care profession, bears the imprint of gender.

Recent years have seen a minor renaissance in the historiography of nursing, a renaissance in keeping with the professional strides in nursing itself as well as the growing interest in and legitimacy of women's history. At the same time, the attention and resources devoted to the history of nursing, as is true of the other "allied" health care professions, pales in comparison to the case of medicine. In large part, of course, that historiographical imbalance reflects physicians' professional dominance in twentieth-century American health care and the accompanying cultural and political authority of medicine and medical science. What might be labeled the "medical phenomenon"—encompassing the astonishing growth of medical science and institutions and the equally astonishing growth of organized medicine in all its manifestations—seized the imaginations of a good many historians and funding agencies and nourished an impressive body of historical scholarship on medicine, scholarship unmatched in nursing or in any of the other health care professions.[2] Hospitals, too, have received significant scrutiny.[3]

For all that, the historiography of nursing is far richer than, say, the historiography of pharmacy or dentistry. In part, that difference reflects the prodigious efforts of nursing's early leaders. Aware perhaps of the importance of their own and their colleagues' achievements, the late nineteenth- and early twentieth-century founders of modern American nursing, most prominently Lavinia L. Dock, M. Adelaide Nutting, and Minnie Goodnow, left a sizable corpus of historical writing.[4] Useful in its own way, that early literature was nonetheless unabashedly inspirational in tone, largely uncritical in perspective, and, in the eyes of today's historians, hopelessly antiquarian in approach and in emphasis. In short, it spoke as much, if not more, about the ideals of those early nursing leaders as it did about nursing history. By and large, that somewhat "whiggish" tradition dominated nursing historiography until well past mid-century; indeed, as late as 1984, one critical reviewer lamented nursing historiography's "comatose state."[5]

A 1959 book by Richard H. Shryock was one of the first to address the history of nursing in an analytical fashion. Shryock was one of the earliest and most prominent of non-physician medical historians, and his work *The History of Nursing* displayed both the strengths and weaknesses of the author's background and interests.[6] On the one hand, it usefully placed nursing in the broader context of medicine and culture. On the other hand, it tilted heavily toward what Shryock knew best, that is, medicine; moreover, it gave scant mention, perhaps a dozen pages, to twentieth-century American nursing. Nonetheless, Shryock's book did grant much needed legitimacy to the history of nursing, and it placed nursing squarely in the domain of the new social history of American health care, a genre that Shryock helped to pioneer.

Several volumes published in the 1970s and 1980s, each markedly different yet each in some sense part of the Shryock legacy, have significantly enriched our understanding of the history of American nursing.[7] Four works in particular have done much to define the shape and texture of current historiographical debate, comprising, by unspoken consensus, a historiographical canon: Jo Ann Ashley, *Hospitals, Paternalism, and the Role of the Nurse* (1976); Barbara Melosh, *"The Physician's Hand": Work Culture and Conflict in American Nursing* (1984); Susan M. Reverby, *Ordered to Care: The Dilemma of American Nursing, 1850-1945* (1987); and Darlene Clark Hine, *Black Women In White: Racial Conflict and Cooperation in the Nursing Profession, 1890-1950* (1989).

Joanne Ashley's contribution, as the title of her book suggests, was to apply feminist history to the subject of nurses and nursing.[8] The result was a stark contrast to the whiggish "history-as-progress" motif prevalent in nursing historiography since the early twentieth century. In Ashley's formulation, the progress of nursing and nurses was in important ways stymied by cultural conventions about women and women's work and by self-serving male hospital administrators and physicians. Taking a quite different approach, Barbara Melosh applied the concepts of labor history to nursing,[9] illuminating the work culture of nursing students, private duty nurses, and hospital staff nurses and highlighting the divisions within the nursing community. Most important, Melosh's approach revealed the yawning differences in outlook between nursing elites and rank-and-file nurses, and she argued that nursing elites' dogged pursuit of professionalism, while eschewing trade unionism, was at the very least ill-advised. In turn, Susan Reverby's *Ordered to Care* was a more synthetic work than either of the above, that is, more detailed, more balanced, and more firmly grounded in both theory and related historiography.[10] Reverby revisited the theme of male-dominated institutions and their influence on the development of nursing and also explored the importance of culture in shaping views about women and women's work, views shared to a considerable extent by women as well as men. Reverby concluded that nurses were "ordered to care" within a culture in which caring—much like today's "family values"—was honored more in rhetoric than in practice.   Taking nursing historiography in a new direction, the last of the four works, Hine's *Black Women in White*, illustrated that divisions grounded in race contributed at least as much to the fragmentation of the nursing community as did divisions based on class and job status.[11]

In addition to those standard monographs, other works in nursing history have much to offer. One example is Vern and Bonnie Bullough, *The Care of the Sick: The Emergence of Modern Nursing*, which provides a brief overview of western nursing from the ancient world through the early modern period as background to developments in the nineteenth and early twentieth centuries.[12] Also, Philip and Beatrice Kalisch have published three editions of their comprehensive survey, *The Advance of American Nursing*, with the most recent edition appearing in 1995.[13] Prior to her untimely death, the University of Iowa's own Teresa Christy was well known in nursing history circles, a champion of historical research and the historical enterprise in general.[14] So, too, is M. Patricia Donahue, who, in addition to her other historical writings, has recently published a second edition of her striking pictorial history of nursing.[15] Meanwhile, other historians have addressed the history of nursing within the broader contexts of social movements and institutional developments. Examples of such literature are Sandra Beth Lewenson's incorporation of nurses in her treatment of the suffrage movement,[16] and Charles E. Rosenberg's observations on the critical importance of nursing in the making of the modern hospital.[17]

While there are, then, several rewarding book-length treatments of nursing history, the current nursing historiography suffers noticeably in the area of article literature. Not surprisingly, the oldest and best established journals in the history of the health professions are heavily weighted toward medicine. For example, a survey of the *Bulletin of the History of Medicine* uncovers just four nursing-related articles from 1980 through 1995, a total that includes one review essay.[18] A survey of the *Journal of the History of Medicine and Allied Sciences* leads to a virtually identical result. To some extent at least, those results reflect the market-driven nature of all scholarly publication and the fact that, at least until quite recently, the scholarly audience for nursing history has been sorely limited. Hence, most of the article literature in nursing history has appeared as occasional pieces in various nursing journals, and the historiography of nursing has thereby suffered on two counts. First, such work is not readily accessible to wider audiences, and, second, much of it has not been subject to the rigorous peer review that most historians would expect. One noteworthy exception is *Nursing History Review*, published annually since 1993 by the American Association for the History of Nursing, an organization that itself dates only to 1980.

As historiographical themes and treatments have evolved in nursing history, so, too, have its practitioners. Indeed, many have argued that the steady influx of non-nurse historians into the field is a principal reason for the history of nursing's recent vitality. While that trend in some sense marks nursing history's emergence as a legitimate field of inquiry, it has not been universally celebrated by nurses, many of whom jealously guard the history of nursing, objecting, first, that only nurses can fully understand their own history and, second, that nursing history should not be used to illustrate some larger, more general argument or principle. In short, such critics argue, nursing history is about nursing and ought to be done by nurses. Having said that, there appear to be exceptions; for example, Charles Rosenberg's sensitive treatment of nursing and its contributions to the modern hospital appears to have been well received.

Of course, nurses are not the first group, nor even the first of the health professions, to face the issue of who "owns" their history. Beginning in the 1960s, physicians confronted a similar unwelcome invasion by professional historians who, in the eyes of physician critics, wrote medical history without medicine, which generally meant that historians focused their attentions on political, cultural, and economic issues in medicine rather than on great men and their great discoveries. In due course, however, physicians and historians reached an accommodation, albeit sometimes uneasy. It seems likely that nurses will, of necessity, do the same.

Like physicians, nurses have routinely deployed professional iconography for didactic reasons. Also like physicians, and rightly so, nurses view professional historians as potential iconoclasts. As a result, the historian of nursing must construct a narrative sufficiently elastic to serve two quite different audiences, namely non-historian nurses and non-nurse historians, each of which brings to the table quite different expectations of what constitutes useful history. In short, nurses must accept that historians are likely to be as impatient with inspirational stories about great women in nursing as they are with tales about great men in medicine; in return, historians must not suppose that traditional academic history is, like spinach, good even for those who find it distasteful. In the end, just as the vitamins in spinach are of no use unless consumed, the only useful history is history that is read by its target audience.

The current historiography of nursing clearly shortchanges some audiences in varying degrees. It is decidedly limited in geographic terms, largely grounded in a few urban areas in the northeastern United States, admittedly a reflection in part of a parallel concentration of scholars and archival resources in the region. The current nursing historiography is also decidedly limited in chronology, concentrating on the seventy-five years from 1875 to 1950, admittedly a critical formative stage in American nursing. Nonetheless, it is also true that historians are reluctant to push the boundaries of interpretation too near the present, whether out of a preference for dealing with people long since departed and issues long since settled or out of an awareness of the inherent risks in drawing hard-and-fast conclusions about recent events.[19] Whatever the case, the limited chronological scope of the nursing historiography leaves a great deal unsaid, at this point roughly half the history of modern American nursing, including the movement of nursing education from hospitals to colleges and universities, the slow but determined growth of nursing research, and profound changes in nursing practice.

At the same time, nursing education overall has received less attention from nursing historians than it surely deserves.[20] Discussion of nursing education prior to the baccalaureate era tends to be general in nature, taking little notice of the disparate nature of diploma programs conducted in institutions ranging from small community hospitals of no more than 50 beds to major teaching hospitals of 500 beds and more.[21] Moreover, the post-World War II explosion in baccalaureate and graduate education has gone largely unremarked, notwithstanding the fact that the integration of nursing into American higher education constituted one of the great watersheds in the history of American nursing. On the one hand, of course, that omission is a simple consequence of the limited chronological scope of current nursing historiography. On the other hand, however, it echoes persistent doubts on the part of some historians and nurses alike regarding nursing elites' determined efforts to emulate the "male" model of professionalism built around state-enforced credentialing and rigorous educational standards. To critics, that strategy was at best naïve or wrong-headed and at worst destructive to the status and interests of rank-and-file nurses and the proud craft tradition they embodied.

The social and economic background of nursing education also deserves at least passing mention. For example, the founding of the University of Iowa Training School for Nurses in 1898 came roughly at the midpoint of the great age of American industrialization. An expansive and loose-fitting label, industrialization embraces a variety of phenomena, all related to one another in some fashion, including an unprecedented surge in population accompanied by unprecedented immigration and urbanization, the spread of mass production and mass marketing techniques and by consolidation in manufacturing and distribution functions, innovations in transportation and communications, an expansion in secondary and post-secondary education, and the advent of state-sanctioned professionalization in many occupations.[22] Professionalization was particularly noteworthy for having been in part a defensive reaction against the rationalizing tendencies of the marketplace—that is, the goal of would-be professionals was not to compete in the marketplace but to stand outside it.[23]

For American women, particularly unmarried women, the industrial transformation of American society during the late nineteenth and early twentieth centuries meant a greater diversity of employment opportunities.[24] In addition to the infamous factory style "sweatshops," industrialization brought new employment for women, particularly young single women, in department stores, in clerical work, in the rapidly expanding communications industry, and in the overtaxed public school system.[25] At the same time and to an increasing extent, the charitable functions of married, middle-class women, such as social work or librarianship, became salaried occupations. Apart from teaching, however, women's opportunities lay primarily in unskilled service occupations, the so-called "pink ghetto"; in particular, the emergent professions almost uniformly denied women anything more than token representation.[26]

At the turn of the century, then, nursing was one of several employment options for young women. Moreover, as a product of the astonishing growth of America's hospital system between the 1870s and 1920s, nursing also owed much, directly and indirectly, to industrialization and its by-products. As historians have abundantly documented, however, nursing was different from most other female occupations in that it was, perhaps even more so than teaching, an extension of women's accepted—and unpaid—domestic roles as caregivers and guardians of morality.[27] For nursing, that connection between domestic roles and professional function was both a blessing and a curse. It imbued nursing with an aura of service and benevolence that nurses have ever since worn with pride; yet it labeled nursing with the stigma of women's work, by definition unpaid or certainly underpaid and undervalued in modern American culture.

Nursing had much in common with other female-dominated professions. For example, women's professional role in education, particularly as elementary school teachers, affords many parallels to that of nurses. As has been well documented, women were the majority of education professionals by the early twentieth century, but they held few positions of real authority, for example, as school principals or superintendents or as faculty in schools of education. However, education was different from nursing in that education, as a recognizable profession, was far older in the American context. Moreover, education was initially a male bailiwick, to which women gained admittance in the nineteenth century because of the demand for large numbers of low-paid teaching personnel resulting from rapid population growth and the increasing acceptance of state-mandated public education.[28]

There are parallels also between nursing and nutrition, social work, and librarianship, professions that, like nursing, emerged

around the turn of the century. As was the case in nursing, nutrition (or dietetics) was a "caregiver" occupation that arose in the
hospital setting and one that held close connections to women's
domestic roles.[29] As a result, nutritionists or dietitians faced resistance to their claims to professional status. In the same way, social
work had its roots in the domestic roles of women, and, like both
nursing and nutrition, its practitioners sought with mixed success to
attain professional recognition in the 1920s and 1930s.[30] Similarly,
librarianship had its origins in the work of untrained women volunteers.[31] Unlike nursing, however, nutrition, social work, and
librarianship developed solid groundings in higher education and, in
varying degrees, in the sciences, although in each case, the academic
sphere was dominated by males. Overall, women in nursing, nutrition, social work, and librarianship faced the same problems of low
public esteem, low pay compared to male-dominated professions,
the threat of competition from untrained or marginally trained
practitioners, and effective subordination to males both in training
schools and often in practice settings.

The care provided by nurses, whether student nurses or graduate nurses, was an indispensable element in the transformation of
the hospital from a nineteenth-century custodial institution to a
twentieth-century institution housing life-saving scientific and technological prowess sufficient to attract a middle-class clientele. In
turn, as Joan Lynaugh attests, the hospital's emergence as the centerpiece of the American health care system was an essential factor
in the development of nursing.[32] Initially, that was so because the
hospital became the seat of nursing education, a role that the hospital assumed partly by design—that is, reflecting its dependence on
the labor of student nurses—and partly by default—that is, the lack
of suitable alternative institutions for the instruction of nurses.
Subsequently, the link between the hospital and nursing strengthened as the hospital's expanded therapeutic capabilities led to an
expanded professional nursing staff. By mid-century, the hospital
had become the principal place of employment for graduate nurses.

The admittedly low status of nurses in the hierarchy of health
care, and especially in the hierarchy of the modern hospital, leads to
the contentious issue of nursing and professionalism. In fact, the
question of professionalism in nursing comes in two parts. The
first is whether or not nursing was or is a profession, and the sec-

ond is whether or not nursing elites' pursuit of the trappings of professionalism was a prudent strategy. In the 1970s and 1980s, many historians of nursing raised doubts about the worth of professionalism to nurses and, thus, questioned the wisdom of a professionalizing strategy. Barbara Melosh, one of the most forceful critics, dismissed the professionalization strategy on grounds that American culture reserved the rewards of professionalism for white males; hence, "nursing by definition cannot be a profession because most nurses are women."[33]

The basic concept of professionalism is itself controversial. In popular usage, the word profession is routinely applied to most any occupational group—from auto mechanics and plumbers to basketball coaches and actors—whose work depends in some measure on a recognizable body of specialized knowledge and/or skill. The concepts of profession and professionalism stirred a good deal of excitement among scholars in the 1960s and 1970s, not just among the sociologists who pioneered the work but among historians and others as well. The literature of professionalism grew rapidly, as scholars aimed primarily to distill the essential attributes of the ideal profession, including a monopoly over occupational practice, a command of specialized knowledge, significant control over the conditions of work, and closely regulated occupational entry.[34] As the archetypal profession, medicine attracted special scrutiny, and historians of medicine, especially historians of more radical bent, readily adapted theories of professionalism to explain the dramatic rise of organized medicine in the twentieth century.[35] In many respects, Paul Starr's benchmark work, *The Social Transformation of American Medicine*, was the high point of that trend, and Starr, a sociologist rather than a historian, began the book with an extended essay on the concept of professionalism, perhaps the best and most persuasive summary on the subject.[36]

Overall, scholars failed to advance our understanding of professions much beyond popular usage.[37] The effort to define professions and professionalism in terms of essential attributes failed miserably in application beyond medicine, which had, of course, inspired the models in the first place. As a result, some scholars, most notably Eliot Freidson, adopted a more functional approach;[38] in turn, others spoke of "semi-professions" and "near professions."[39] However, such approaches failed to resolve the essential ambiguities surrounding the concept of professionalism. At the same time, it became increasingly apparent that concepts of professions and professionalism were not static, but varied over time in accordance with a range of internal and external circumstances. Finally, by the middle to late 1980s, a variety of political and economic forces—from consumer activism and health care cost containment efforts to the decline of the entrepreneurial model of medical practice and the expansionist claims by other health care professions—had significantly diminished the professional "sovereignty" of medicine, the very principle on which the entire edifice of professionalism had initially been erected.

Coming in 1988, Andrew Abbott's work, *The System of Professions: An Essay on the Division of Expert Labor*, offered a minimalist political-legal formulation of professionalism centered on the concept of professional "jurisdiction" continuously redefined in the rough-and-tumble of legislative politics.[40] Borrowing from Abbott, then, while professionals routinely couch their jurisdictional claims in the language of public welfare, professionalism is, at heart, a political construct, defined and regulated in the American context principally by state legislatures and state regulatory agencies and, in more limited ways until quite recently, by the federal government. Thus, in some sense, professional occupations are those designated as such by state or federal enactments that define the boundaries of professional practice, regulate occupational entry, and recognize a body of specialized knowledge. In Iowa, for example, state examining boards currently regulate the practice of more than a dozen health-related occupations in addition to nursing, dentistry, pharmacy, and medicine. Critics might argue that occupations such as nursing home administration, social work, and optometry are not professions, but, notwithstanding all the words written by scholars on the topic, one would be hard pressed to mount a persuasive argument why they are not.

Nurses' and nursing historians' disappointment with professionalism is understandable; professionalism clearly did not deliver the benefits to nurses that it did, for example, to physicians. Still, the debate over nursing's professional status and especially over nursing elites' professionalizing strategy is at best counterproductive and at worst an intellectual dead-end. Was there a viable alternative to professionalization in nursing? One possibility, of course, was a trade unionist strategy, what Daniel Walkowitz, in his article on social workers called the "professional worker" strategy, as distinct from the "woman professional" strategy.[41] In the case of nursing, Barbara Melosh has argued in favor of a trade unionist approach, an approach grounded in the craft tradition that prevailed in nursing early in this century.

To be sure, trade unionism might have fostered a greater solidarity across what became a very fragmented nursing community; likewise, trade unionism might have been a more effective means for negotiating higher pay and perhaps also for pressing some of nurses' claims to authority in the workplace. Yet it is easy to romanticize the potential of trade unionism and thereby to ignore its weaknesses. First, recognizing the deeply ingrained skepticism of the labor movement generally within American culture, it is hard to see how identification with a trade union mentality could have enhanced the public image of nurses and nursing. Second, the labor movement was—and still remains—notoriously apathetic toward women workers and their problems, while women workers themselves are just as notoriously difficult to organize into collective bargaining units.[42] Third, looking backward from the 1990s, the apparent power of organized labor, a topic of much discussion in the 1950s and 1960s, appears to have been largely illusory, the result not of the power of trade unions but of American industry's dominance of both domestic and global economies. Fourth, the rudimentary system of apprenticeship training, a centerpiece of the craft tradition, was thin stuff from which to elaborate the science-based language needed to claim recognition for nursing in a health care system increasingly ordered by science and by scientific credentials.[43]

It is important, too, that nurses were not the only health care professionals to experience frustration with the limits of professionalism, frustrations almost universally attributed to physicians' professional dominance of the health care system. Indeed, viewing nursing within the larger context of the health care professions raises questions about the extent to which physicians' negative responses to the professional ambitions of nurses and nursing were predicated on gender. The fact that physicians used the gender issue against nurses is hardly open to dispute, but that observation begs the question whether or not physicians would have responded with substantially less hostility if nursing had been a male-dominated profession. On that score, the even longer and sometimes more rancorous history of professional relations between physicians and pharmacists suggests that animosity between medicine and other health care professions was and is the rule rather than the exception. Additional evidence might be taken from the history of relations between physicians and chiropractors, between physicians and optometrists, between physicians and podiatrists, or between physicians and physical therapists. Likewise, nursing was scarcely alone in its internal divisions. As Richard H. Shryock observed in a 1968 article, one could scarcely argue that nursing is more fragmented than medicine, whether judged in terms of the diversity of practice specialties or in terms of levels of training.[44] The same is true of pharmacy, a profession rightly noted for its ceaseless internal bickering.

The central problem facing nursing elites from the early twentieth-century was that much of patient care was low-skilled work; making beds, dusting furniture, and emptying bed-pans was not the work of professionals, however one might define the term. In that light, whether or not to pursue a strategy of professionalization was not the fundamental issue in nursing; rather, the issue was how to define nursing so as to make it an occupation deserving of the respect and status that nursing elites and most nurses sought. From the Progressive Era onward, a period in which American society placed great store in science-based education and expert knowledge, the path to respectability for nurses, as for all professions and would-be professions, lay in higher education and associated certification. For nurses, that could only mean escape from stifling hospital-based diploma schools where the chief admissions requirements were "health and strength."[45] The cost of such a strategy, of which nursing elites were well aware, was an inevitable differentiation within the community of nurses, a differentiation grounded in levels of skill and education.

In the half-century from 1870 to 1920, the American teaching-research university became the chief locus for the "discovery and diffusion of knowledge."[46] The state universities were among the noteworthy developments of the era, and the University of Iowa was a case in point. Founded in 1847, the university limped through its early decades, beset by low enrollments, inadequate funding, mediocre leadership, and occasional political turmoil, but from the 1890s, the university blossomed.[47] University enrollments reached some 7,000 by the early 1920s and state appropriations multiplied in proportion. In Iowa as elsewhere, however, the exponential growth of university-based higher education passed nursing by. While baccalaureate education became the norm in medicine, pharmacy, and dentistry, apprenticeship training—its inadequacies laid bare in long experience in the other health care professions—became institutionalized in nursing. Thus, nursing's status as a "near profession" was, in no small part, a direct consequence of the "near education" of nurses, the latter in turn a consequence of nursing education's dependence on the hospital.

Standard works on women in higher education—most of those works focused on the period prior to World War II—offer penetrating analyses of women's opportunities to pursue higher education, the demographics and content of women's education, and the obstacles confronting women who then sought careers in higher education.[48] Not surprisingly, such works have little to say about nursing, since nursing did not, until after World War II, have a significant foundation in higher education. Nursing is missing also from works specifically about women in the professions and sciences, works that deliver much the same sad verdict about educated women's career prospects apart from women's colleges and "women's professions" such as social work and elementary school teaching and administration.[49] Even in the latter cases, as earlier noted, men predominated in positions of authority.[50]

In that light, the rapid post-World War II expansion of baccalaureate programs in nursing, and the accompanying decline in hospital diploma schools, was not only a major chapter in the history of nursing but also a major chapter in the long and difficult history of women in higher education. Nursing colleges represented women's first independent institutional base within the modern university structure, a base within which female leaders constructed an educational curriculum of their own design and in which they began, however haltingly, to elaborate a body of specialized professional knowledge.

Critics of baccalaureate education in nursing might argue that the hospital-based diploma schools, in their own way, defined a "separate sphere" in which women could exert a measure of control over their own activities.[51] However, as Martha Vicinus has argued, early nursing schools, whether British or American, were not comparable to the nineteenth-century convents and religious sisterhoods, which were self-enclosed and self-governed communities.[52] Women's autonomy in the hospital diploma schools was severely circumscribed; nurses exercised direct control only over other women, specifically over nursing students, and not, for the most part, over the hospital itself or even over the nursing curriculum they implemented. At the University of Iowa, for example, the medical faculty effectively controlled the nursing curriculum and also provided the bulk of classroom instruction; at the same time, the dean of the College of Medicine held ultimate administrative authority over the nursing school and spoke for the school in university councils. Surely, then, whatever the traditional diploma school may have offered in the way of solidarity must be balanced against the high cost of nurses' more or less effective exclusion from decision-making at all levels and also their exclusion from the hospital's reward system.

Nursing moved much more slowly into the university setting than did other female-dominated professions or would-be professions.[53] No doubt that was so because nursing education was already well entrenched in hospitals by the time that baccalaureate education in nursing became a significant issue. In addition, the slow advance of baccalaureate education in nursing reflected the almost universal opposition of physicians and hospital administrators, who, each for different reasons, took jaundiced views of any scheme to upgrade nursing education and, by implication, nursing practice. Finally, like practicing physicians in an earlier era, many rank-and-file nurses also opposed attempts to upgrade professional education, fearing the depreciation of the market value of their own skills.

Against that backdrop, the forging of links between nursing and higher education in America was slow.[54] The first successful, if still limited, effort to bring nursing education into the university came in 1909 at the University of Minnesota; however, that program—a three-year diploma program conducted by the university— was in most respects indistinguishable from programs conducted by "the better hospital training schools."[55] In one account, Indiana University in 1914 was the first institution to offer a baccalaureate degree along with the nursing diploma; in another account, the University of Cincinnati in 1916 was the first institution to offer such a combined program.[56] In any event, similar programs followed at the University of California and at Presbyterian Hospital in New York, the latter program affiliated with Columbia University Teachers College. By 1923, seventeen schools, including the University of Iowa, offered combined baccalaureate-diploma programs, with two years of university instruction added to the customary three-year apprenticeship training in nursing. However, few students chose to invest five years rather than three in their educations, a consequence both of the limited rewards accruing to better educated nurses and to the limited ambitions of most nursing students. Meanwhile, the first true collegiate nursing programs were begun at Western Reserve University in 1923, at Yale University in 1924, and at Vanderbilt University in 1930, all of them subsidized by private philanthropy.

For nurses and nursing, the slow pace of educational advance hindered the attainment of professional standing. Certainly, the pre-1920 graduates of the University of Iowa Training School for Nurses and of other institutions like it could hardly be counted as professionals, even in the loosest sense of the word. Yet, by the 1930s, and notwithstanding the still limited nature of their education, the graduates of the renamed University of Iowa School of Nursing appear, in many cases at least, to have thought themselves professionals, and such perceptions are not an insignificant part of the phenomenon of professionalization. Nonetheless, in the 1930s, nurses still lacked an educational curriculum thoroughly grounded in relevant sciences; they lacked the degree of autonomy, especially in their educational institutions, normally associated with professions; and they possessed only the most rudimentary base of specialized nursing knowledge. It was only in the collegiate setting that nurses could hope to attain all the accouterments of a true profession; the first post-World War II generation of collegiate nursing leaders—women like the University of Iowa College of Nursing's first dean, Myrtle Kitchell [Aydelotte]—understood that nurses could not base their claims to status on diploma school educations. Instead, that new generation of nursing leaders believed strongly that academic credentials, including graduate degrees, were the only viable path for nursing in the highly professionalized universe of

American health care, particularly as it existed in the rapidly expanding hospital system. Moreover, in Iowa at any rate, a good many diploma nurses held to the same position and gave their wholehearted support to the baccalaureate movement.

Nursing's path to academic respectability was not a smooth one, as the present study shows all too well. First, the development of academic nursing was stunted by the dearth of nurses holding baccalaureate and advanced degrees, a legacy of the long tradition of apprenticeship training in nursing. As a result, diploma nurses played major roles in building the postwar colleges of nursing. Second, until the 1980s, nursing research was shackled by limited funding and by difficulties in building a research culture among faculty with limited commitments to and limited backgrounds in scientific research. Third, colleges of nursing and their deans were upstarts in the long established institutional order of higher education, an order in which competition for limited resources was customarily fierce and in which women operated under significant handicaps. To a considerable extent, then, the academic success of nursing depended upon the quality of individual leadership, especially so in the early postwar decades. On that score, the University of Iowa College of Nursing was perhaps better served than most. Two University of Iowa presidents, Virgil Hancher and Howard Bowen, provided support to the college at critical moments and on critical issues, while the forceful leadership of Deans Myrtle Kitchell and Laura Dustan shaped the college in ways still apparent today.

This case study of nursing education at the University of Iowa cannot stand for nursing education everywhere in America; nor is that its purpose. However, it can perhaps help to illuminate salient issues associated with nursing education in the twentieth century. It addresses the problems and limitations inherent in the hospital-based diploma school, even one associated with a university academic medical center; the difficult and sometimes painful transition from diploma to baccalaureate programs; and, finally, the fundamental—and occasionally explosive—divisions that developed within academic nursing over issues surrounding faculty credentials, tenure, and promotion. Moreover, like nursing history in general, this case study is a narrative of nurses' struggles to achieve professional recognition over external and internal opposition.

Notes

1. For more than a century, that is, from the mid-nineteenth century to the mid-1960s, what is now the University of Iowa was known as the State University of Iowa. For simplicity, the name University of Iowa is used throughout.

2. Among the best examples of the medical historiography are Rosemary Stevens, *American Medicine and the Public Interest* (New Haven, CT: Yale University Press, 1971); Paul Starr, *The Social Transformation of American Medicine: The Rise of a Sovereign Profession and the Making of a Vast Industry* (New York: Basic Books, 1982); John S. Haller, *American Medicine in Transition, 1840-1910* (Chicago and Urbana: University of Illinois Press, 1981); William G. Rothstein, *American Medical Schools and the Practice of Medicine: A History* (New York: Oxford University Press, 1987); Kenneth M. Ludmerer, *Learning to Heal: The Development of American Medical Education* (New York: Basic Books, 1985).

3. See Morris J. Vogel, *The Invention of the Modern Hospital: Boston, 1870-1930* (Chicago: University of Chicago Press, 1980); Charles E. Rosenberg, *The Care of Strangers: The Rise of America's Hospital System* (New York: Basic Books, 1987); Rosemary Stevens, *In Sickness and In Wealth: The American Hospital in the Twentieth Century* (New York: Basic Books, 1989); Joel D. Howell, *Technology in the Hospital: Transforming Patient Care in the Early Twentieth Century* (Baltimore, MD: The Johns Hopkins University Press, 1995).

4. See M. Adelaide Nutting and Lavinia L. Dock, *A History of Nursing: The Evolution of Nursing Systems from the Earliest Times to the Foundation of the First English and American Training Schools for Nurses*, 2 vols. (New York: G. P. Putnam's Sons, 1907), with two more volumes published in 1912; and Minnie Goodnow, *History of Nursing* (Philadelphia: W. B. Saunders, 1916), a work that subsequently appeared in more than a dozen editions with various author-editors.

5. Janet Wilson James, "Writing and Rewriting Nursing History: A Review Essay," *Bulletin of the History of Medicine* 58 (Winter 1984), p. 568. For other insightful discussions of nursing historiography in its various stages of development, see Ellen Condliffe Lagemann, "Nursing History: New Perspectives, New Possibilities," in Lagemann, ed., *Nursing History: New Perspectives, New Possibilities* (New York: Teachers College, 1983); and Ellen D. Baer, "Nurses," in Rima D. Apple, ed., *Women, Health, and Medicine in America: A Historical Handbook* (New Brunswick, NJ: Rutgers University Press, 1992).

6. Richard H. Shryock, *The History of Nursing: An Interpretation of the Social and Medical Factors Involved* (Philadelphia: W. B. Saunders, 1959).

Shryock's bibliography in the history of medicine was extensive, comprising dozens of articles and books and spanning roughly four decades to the 1960s; among his best known works is *The Development of Modern Medicine: An Interpretation of the Social and Scientific Factors Involved*, 2nd ed. (New York: Alfred A. Knopf, 1947).

7. There are also excellent examples of British nursing historiography; see, as examples, Celia Davies, ed., *Rewriting Nursing History* (London: Croom Helm, 1980); and Christopher J. Maggs, *The Origins of General Nursing* (London: Croom Helm, 1983). The Davies work also contains a good general discussion of nursing historiography, pp. 11-17. For an interesting comparative look at British and American nursing, see Joanne McCloskey, "The Professionalization of Nursing: United States and England," *International Nursing Review* 28 (1981), pp. 40-47.

8. Jo Ann Ashley, *Hospitals, Paternalism, and the Role of the Nurse* (New York: Teachers College Press, 1976).

9. Barbara Melosh, *"The Physician's Hand": Work Culture and Conflict in American Nursing* (Philadelphia: Temple University Press, 1982).

10. Susan M. Reverby, *Ordered to Care: The Dilemma of American Nursing, 1850-1945* (New York: Cambridge University Press, 1987).

11. Darlene Clark Hine, *Black Women in White: Racial Conflict and Co-operation in the Nursing Profession, 1890-1950* (Bloomington, IN: Indiana University Press, 1989).

12. Vern Bullough and Bonnie Bullough, *The Care of the Sick: The Emergence of Modern Nursing* (New York: Prodist, 1978).

13. Philip A. Kalisch and Beatrice J. Kalisch, *The Advance of American Nursing*, 3rd ed. (Philadelphia: J. B. Lippincott, 1995).

14. See, for example Teresa Christy, *Cornerstone for Nursing Education: A History of the Division of Nursing Education of Teachers College, Columbia University, 1899-1947* (New York: Teachers College Press, 1969); see also her series on nursing leaders in *Nursing Outlook* 17, 18 (1969).

15. M. Patricia Donahue, *Nursing, The Finest Art: An Illustrated History*, 2nd. ed. (St. Louis, MO: Mosby, 1996).

16. Sandra Beth Lewenson, *Taking Charge: Nursing, Suffrage, and Feminism in America, 1873-1920* (New York: Garland Publishing, 1993).

17. Rosenberg, *The Care of Strangers*, Chapter 9, "Healing Hands: Nursing in the Hospital," pp. 212-236.

18. Janet Wilson James, *op. cit.*; Nancy Schrom Dye, "Mary Breckenridge, the Frontier Nursing Service, and the Introduction of Nurse-Midwifery in the United States," 57 (Winter 1983), pp. 485-507; Diane Hamilton, "The Cost of Caring: The Metropolitan Life Insurance Company's Visiting Nurse Service, 1909-1953," 63 (Fall 1989), pp. 414-434; Douglas O. Baldwin, "Discipline, Obedience, and Female Support Groups: Mona Wilson

at the Johns Hopkins Hospital School of Nursing, 1915-1918," 69 (Winter 1995), pp. 599-619.

19. The authors well remember, as will many other historians, graduate school professors who solemnly warned that events within one's memory lie outside the bounds of history.

20. Two examples of note are Margene O. Faddis, *A School of Nursing Comes of Age: A History of the Francis Payne Bolton School of Nursing, Case Western Reserve University* (Cleveland: The Alumnæ Association of the Francis Payne Bolton School of Nursing, 1973); James Gray, *Education for Nursing: A History of the University of Minnesota School* (Minneapolis, MN: University of Minnesota Press, 1960).

21. For a history of one of the nation's premier hospital schools, see Sylvia Perkins, *A Centennial Review: The Massachusetts General Hospital School of Nursing, 1873-1973* (Boston, MA: School of Nursing, Nurses Alumnæ Association, 1975).

22. Two standard interpretive surveys are Robert Wiebe, *The Search for Order, 1877-1920* (New York: Hill and Wang, 1967); and Olivier Zunz, *Making America Corporate, 1870-1920* (Chicago: University of Chicago Press, 1990).

23. In Max Weber's terminology, professionals are generally not "rational-economic monopolists" seeking privileged positions through market competition but ""status monopolists" who claim privilege on other grounds. See "Class, Status, Party," in H. H. Gerth and C. W. Mills, eds., *From Max Weber: Essays in Sociology* (New York: Oxford University Press, 1958), pp. 180-195.

24. Still one of the best general works on the subject is Alice Kessler-Harris, *Out to Work: A History of Wage-Earning Women in the United States* (New York: Oxford University Press, 1982).

25. See, as examples, Margery Davies, *Women's Place Is at the Typewriter: Office Work and Office Workers, 1870-1930* (Philadelphia, PA: Temple University Press, 1982); Susan Porter Benson, *Counter Cultures: Saleswomen, Managers, and Customers in American Department Stores, 1890-1940* (Urbana, IL: University of Illinois Press, 1986).

26. The story of women in medicine is the best documented; see, as examples, Mary Roth Walsh, *"Doctors Wanted, No Women Need Apply": Sexual Barriers in the Medical Profession, 1835-1975* (New Haven, CT: Yale University Press, 1977); Regina Markell Morantz-Sanchez, *Sympathy and Science: Women Physicians in American Medicine* (New York: Oxford University Press, 1985).

27. The gendered structure of labor resulting from the movement of economic production out of the home or family business as a consequence of industrialization is a theme in Jeanne Boydston, *Home and Work: House-*

work, Wages, and the Ideology of Labor in the Early Republic (New York: Oxford University Press, 1990).

28. See Carl Kaestle, *Pillars of the Republic: Common Schools and American Society, 1780-1860* (New York: Hill and Wang, 1983); Elisabeth Hansot and David Tyack, *Managers of Virtue: Public School Leadership in America, 1820-1980* (New York: Basic Books, 1982); Maris Vinovskis and Richard Bernard, "The Female School Teacher in Ante-Bellum Massachusetts," *Journal of Social History* (March 1977), pp. 332-342.

29. For description of the creation and growth of the Department of Nutrition at the University of Iowa Hospitals, see Lee Anderson, *Internal Medicine and the Structures of Modern Medical Science: The University of Iowa, 1870-1900* (Ames, IA: Iowa State University Press), pp. 72-77.

30. See Daniel J. Walkowitz, "The Making of a Feminine Professional Identity: Social Workers in the 1920s," *American Historical Review* 95 (October 1990), pp. 1051-1075; see also, Linda Gordon, "Social Insurance and Public Assistance: The Influence of Gender in Welfare Thought in the United States," *American Historical Review* 97 (February 1992), pp. 19-54.

31. Joanne Passet, "Entering the Professions: Women Library Educators and the Placement of Female Students, 1887-1912," *History of Education Quarterly* 31 (Summer 1991), pp. 207-228.

32. Joan E. Lynaugh, "Riding the Yo-Yo: The Worth and Work of Nursing in the 20th Century," *Transactions and Studies of the College of Physicians of Philadelphia* 11 (1989), pp. 201-217.

33. Melosh, *"The Physician's Hand,"* p. 20.

34. Some of the classic pieces were William J. Goode, "Community Within a Community: The Professions," *American Sociology Review* 22 (1957), pp. 194-201; Harold Wilensky, "The Professionalization of Everyone?" *American Journal of Sociology* 70 (1964-65), pp. 137-158; Talcott Parsons, "Professions," *International Encyclopedia of the Social Sciences*, 1968; Howard M. Vollmer and Donald L. Mills, eds., *Professionalization* (Englewood Cliffs, NJ: Prentice-Hall, 1966); and Magali Sarfatti-Larson, *The Rise of Professionalism: A Sociological Analysis* (Berkeley, CA: University of California Press, 1979).

35. See, for example, E. Richard Brown, *Rockefeller Medicine Men* (Berkeley, CA: University of California Press, 1979). For criticisms of such works, see Renee C. Fox, "The Medicalization and Demedicalization of American Society," *Daedalus* 106 (1977), pp. 3-22.

36. Starr, *The Social Transformation of American Medicine.*

37. See Bernard Barber, "Some Problems in the Sociology of the Professions," *Daedalus* 56 (1963), pp. 669-688; Robert Dingwall, "Accomplishing Profession," *Sociological Review*, n.s. 24 (1976), pp. 331-349; Terence Johnson, *Professions and Power* (London: Macmillan Press, 1972).

38. See Eliot Freidson, *The Profession of Medicine* (New York: Harper and Row, 1970), as well as his subsequent publications.

39. As an example, see Amitai Etzioni, ed., *The Semi-Professions and Their Organization* (New York: The Free Press, 1969).

40. Andrew Abbott, *The System of Professions: An Essay on the Division of Expert Labor* (Chicago: University of Chicago Press, 1988).

41. Walkowitz, "The Making of a Feminine Professional Identity."

42. Heidi Hartmann, "Capitalism, Patriarchy and Job Segregation by Sex," in Martha Blaxall and Barbara Reagan, eds., *Women and the Workplace: The Implications of Occupational Segregation* (Chicago, IL: University of Chicago Press, 1976), pp. 137-169; Alice Kessler-Harris, "Where Are the Organized Women Workers?" in Linda K. Kerber and Jane DeHart Matthews, eds., *Women's America: Refocusing the Past* (New York: Oxford University Press, 1982), pp. 225-242; Ruth Milkman, "Organizing the Sexual Division of Labor: Historical Perspectives on 'Women's Work' and the American Labor Movement," *Socialist Review* 10 (January/February 1980), pp. 95-150.

43. For an insightful essay on the importance of professional language, see JoAnne Brown, "Professional Language: Words That Succeed," *Radical History Review* 34 (1986), pp. 33-51.

44. Richard Harrison Shryock, "Nursing Emerges as a Profession: The American Experience," *Clio Medica* 3 (1968), pp. 131-147.

45. Susan M. Reverby, "The Search for the Hospital Yardstick: Nursing and the Rationalization of Hospital Work," in Judith Walzer Leavitt and Ronald L. Numbers, eds., *Sickness and Health in America* (Madison, WI: University of Wisconsin Press, 1985), pp. 206-216.

46. Edward Shils, "The Order of Learning in the United States: The Ascendancy of the University," in Alexandra Oleson and John Voss, eds., *The Organization of Knowledge in Modern America, 1860-1920* (Baltimore, MD: Johns Hopkins University Press, 1979), pp. 19-47. See also, Burton Bledstein, *The Culture of Professionalism: The Middle Class and the Development of Higher Education in America* (New York: W. W. Norton, 1976).

47. See Stow Persons, *The University of Iowa in the Twentieth Century: An Institutional History* (Iowa City, IA: University of Iowa Press, 1990).

48. See, as examples, Barbara Miller Solomon, *In the Company of Educated Women: A History of Women in Higher Education in America* (New Haven, CT: Yale University Press, 1985); Lynn Gordon, *Gender and Higher Education in the Progressive Era* (New Haven, CT: Yale University Press, 1990).

49. See Barbara J. Harris, *Beyond Her Sphere: Women and the Professions in American History* (Westport, CT: Greenwood Press, 1978); Margaret Rossiter, *Women Scientists in America: Struggles and Strategies to 1940*

(Baltimore, MD: Johns Hopkins University Press, 1982); Rosalind Rosenberg, *Beyond Separate Spheres: Intellectual Roots of Modern Feminism* (New Haven, CT: Yale University Press, 1982).

50. See Robyn Muncy, *Creating a Female Dominion in American Reform, 1890-1935* (New York: Oxford University Press, 1991); Ellen Fitzpatrick, *Endless Crusade: Women Social Scientists and Progressive Reform* (New York: Oxford University Press, 1990); Gordon, "Social Insurance and Public Assistance."

51. The classic work is Nancy Kott, *The Bonds of Womanhood: 'Woman's Sphere' in New England, 1780-1835* (New Haven, CT: Yale University Press, 1977).

52. Martha Vicinus, *Independent Women: Work and Community for Single Women in England, 1850-1920* (Chicago, IL: University of Chicago Press, 1985).

53. For general discussion, see Bullough and Bullough, *The Care of the Sick*, pp. 154-165; Bullough and Bullough, "Collegiate Nursing in the United States, *International Nursing Review* 10 (January/February), 1963), pp. 41-47.

54. Nursing education in Canada followed much the same path; see Rondalyn A. Kirkwood, "Discipline Discrimination and Gender Discrimination: The Case of Nursing in Canadian Universities, 1920-1950," *Atlantis* 16 (1990), pp. 52-63.

55. Bullough and Bullough, *The Care of the Sick*, p. 159.

56. Beatrice J. Kalisch and Philip A. Kalisch, "Slaves, Servants, or Saints?: An Analysis of the System of Nurse Training in the United States, 1873-1948," *Nursing Forum* XIV (1975), p. 237; Bullough and Bullough, *Ibid.*

Chapter One

Defining a Profession, 1898-1928

Throughout most of the nineteenth century, health care in Iowa and in much of America was an integral part of the domestic economy, and nursing performed by wives and mothers or by female relatives and neighbors lay at the heart of domestic health care.[1] In the last decades of the century, however, a combination of factors—most importantly, rapid population growth, industrialization, urbanization, and accompanying changes in political and cultural environments—dramatically transformed Iowa's economy and society, with profound implications for most Iowans' health care expectations and behaviors. Indeed, one of the most striking, if seldom appreciated, developments of the late nineteenth and early twentieth centuries in Iowa and elsewhere in the United States was the movement of a significant part of health care out of the home and into the marketplace and the emergence of the modern health care professions.

Iowa's population exploded from 96,000 in 1846, when Congress granted statehood, to nearly 1.2 million in 1870 and to more than 2.2 million in 1900. Also in 1900, the number of Iowans living in cities and towns with populations of 2,500 or more surpassed a half million, up from just 10,000 in 1850, while Iowa's farm population had already begun its long decline. At the same time, railroads and telephone and telegraph lines criss-crossed the state in crazy-quilt patterns, linking Iowans, rural and urban alike, to national and global networks of commerce and communication.

The combined forces of industrialization and urbanization fostered the growth of a modern middle class in Iowa, one that valued education and science as remedies for many of society's evils and one that brought the state's police power to bear upon the rapidly expanding and remarkably chaotic market for health care goods and services. In 1880, the Iowa general assembly passed two landmark pieces of health related legislation. The first created a State Board of Health empowered "to act for the preservation or improvement of the public health," including the compilation of vital statistics, the control of contagious disease, and the registration—though not yet the licensing—of medical practitioners and midwives. The second defined the practice of pharmacy and set in place a licensing system prescribing educational standards, restricting entry into the profession, and regulating professional conduct. In 1882, the general assembly passed similar legislation to regulate the practice of dentistry, and in 1886, after many years of contentious debate within the medical profession itself, the general assembly passed Iowa's first medical practice act. In contrast, legal recognition of the nursing profession came only some two decades later, a time lag reflecting the difficulties in arriving at a politically acceptable definition of nursing practice and the problems in mobilizing nurses behind the ideals of professionalization.

The University of Iowa Nurse Training School and the Growth of Nursing

The professional development and recognition of nursing in Iowa hinged upon the belated development of the modern hospital, which became the home of nursing education and, eventually, the principal focus of nursing practice. Prior to the last two decades of the nineteenth century, hospitals were virtually unknown in Iowa, apart from the "pest houses" erected by communities in response to sporadic outbreaks of epidemic disease and used primarily to quarantine indigent victims. The first recognizable hospital in Iowa appears to have been the rudimentary teaching facility opened in 1851 by the Keokuk College of Physicians and Surgeons, a proprietary medical school that served at the time as the "Medical Department" of the University of Iowa. Like the school itself, that hospital—known hopefully as "University Hospital"—was a shoestring operation, and it served as little more than a modest warehouse for the indigent sick who were the convenient, albeit sometimes unwilling, objects of indifferent clinical education. Iowa was not alone in its lack of hospital facilities. One observer counted just 178 hospitals in all of America in 1873, a figure that included mental institutions like the state hospital for the insane established in Mt. Pleasant, Iowa, in 1861.[2]

The opening of the University of Iowa Medical Department on the university's Iowa City campus in 1870 superseded the affiliation between the university and the Keokuk College of Physicians and Surgeons. Like virtually all medical schools of the time, the university's new Medical Department suffered serious deficiencies in curriculum and facilities, particularly in the area of clinical instruction. In 1873, the university's governing Board of Regents designated the Mechanics Academy, a small and somewhat dilapidated building, for use as a hospital for the clinical training of medical students. Medical Department Dean Washington F. Peck arranged with the Sisters of Mercy to send a mission from their Davenport convent to administer this second "University Hospital" and to provide nursing care.[3] In 1886, after more than a decade of squabbles with the Medical Department, the Sisters of Mercy opened an independent Mercy Hospital in a renovated home near the campus, which largely replaced the old Mechanics Academy as a site for clinical instruction.

Relations between the Sisters of Mercy and the faculty of the Medical Department remained troubled on several counts, not least by jurisdictional disputes and by conflict over the primary function of the hospital. As a result, university officials and the Board of Regents resolved by the late 1880s to build a hospital designed specifically to serve the needs of medical education. That decision led to a long and arduous campaign to win approval and funding from the state general assembly, a campaign spearheaded by University of Iowa President Charles Ashmead Schaeffer and a small handful of political allies. In Schaeffer's view, the need of a university hospital was obvious to one and all, given that "the state needs a body of trained physicians and a thoroughly equipped Hospital is a necessary adjunct to a school of medicine."[4]

It was not until 1896 that Schaeffer and his backers won approval of the project from the state legislature, and not until January 11, 1898, that the new University Hospital opened and the first twelve patients were admitted. For its time, the hospital, although smaller than initially envisioned, was no mean enterprise. Boasting sixty-five beds, a modern surgical amphitheater, steam heat, and electric lighting, it was, the university's Board of Regents boasted, "one of the most complete hospitals in every particular west of Chicago."[5]

Though always a secondary concern, nursing education was a necessary adjunct to medical education at the University of Iowa Hospital. Formal nursing education in the United States dated to the early 1870s, but its subsequent growth had been both explosive and haphazard.[6] In 1880, there were only some fifteen nursing schools; by 1900 there were 432.[7] Moreover, it was no accident that the rapid growth in the number of nurse training programs in the 1880s and 1890s paralleled the equally rapid growth in the numbers of American hospitals; for early nursing schools, whatever their shortcomings, were important elements in the transformation of the hospital from an undifferentiated indigent care institution to the modern symbol of scientific health care.

While, in many cases at least, hospital administrators and governing boards undertook nursing education largely as an expedient, they had, by the late 1890s, discovered the virtues of nurse training programs as a source of inexpensive and relatively pliant hospital labor. In short, it was cheaper and more convenient to conduct in-house training courses—providing student nurses "full maintenance," that is, room, board, and laundry—and to employ those students on the wards than to hire trained graduate nurses. So it was at the University of Iowa Hospital, where the University of Iowa Training School for Nurses began operation in 1898, its two-year nursing program enrolling an initial class of five students.[8]

American nursing echoed to some extent the ideals and evangelistic zeal of Florence Nightingale, a larger than life Victorian presence whose iconic standing—judging from past and present nursing literature—is unmatched in any other profession, indeed exceeding even that of William Osler in medicine. Yet, to an outsider at least, Nightingale's legacy was ambiguous. On the one hand, Nightingale made nursing a respectable occupation for middle-class women; she imbued nurses and nursing with a worthy mission; and she helped to transform the hospital from a holding pen for society's unfortunates to a temple of cleanliness, if not of science. On the other hand, Nightingale's emphasis on discipline and cleanliness bequeathed to nursing a moral language that was, by the early twentieth century, eclipsed both in the public imagination and in hospital practice by the language of scientific medicine, born chiefly of the germ theory of disease. Nightingale, then, bears some responsibility, along with patriarchal physicians and hospital administrators, for the slow development of a scientific element in nursing and also for nursing's ongoing focus on housekeeping and elementary caregiving functions.

In any event, American nursing education did not, as Nightingale might have hoped, develop an independent institutional base alongside the hospital, but developed within the hospital, an outcome that posed serious long-term problems. Ironically, too, just as the proprietary medical schools—many of them known then and since as "diploma mills"—disappeared from the landscape of medical education, an enterprise sharing many of the same characteristics came to command the field of nursing education and was generally welcomed by the same medical elites who rightly cheered its demise in their own field. By and large, of course, the relationship between the nursing profession and increasingly male-directed hospitals echoed the patriarchal nature of American society at large. At the same time, there was no likely educational alternative to the hospital nurse training school. Also, as was true of nineteenth-century proprietary medical schools, the nursing education afforded by hospital "diploma programs" was not inevitably of poor quality, but varied widely from one institution to another.

At the University of Iowa, the dean of the Medical Department, which became the College of Medicine in 1901, held authority over the University Hospital, aided by a medical director elected from among the medical faculty and a hospital superintendent responsible for day-to-day hospital operations as well as nursing care. In keeping with nineteenth-century tradition, women held the superintendent's position for the first several years of the hospital's existence; Jennie Cottle served as superintendent at the hospital's opening in 1898. One local newspaper account incorrectly named Cottle as a graduate of the nurse training course at Massachusetts General Hospital; in fact, however, she was a product of the Farrand Training School for Nurses at Harper Hospital in Detroit, one of the more progressive nursing schools of the era. In addition to her other duties, Cottle also had charge of the nursing school, known until 1919 as the Training School for Nurses and thereafter as the School of Nursing.

The hospital superintendent's position was complicated and demanding; her broad responsibilities entailed divided and some-

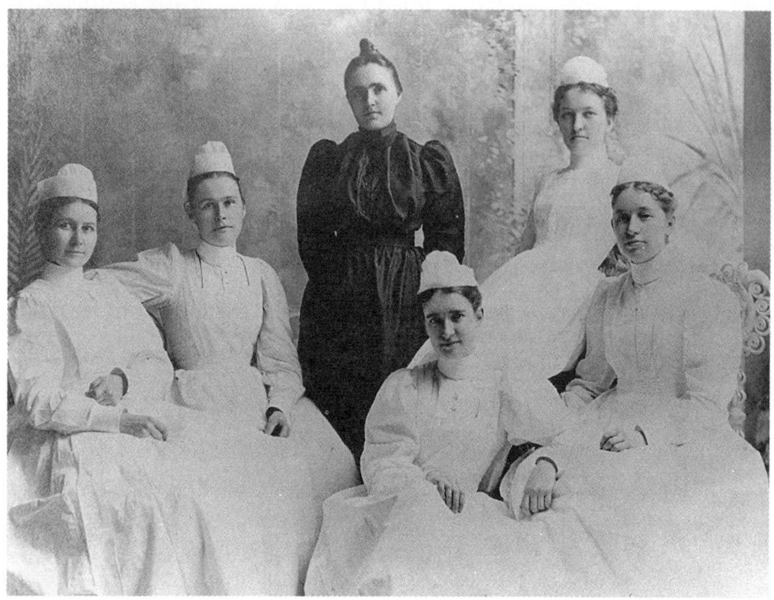

Fig. 1.1. The first graduating class of the University of Iowa Nurse Training School, 1900 (UI College of Nursing Collection). From left: Laura Lang Williams, Mary Holden Lamb, Superintendent Jennie Cottell, Olive Honie Ray, Emma Thomas, Antonia Epeneter.

times incompatible professional loyalties, balancing nursing education, the provision of competent nursing care to the patients in her charge, and the efficient and economic operation of the hospital. Also, both as head of the hospital and as head of the Nurse Training School, she faced major jurisdictional ambiguities, since the College of Medicine, and ultimately the dean of medicine, claimed final authority in both areas. In a real sense, then, the hospital superintendents served at the dean's pleasure. Perhaps because of the inherent ambiguities in her position, Jennie Cottle's tenure at the University of Iowa Hospital was short. Her resignation came in January 1900, and she became chief nurse at a new 200-bed hospital in Pueblo, Colorado, a facility built and operated by the Colorado Fuel and Iron Company. Florence E. Brown succeeded Cottle as superintendent, her tenure lasting until 1905.

The two-year nurse training program instituted in 1898 became a three-year program in 1902, and the hospital also added a principal—a job title adapted from the public schools—to take charge of the Nurse Training School, a position held by Susan G. Parrish from 1900 to 1903, Antonia Epeneter in 1903-1904, and Bertha Wilkinson in 1904-1905. After graduating in the training school's first class in 1900, Epeneter had subsequently followed Jennie Cottle to Colorado.

Driven chiefly by the growth in the hospital's patient admissions, training school enrollments expanded rapidly in the early twentieth century, numbering fourteen in 1900, eighteen in 1905, and forty-six in 1910. From today's perspective, the school's curriculum was an indifferent one, since nursing education was a secondary concern for the physicians in charge of the hospital. In theory, the curriculum spanned three years; in practice, it was for several years an ungraded course in which students in first, second, and third-years repeated essentially the same course of instruction—a pattern modeled on earlier proprietary medical schools.

Student nurses' classroom instruction included a series of lectures by medical faculty embracing the rudiments of the basic sciences, anatomy, physiology, materia medica, and bacteriology. The curriculum also included a clinical component consisting of obstetrics/gynecology, surgery, ophthalmology/otolaryngology, and pediatrics. In addition, nursing students received some instruction in dietetics, massage, and administration. As was universally the case at such schools, practical experience on the hospital wards was the primary purpose of the training program, pushing lectures into the late afternoon and evening hours. And students had much to learn, since the nurse was of necessity a Jill-of-all-trades, given the limited differentiation in the hospital's occupational structure. Dressed in mandatory ankle-length skirt, black hose, and high-top shoes, student nurses scrubbed the rooms and wards from top to bottom, prepared and served meals to patients, changed bed linen, and generally performed the sundry housekeeping tasks associated with patient care. In the early years, the University of Iowa Hospital also on occasion assigned students to private duty, with fees paid to the hospital.[9]

In important respects, the emphasis on discipline and moral rectitude extended beyond the classrooms and hospital wards. Nursing supervisors placed a heavy emphasis on the general deportment and moral instruction of their charges, both of which were crucial factors in enhancing the professional image of nursing.

Those were likewise crucial considerations to hospital administrators bent upon enhancing the public image of early twentieth-century hospitals, institutions of dubious heritage and reputation. Anxious to attract middle-class, paying patients, for example, the University of Iowa Hospital early on refused admission to patients with "diseases of an offensive nature," notably venereal diseases.

Indigent patients made up nearly the entire caseload in the early years of the University Hospital. Lacking the resources to pay for professional care, indigent patients came to the hospital on the basis of a referral from local officials or pastors to serve as clinical material for the training of physicians and, secondarily, for the training of nurses. In a society in which poverty was understood as a mark of moral failure, indigent patients were deeply suspect, viewed by hospital officials as misguided children, likely to misbehave and in need of firm guidance. Much of the responsibility for that guidance fell upon nurses, and, by all accounts, nursing supervisors took their moral responsibilities very seriously and ensured that their student charges did so as well. For various reasons, then, as one historian has pointed out, nursing elites in America sought to emulate the British emphasis on "rigid discipline, hierarchical authority, efficient organization, and autonomy of nursing service,"[10] although the last of those goals was severely compromised by the housing of nursing education in hospitals.

The emphasis on discipline and moral development lent a military or monastic cast to the life of the student nurse. Nursing students at the University of Iowa, like the medical interns who appeared on the scene in increasing numbers in the first two decades of this century, lived near the hospital, first in single-family residences converted to serve as dormitories and, from 1914, in Eastlawn, a building constructed specifically for use as a nurses' dormitory. The off-duty lives of nursing students were subject to close regulation and scrutiny, and a fixed schedule for the routines of daily life prescribed evening curfews and strict standards for dress and overall decorum. One early nurse supervisor proudly recalled that "during my administration no SUI nurse was ever guilty of a grave indiscretion,"[11] but left the definition of "grave indiscretion" to the imagination of the reader.

The personal notes of a University Hospitals supervisory nurse, Bertha Kampmeier, lend insight into the stern moral tone of

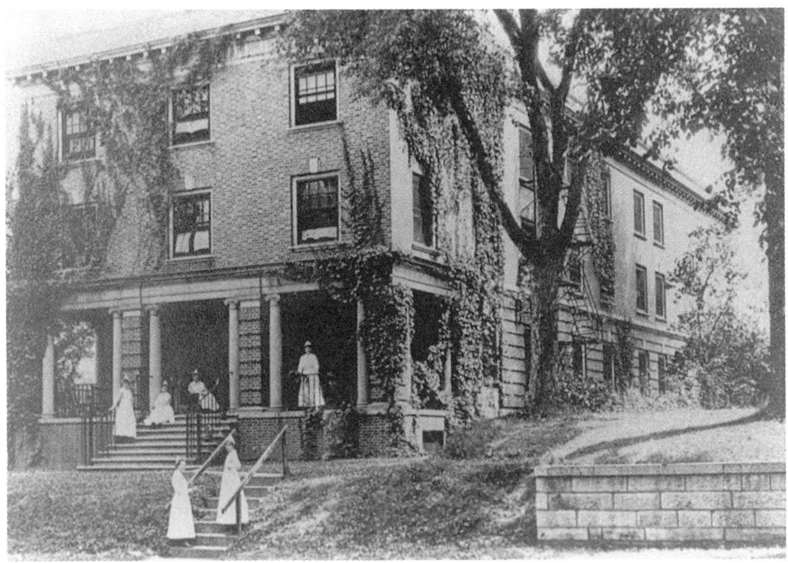

Fig. 1.2. Nurses' residence at Eastlawn, c. 1920 (College of Nursing Collection).

early twentieth-century nursing at the University of Iowa Hospital. In 1920, Kampmeier was nurse supervisor in the orthopædic operating theatre, one of thirty-four supervisory nurses in the hospitals, and her duties included the instruction of senior nursing students, each of whom spent two weeks in her charge. Kampmeier's notes make clear that she gave meticulous instruction to students on preparing patients for surgery, assisting surgeons during surgical procedures, sterilizing instruments, and the general care and cleaning of the operating theatre. Pasted into one of Kampmeier's handwritten books of procedure was a quotation—source unknown—extolling the satisfaction the individual derived "in doing perfectly, or at least to the best of one's ability, everything he attempts to do." Thus, "a work which is rounded, full, exact, complete in all its parts," the quotation continued, was the source of a "completeness" that "turns work into art."[12]

The early development of nursing education at the University of Iowa took place against a backdrop, both local and national, of broader professional movements in nursing. Two major national nursing organizations emerged in the 1890s and a third early in the twentieth century. In 1893, aiming to improve the hospital training schools of the era, Isabel Hampton Robb and her colleagues founded the American Society of Superintendents of Training Schools for Nurses, which became the National League of Nursing Education in 1912.[13] In 1896, Robb was again a principal in founding the Nurses' Associated Alumnæ of the United States and Canada, the name changed to the American Nurses Association in 1911, a professional organization intended to further the interests of graduate nurses. Finally, in 1912, public health nurses, an occupational specialty that grew out of the settlement house movement, created the National Organization for Public Health Nursing.

The opportunities afforded by the rapid multiplication of nurse training schools and the birth of professional organizations were limited by race.[14] Echoing the prevalent racial prejudice and segregation in American society at large and the consequent limitations—de jure and de facto—on African-American women's citizenship rights, the training and professional development of white and African-American nurses diverged sharply. In northern states, few nurse training schools accepted African-American students, and separate African-American schools existed only in a handful of major cities, including New York, Chicago, and Philadelphia. In southern states, the exclusion of African-American students from existing nurse training schools was virtually complete, and a lack of resources stunted the development of parallel African-American schools. At the same time, African-American nurses' systematic exclusion from existing state professional organizations in southern states, along with their small numbers in northern states, meant that African-American nurses were effectively excluded from national nursing organizations as well. Moreover, white nursing elites, by and large, disparaged the professional competence of their African-American counterparts. As a result, African-American graduate nurses, like African-American physicians, formed their own professional organizations, beginning with the National Association of Colored Graduate Nurses established in 1908. The treatment accorded African-Americans in Iowa was no different from elsewhere. The University of Iowa Training School for Nurses, like other nursing schools, appears to have discouraged African-American applicants, and there is no record of African-American or other ethnic minority enrollments prior to World War II.

The first professional organization for nurses in Iowa appeared in January 1904 when a small group of graduate nurses representing some of the state's larger hospitals convened in Des Moines to create a state association "for the purpose of improving the profession and securing state registration of nurses."[15] Adoption of a constitution signed by the twenty-nine inaugural members and the election of Rachael Estella Campbell as president marked the beginning of the Iowa State Graduate Nurses Association, renamed the Iowa State Association of Registered Nurses, or ISARN, in 1909. In 1906, the association counted forty-eight members, and in the same year members voted to affiliate with the national Associated Alumnæ. Adding from fifty to 100 new members each year, the association claimed 420 members in 1914, accounting for just over forty percent of Iowa's 1,020 registered nurses.

One of the first acts of the new association in 1904 was appointment of a legislative committee to draft a professional practice act. By the first decade of the twentieth century, the growing numbers of nurse training schools and of graduate nurses and the growing visibility and importance of nursing care fueled efforts in many states to devise licensing requirements for graduate nurses similar to those already operative in other health care professions. In 1903, legislatures in North Carolina, Virginia, New York, and New Jersey enacted the first licensing statutes in America to impose standards on nursing education and practice.[16] In Iowa, members of the state association debated and approved draft legislation in 1905 and voted to submit the proposed act to the state legislature with Alice Isaacson, superintendent of St. Luke's Hospital in Cedar Rapids, charged with shepherding the bill through the legislative process. The state legislature approved Iowa's Nurse Practice Act in March 1907, creating a Board of Nurse Examiners—made up of three physicians and two nurses operating under the auspices of the State Board of Health—to implement a system of registration of graduate nurses. For the first year, until July 1908, graduate nurses already in practice registered without examination, a total of 748 registrations by the close of that initial registration period. Thereafter, registration was by examination, open only to graduates of schools accredited by the board under the terms of minimum accreditation requirements first issued in April 1908.

Like the statutes enacted in other states in the same period, the Iowa Nurse Practice Act of 1907 had significant faults. First, unlike licensing laws regulating other health professions, such as medicine and pharmacy, Iowa's Nurse Practice Act did not reserve nursing practice to individuals possessing specific qualifications defined by the statute and by the examining board. Indeed, the act made no effort to define the practice of nursing, but reserved to qualified practitioners only the right to use the appellation "registered nurse." Thus, so-called practical nurses, with little or no formal training, were scarcely affected by the law; moreover, many graduate nurses, echoing earlier experience in both medicine and pharmacy, refused to comply with the registration provisions. Second, the law provided no mechanism for the physical inspection of nurse training schools; instead, the Board of Nurse Examiners based its accreditation decisions on materials submitted by the schools. Finally, the Graduate Nurses Association lobbied hard but failed to achieve an independent state nursing board, which would put nursing on the same regulatory footing as medicine, pharmacy, and dentistry. Amendments to the nurse practice law in 1909 and 1911 did not alter those fundamental problems but did strengthen registration requirements and broaden the examining board's powers.

The "Flexner Revolution" and Nursing Education at the University of Iowa

Abraham Flexner's two 1909 visits to the University of Iowa carried important ramifications for the Nurse Training School.[17] Flexner's aim, now more than adequately documented, was to reshape American (and Canadian) medical education, a project he undertook for the Carnegie Endowment for the Advancement of Teaching and with the endorsement of the American Medical Association. Flexner's opinion of the University of Iowa College of Medicine was not a happy one. Flexner's initial report, which arrived in mid-June 1909, praised basic science instruction as "generally good and in some points excellent," but he found the situation in the clinical departments "of a different order altogether." Flexner charged that the University Hospital was, "in its teaching aspects, headless" and that hospital operations were a shambles, with pitiful patient records making it "impossible to say what ground the clinical teaching has actually covered."[18] Later in the year, Flexner returned for a second tour, but his opinion was little changed.

Abraham Flexner's indictment of medical education at the University of Iowa, accompanied by the thinly veiled suggestion that medical students and the state of Iowa would be best served by closing both the College of Medicine and the University Hospital, sparked a determined effort on the part of university officials and the Iowa State Board of Education,[19] aided by an enlarged commitment from the Iowa legislature, to salvage the college and the hospital. The results were an immediate upgrading of the medical curriculum, with particular attention to clinical education, the addition of new medical faculty recruited from respected schools in Chicago and the East, and expansion of the University Hospital's physical plant—to more than 300 beds in 1915—coupled with significant improvements in hospital procedures.

Although never foremost among the concerns of university administrators, the hospital nursing service and the Nurse Training School, boosted by pressures from nurses themselves, also profited from the general reform of the College of Medicine and University Hospital. The number of graduate nurse supervisors, whose duties included both patient care and the practical instruction of student nurses, rose from just two in 1900 to four in 1910 and to thirteen by the fall of 1915; in comparison, the University of Michigan in 1915, with a hospital of similar size, boasted a staff of twenty graduate nurses.[20] In 1915, the nursing administration at the University Hospital consisted of Superintendent Josephine Creelman, who served also as director of the Nurse Training School; a hospital matron, whose responsibilities included patient admissions, the assignment of patients to appropriate clinical services, and the settling of patient accounts; a head nurse generally in charge of coordinating all hospital nursing services; head nurses in each of the four major clinical departments—surgery, medicine, obstetrics-gynecology, and "head specialties," or eye-ear-nose-and-throat; a head nurse in the hydrotherapeutic department; a night supervisor; and a nurse-dietitian.

Meanwhile, enrollments in the Nurse Training School rose to seventy in 1915. In that period, admissions standards were yet

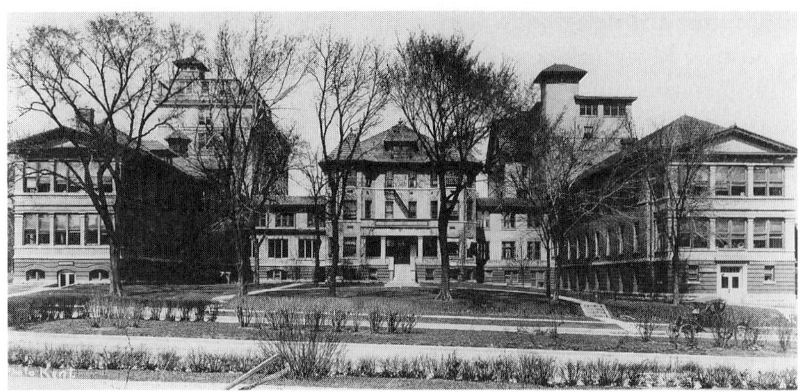

Fig. 1.3. University of Iowa Hospital, c. 1920 (College of Nursing Collection).

minimal; specifications in 1915 required only that students should be twenty to thirty years of age and possess a grammar school education, although those with high school diplomas were promised preference in admissions. By 1915 the three-year nursing curriculum was divided into freshman, junior, and senior years, each year with its allotted courses, a curriculum still largely organized and conducted by the medical faculty. The first year curriculum introduced nursing students to anatomy, physiology, bacteriology, pathology, and gynecology; the second year covered general medicine, materia medica, toxicology, hygiene, and anesthetics; and third-year students studied general surgery, eye-ear-nose-and-throat, obstetrics, bandaging, pediatrics, and urinalysis.

Textbooks were standard works for the time, most of them written specifically for nursing students in accordance with guidelines of the National League of Nursing Education and the Training School Committee of the American Hospital Association. Titles in use at the University of Iowa included Minnie Goodnow's *First-Year Nursing: A Textbook for Pupils During Their First Year of Hospital Work*, Isabel Robb's *Nursing Ethics: For Hospital and Private Use*, and Diana Clifford Kimber and Caroline E. Gray's *Textbook of Anatomy and Physiology*. Goodnow's book in particular lends insight into the world of nursing in the first decades of this century. Early chapters on cleaning, bed-making, preparing and serving meals, bathing the patient, and undressing, turning, and lifting patients described practices little changed from the turn of the century; however, later chapters on record-keeping, vital signs and symptoms, and drug therapy had a more modern flavor. In 1915, a College of Medicine faculty committee recommended creation of a library at the nurses' residence, and the full medical faculty forwarded the request to the University Library Board. However, it was only the intercession of Campbell Howard of the Department of Internal Medicine that finally—a year later—pried loose the necessary funding from the close-fisted library board. Despite undoubted improvements in the didactic portions of the curriculum, the bulk of instruction was yet practical in nature, learned through long, arduous hours on the wards—five eight-hour days and two-four hour days per week.

An important consequence of the "Flexner revolution" at the University Hospital was the expansion and regularization of the indigent care service for the purpose of providing adequate clinical material for the instruction of medical students. From the outset, local indigents—their care subsidized by Johnson County authorities—had made up the bulk of the hospital's patient population; however, prompted by an indigent care law passed by the Michigan legislature in 1913, University of Iowa officials pressed the Iowa legislature to enact legislation providing state-subsidized care at University Hospital for indigent children under the age of sixteen. That law, passed in 1915 and known as the Perkins Law, soon brought hundreds of children, as well as smaller numbers of adults held in other state institutions, to the hospital for treatment at state expense. A second law, passed in 1919 and known as the Haskell-Klaus law, extended care to indigent adults. Thanks to the indigent care laws, hospital admissions rose from 2,362 in 1915 to 7,268 in 1920 and to some 10,000 by 1927,[21] with state indigent patients comprising two-thirds of the total.

The influx of indigent patients had a striking effect on both the hospital nursing service and the Nurse Training School, later the School of Nursing. The hospital's roster of graduate nurses grew from the thirteen of 1915 to thirty-four in 1920 and to forty-two in 1925.[22] No daily hospital census records survive from the early 1920s; however, the ratio of patient admissions to graduate nurses stood at 217 in 1927, down from 355 in 1910, reflecting the significant increase in graduate nurse staffing levels. Not surprisingly, the organization of the nursing service became more complex as well. In 1924, Josephine Creelman, who returned for a second stint as superintendent of nurses and principal of the renamed School of Nursing from 1922 to 1925, supervised first and second assistant superintendents of nurses, an educational director, a practical instructor, a night supervisor, and thirty-five head nurses and supervisors. Twenty-two of those graduate nurses had received their training at the University of Iowa; four others held diplomas from the Army School of Nursing, established in 1918.

Following much the same pattern, enrollments in the Nurse Training School/School of Nursing nearly doubled from 1915 to 1920, reaching 137 in the latter year. Nationally, some 1,750 nursing schools enrolled 55,000 students in 1920, putting the University of Iowa well above the national average of 31.4 students per school. By 1924, reflecting the continued growth in patient admissions and also the slow but certain specialization in clinical services, enrollments in the University of Iowa School of Nursing swelled to 209. Also in 1924, the school of nursing enrolled forty-four "affiliated students" in a program begun in 1920 to provide broader experience to students from smaller hospital training schools.

The maturation of the American hospital during the first two decades of the twentieth century brought major changes in hospital administration—most importantly in this context, the demise of the female nurse-superintendent, which had been a carryover from nineteenth-century practice. By the mid-teens, hospital administration was a recognized occupational specialty, with its own professional organization and its own professional journal, *The Modern Hospital*. Moreover, the new professional superintendent that emerged at most major hospitals was a male, often a physician. At the University of Iowa Hospital, Josephine Creelman, superintendent from 1912 to 1916, was the last female and the last nurse to hold that position. In 1914, the University of Iowa medical faculty approved a report from two outside experts recommending a substantially enhanced administrative role for the superintendent and also recommending recruitment of a physician to fill the position.[23] In September 1915, the finance committee of the State Board of Education proposed hiring "a male superintendent of the University Hospital, if the right man could be secured at a reasonable rate."[24] On January 1, 1916, William T. Graham, a physician and former superintendent of Methodist Hospital in Des Moines, became hospital superintendent at a salary of $2,750, well below the amount recommended in the 1914 report but well above the $1,800 paid Josephine Creelman as hospital superintendent and principal of the Nurse Training School. Creelman's successor, Mary C. Haarer, was formally superintendent of nursing and principal of the training school, reporting both to the hospital superintendent and the dean of the College of Medicine, the latter maintaining control over the hospital superintendent as well.

World War I and Nursing Education

When the United States entered World War I in April 1917, the Army and Navy Nurse Corps—created by acts of Congress in 1901 and 1908 respectively—expanded sharply, raising concerns over the availability and quality of nurses for both military and civilian service. In Iowa, the National Committee on Red Cross Nursing Service had established four enrollment districts already in 1914, and from 1917 those Red Cross enrollees constituted part of the reserve for the Army Nurse Corps, by far the larger of the two military nursing services.[25] Formal American entry into the war spurred renewed activity and the implementation of new machinery for the recruitment of nurses to the war effort. In November 1917, for example, the Iowa State Association of Registered Nurses held a special convention to hear a presentation from the director of the Central Division of the Red Cross Nursing Service. By Red Cross estimates, Iowa's fifty-four accredited nursing schools, producing some 3,275 graduate nurses annually, suggested a target enrollment of 416 nurses for wartime service, and an Iowa Red Cross field secretary began a recruiting tour of nurse training schools in May 1918. An unknown number of University of Iowa nursing students joined the Red Cross; however, one of them, Mabel Inez Sherburne, received an early release, with her diploma, in order to do so.[26] By the November 11, 1918, European armistice, 556 Iowa nurses had enrolled in the Red Cross Nursing Service. Most of those were in military service, and nine Iowa nurses died while in service.[27]

At the height of the war during 1917 and 1918, a massive nationwide campaign to recruit nursing students led to a twenty-five percent increase in nurse training school enrollments.[28] At the University of Iowa, however, there was no wartime enrollment bubble, as total enrollments stood at eighty in 1916-17 and eighty-two in 1917-18, despite what appears to have been a vigorous recruitment campaign by the Nurse Training School. A 1917 circular letter from Superintendent of Nursing Mary Haarer, for example, solicited the aid of high school officials in recruiting young females to nursing, and the May 1, 1918, edition of the *Bulletin of the State University of Iowa* included a rousing appeal to women to help the country in time of war by becoming trained nurses.

In addition to the existing Nurse Training School, the University of Iowa operated a special nurse training unit (#587) that recruited nurses—screened for physical and professional suitability—for assignment to hospitals on the home front. In the summer of 1917, the Nurse Training School also offered a series of preparatory courses—open to women and girls over age sixteen—to train Red Cross volunteers to provide elementary nursing services in homes and communities.[29] The following year, the University of Iowa was one of five university training schools to offer a preparatory course—part of an accelerated course of instruction known as the "Vassar Plan"—designed to attract college women to nursing, with the promise that recruits would obtain the nursing certificate in two years and three months rather than the standard three years.[30] Overall, local and national efforts to train more nurses for wartime service stood in striking contrast to the belated acceptance of accelerated instruction in medicine, which the American Medical Association and Association of American Medical Colleges resisted through 1917 on the basis of the need to preserve hard-won educational standards.

The influenza epidemic of the autumn of 1918 was one of the most memorable wartime experiences at the University of Iowa, one that placed extraordinary demands upon the hospital staff and student nurses.[31] By the opening of the 1918-1919 academic year, the war effort had transformed the university campus into a military camp, with some 2,000 male students enrolled in the Student Army Training Corps and housed in a mix of university facilities and hastily constructed barracks. When influenza struck the campus in September, the flood of patients soon swamped the University Hospitals, and in October Nursing Superintendent Haarer organized an effort by university and community leaders to provide patient care in a variety of public and private facilities, to which

Haarer, accompanied by the dean of the College of Medicine and the heads of internal medicine and surgery, made daily visits. By early October, a siege mentality gripped the community, as armed soldiers enforced quarantine regulations, university authorities barred Army Training Corps cadets from classes, and Iowa City churches, public and private schools, and theaters were closed. On October 5, University of Iowa President Walter Jessup reported some 480 cases quarantined, including thirty female students. By the end of October, however, the crisis was over, departing as rapidly as it had arrived. On average, seven student cadets died each day at the peak of the epidemic; overall, influenza struck seventy-six nurses, claiming the lives of one supervisor and five students.

Educational and Professional Reform Efforts

As nursing school enrollments expanded both locally and nationally through the 1920s, pushing the total of graduate nurses nationwide from fewer than 12,000 at the turn of the century to more than 149,000, nursing elites redoubled their efforts at professional reforms aiming to raise professional standards, to curtail entry into the profession, and to enhance the professional status of nursing.[32] Early in the century, Lavinia L. Dock had warned that licensing laws were not an "automatically working machine" and that nursing's status and jurisdiction could be defended and augmented only through "a recognized standard of professional education."[33] Accordingly, in 1917, the Education Committee of the National League of Nursing Education provided the first such effort in its *Standard Curriculum*, a comprehensive guide to curriculum content and objectives.[34] Six years later, the so-called "Goldmark Report"—initiated by Adelaide Nutting, funded by the Rockefeller Foundation, and compiled by the nineteen-member Committee for the Study of Nursing Education—made a powerful call for the reform of nursing education.

Taking the name of committee secretary Josephine C. Goldmark, that first national survey of nursing education documented programs at twenty-three nurse training schools across the United States.[35] Like Abraham Flexner's 1909 report on medical education,[36] the Goldmark Report was less noteworthy for its specific content, most of which was already common currency among nursing elites, than for the authority that the Rockefeller imprimatur conferred upon the committee's reiteration of the all-too-obvious shortcomings in existing hospital-based nurse training schools like that at the University of Iowa. In short, the committee concluded, nursing education in the common diploma program fell well below prevailing standards in other health care professions, the fault in general of too little emphasis on formal instruction and too long hours on the wards.

The solution to that problem, in the minds of committee members, was to make nursing education, like medical education, a university academic program. A 1923 article in *The Modern Hospital* offered much the same advice, exhorting hospital administrators to recognize that "the teaching hospital exists primarily for educational ends."[37] However, parallels between the Goldmark Report and the Flexner Report foundered, first, on the lack of resources to effect the recommended transformation in nursing education and, second, on the stiff resistance—from hospitals, from physicians, from university administrators, and from graduate nurses and student nurses themselves—to the implementation of higher educational standards. As a result, although Yale University opened its school of nursing as an independent university department in the wake of the Goldmark Report, the hospital nurse training schools survived largely unscathed, while a handful of universities began combined programs offering a bachelor of science degree and a nursing certificate or diploma.

In most respects, Iowa experience mirrored the mixed results of national efforts at nursing reform. In 1913, the Iowa State Association of Registered Nurses approved a modest set of educational recommendations, including adequate living quarters and classrooms in nursing schools, a maximum of fifty hours duty per week for students, and employment of a nurse inspector by the Board of Nurse Examiners to conduct on-site inspections of nursing schools.[38] In March 1914, a group of Iowa nurse training school superintendents established the Iowa State League of Nursing Education, an organization that soon affiliated with the National League of Nursing Education. With authorization from the state legislature, the Iowa Board of Nurse Examiners in 1917 adopted more stringent requirements for the fifty-plus nurse training schools in the state, and in the 1920s the board employed a state education director—a position subsidized by the state nurses association until the legislature appropriated funds for the purpose in 1929.

A 1924 state government reorganization renamed the Iowa State Board of Health the State Department of Health, and the professional licensing boards for medicine and nursing previously a part of the State Board of Health gained a significant measure of autonomy. In particular, the reorganization reduced the Board of Nurse Examiners from five members to three, all of them nurses, giving the board the independent status that nurses had initially envisioned. At the same time, however, the statute excluded from board membership all nurses associated with training schools. Intended to preclude the politicization of the examining board, a problem that had surfaced with regard to the board of medical examiners in the late nineteenth-century, the exclusion of educational elites from service on the Board of Nurse Examiners sorely limited the board's appetite for reform of education and practice standards.

The early postwar period also saw a restructuring of the Iowa State Association of Registered Nurses. In November 1919, during the presidency of Mary C. Haarer, association members reorganized the association in line with recommendations from the recently reorganized American Nurses Association.[39] The 1919 articles of incorporation and by-laws designated the Iowa association as an ANA affiliate and dedicated the organization to "secure legislation for nurses" and "to advance all other interests of the profession." The reorganized association rested upon a base of local alumnæ associations, although membership was also open to all registered nurses practicing in Iowa. In turn, alumnæ associations were represented in ten district associations, each of those allotted representation at the state level on the basis of district membership. Finally, the association's new articles of governance provided for seven standing committees: credentials, legislation, publication and press, program, nominations, Nurses Relief Fund of the ANA, and Red Cross.

In 1920, University of Iowa School of Nursing administrators implemented a combined program leading to the bachelor of science degree and graduate nurse certificate, a program entailing three years' study in the college of liberal arts followed by two years in nursing. However, the University of Iowa's combined program, like similar programs at other schools, attracted relatively few students since the market placed no premium on the bachelor's degree. In the mid-1920s, some two dozen combined programs nationwide enrolled fewer than 400 students.

A far more radical proposal surfaced in the early 1920s at the University of Iowa, one containing a blueprint for an independent college of nursing.[40] Arguing that higher nursing education standards would benefit the public health, the unsigned report envisioned a college set up much like the medical college, with the dean and faculty—who would hold clinical status in the University Hospitals— responsible for student admissions and instruction as well as selection and assignment of the hospitals' nursing staff. An operating budget accompanying the proposal called for an additional $49,000 above the current budget of $176,000 for hospital nursing services, most of the additional revenues applied to higher salaries for staff nurses and an hourly wage for student nurses. As might be imagined, that proposal went nowhere; nonetheless, it was indicative of nursing elites' frustrations with the hospital diploma school and, perhaps especially, physicians' continuing control over nursing education and hospital nursing practice.

From 1920 to 1925, working through the university extension service, the School of Nursing offered a two-semester course in public health nursing open to graduate nurses. The public health nursing course encompassed one semester of classroom courses from various colleges and departments of the university and a semester's field experience in visiting nursing, school nursing, industrial nursing, social service, and infant health clinics. The School of Nursing also offered postgraduate courses in "nursing administration and instruction," a curriculum consisting of required courses in psychology, institutional administration and management, and the teaching of nursing principles and methods in addition to a menu of electives in areas such as the sciences, education, psychology, and economics.

In the mid-1920s, the regular undergraduate curriculum in the School of Nursing began with a four-month preparatory term that included introductory work in the basic science areas as well as instruction in the rudiments of hospital economy, history of nursing, ethics of nursing, and physical education. Success in those preparatory subjects earned the student nurse the right to begin work on the wards and to participate in the "capping" ritual, marking her formal initiation into the nursing profession. The overall classroom curriculum had expanded substantially in the previous decade; in the course of the three-year program, student nurses attended a total of 440 hours of lectures—122 hours for freshmen, 213 hours for juniors, and 105 hours for seniors.

Nonetheless, the emphasis in training remained in the wards of the various clinical services, including three months in internal medicine, two months each in orthopædics, obstetrics, and surgery, and one month each in neurology, communicable diseases, gynecology, urology, and eye-ear-nose-and-throat. Standards of admission had also risen, requiring a high school education, evidence of physical fitness, and information on employment experience, financial resources, ethnic background, church membership, and marital status. Application materials warned prospective applicants that there had been "some trouble" in the past with "indiscretions" on the part of married, divorced, and widowed students, and the superintendent had no wish to repeat those unspecified experiences.

The August 1927 *Bulletin of the State University of Iowa* declared the student nurse's role "a high privilege and a sacred duty" leading to "unlimited opportunities" in a rapidly expanding profession.[41] Likewise, the School of Nursing counted among its missions the need "to institute and maintain the highest standards of nursing education."[42] Clearly, however, there was considerable dissonance between official rhetoric and both students' expectations and the harsh realities of the nursing profession. In the 1920s, most graduates still faced a future in the catch-as-catch-can world of private duty nursing, and barely more than half the School of Nursing's graduates in fact found a lifelong career in the nursing profession. In that respect, the career patterns of Iowa graduates approximated national averages. A survey of 420 nursing schools published in 1928 by the Committee on the Grading of Nursing Schools found just sixty percent of 1922 graduates actively engaged in nursing five years after graduation.[43]

Clearly, too, there was dissonance between official rhetoric and the immediate experience of student nurses, experience that found students squeezed between, on the one hand, rising academic expectations and, on the other hand, demanding work schedules imposed by hospital administrators more interested in labor productivity than in education. Not surprisingly, indeed in part by design, attrition rates among nursing students were high; of the ninety-two first-year students admitted to the University of Iowa School of Nursing in 1924, for example, just fifty-two received graduation certificates in 1927.

In the face of those realities, student nurses in the early twentieth century were not always the passive participants in an academic and professional culture that hospital administrators, staff physicians, and nurse instructors would have preferred. Instead, student nurses often sought to create an acceptable culture of their own, whether on the wards, in the classroom, or in the dormitory. As other observers have noted, frictions between nursing students and their instructor/supervisors were common, reflecting the stresses inherent in the student nurses' role, differences in social class and in cultural outlook, and generational differences, the last perhaps especially important in the "roaring twenties."[44]

It may well be that the University of Iowa School of Nursing's recruits, a high proportion of whom were daughters of farm families, were more accustomed to hospital-style work discipline than was true in many other areas of the country. Whatever the case, surviving evidence suggests only isolated incidents of student rebellion. In 1918, superintendent Haarer dismissed—and later reinstated—one student for having "bobbed" her hair, in violation of School of Nursing rules requiring either long hair or the wearing of a hairpiece or "switch." A few years later, in perhaps the most memorable instance of student self-expression, one student, Carmelita Calderwood, who later earned significant national recognition in nursing, repainted her Westlawn room in bright colors to hide the notorious "battleship gray" that coated the walls of the entire University Hospitals complex.[45]

University of Iowa student nurses in 1919 organized a student council to "present any subject or problem...as a composite whole and not as a collection of individual factions." Immediately, a delegation from the newly constituted council met with Nursing Superintendent Mary Haarer to apprise her of their organization and its aims and to discuss a pending disciplinary matter.[46] In subsequent years, the student nurses, acting through their council, sought relief on various fronts from what the students characterized as "the military discipline of the Training School." Most student concerns revolved around strictures on their social lives, including rules designed to limit fraternization with males and to discourage smoking, card-playing, and dancing. November 1920 resolutions, for example, demanded elimination of the Friday night curfew, institution of parlor visitations—presumably by males—after 10:00 PM on Saturdays, and dances with live music one Friday night each month.

Detailed rules still governed the lives of student nurses.[47] The day began with the ringing of the "rising bell" at 6:00 AM and breakfast at 6:20. Dinner came at noon and supper at 5:30 PM; eating "outside of the stated hours" was prohibited. Study hours began at 8:00 PM for freshman students and 9:00 PM for juniors. The dormitory was locked at 10:00 PM, with lights out at 10:45, except for Friday and Saturday nights. Each student was entitled to one late leave—until 12:20 AM—per week. Rules also required the student each morning to "make her bed, dust, and arrange her room, leaving it in good order." Each student enjoyed a weekly laundry quota of two uniforms, seven aprons, "two colored skirts," one cap, four collars, and four pieces of underwear; excess articles and those "requiring unusual time to iron" were "returned unlaundered." Students were "not to be seen in the hospital in street clothes." Conversely, they were not to "sit in autos" in front of the nurses dormitory while in hospital uniform.

In addition to pleasing their nursing supervisors, student nurses also learned to deal with physicians. Although physicians' views of nurses no doubt varied widely; most appear to have viewed the graduate nurse at best with ambivalence and often saw student nurses as barely more than menials. One nurse described an incident in which College of Medicine Dean Lee Wallace Dean ordered graduate nurses and students alike to undergo throat cultures, on the assumption that nurses were apt to be carriers of dangerous communicable diseases. When, to no one's surprise, virtually all proved to be harboring disease organisms, the dean jammed the hospital's isolation wards with designated nurse-carriers, leaving only "a foreign girl dishwasher" and a few nurses "to run the hospital."[48] Likewise illustrative of physician attitudes, one University of Iowa medical faculty member counseled student nurses to pledge "instant, constant and faithful service" to "kind-hearted and helpful physicians" whom it was their "privilege and duty to serve."[49] The same physician lectured student nurses, "Never act upon impulse, and as infrequently as possible upon your own judgment."[50] It should perhaps be noted, however, that those words bore an uncanny resemblance to some of Florence Nightingale's own observations on nurses and their duties.

A New Medical Campus: Triumph and Turmoil

Plans for a new University of Iowa medical campus on the west bank of the Iowa River were firmly in place prior to 1920, driven by the upward spiral in hospital admissions and the rapid growth in enrollments in the College of Medicine and the Nurse Training School. The vision of the new campus included a 1,000-bed general hospital, a children's hospital, a psychiatric hospital, a medical laboratories building, and a nurses' dormitory, a project begun with the Children's Hospital and Westlawn nurses' dormitory that opened in 1919 and 1921 respectively. Ironically, Abraham Flexner, whose 1909 report had savaged the University of Iowa College of Medicine and the University Hospital, not only embraced the plan put to him by university officials at a 1920 meeting; he also pledged "to put the entire reorganization through at once" with the help of funding from the Rockefeller Foundation and the General Education Board.[51]

Although events did not proceed at the pace Flexner and university planners initially hoped, the two Rockefeller foundations, under intense lobbying from Flexner, agreed in late 1922 to commit $1,125,000 each to the project, with a matching appropriation of $2,250,000 from the Iowa legislature. Construction of the new medical complex began in 1924, and the three-day dedication of the new General Hospital and Medical Laboratories in November 1928 attracted a cross-section of America's medical elite and marked the culmination of nearly two decades of dynamic growth for the University Hospitals, the School of Nursing, and the College of Medicine. Symbolic of nursing's professional marginalization, the dedication program did not recognize the occasion as one of special significance in the history of nursing education at the university. Indeed, the long list of distinguished guests did not include any representation from nursing, and nurses and nursing played little part in the festivities apart from an "informal reception and tea" hosted at the nurses' dormitory by Nursing Superintendent Lois B. Corder.

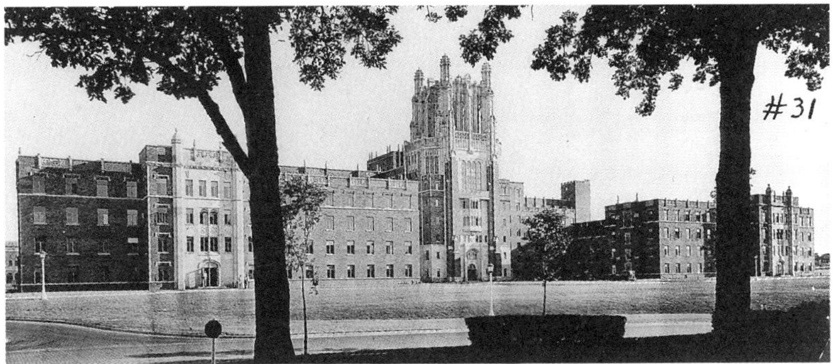

Fig. 1.4. New University of Iowa General Hospital, 1928 (College of Nursing Collection).

At the time of the hospital dedication, Lois Blanche Corder in fact had been nursing superintendent barely more than a year. A University of Iowa diploma graduate, later operating theater supervising nurse, then assistant superintendent of nursing and, in 1925-26, acting superintendent, Corder's permanent elevation to the superintendency was the result of a spring 1927 blowup that rocked both the University Hospitals and the College of Medicine. Directly at issue for all concerned in the dispute was the administrative style of College of Medicine Dean Lee Wallace Dean, who had, with the support of successive university presidents, forged a tightly centralized administration that gave him a firm grip on the College of Medicine and the University Hospitals. Over the course of more than a decade in office, Dean's ambitions and his alleged favoritism toward his own department of head specialties had alienated many of his colleagues, ranging from department heads and junior faculty to the hospital superintendent and the superintendent of nursing.

The storm broke in April 1927 with a banner headline in the local newspaper declaring "Three Resign Posts on Iowa 'Medic' Staff," a reference to the resignations of surgery head Charles J. Rowan, acting internal medicine head Frank J. Rohner, and hospitals Superintendent Jesse L. MacElroy. "I have resigned," Rohner wrote, "because I have no confidence in, or respect for the present head of the medical school."[52] As events unfolded, it became clear that Rohner's sentiments applied to a good many others upset with Dean's "high-handed," "one-man" rule and his "insincerity" and "duplicity."[53] In early May, the State Board of Education accepted

Lee Wallace Dean's resignation from the deanship. Under continued faculty pressure, Dean shortly thereafter resigned his faculty position as well.

Among the casualties of the affair was Superintendent of Nursing Mae MacArthur, who had come to the job only in 1926. MacArthur joined the protest against the dean by submitting her resignation within a few days of the initial round of resignations, at which time Lois Corder became nursing superintendent. Thus, the end of the first three decades of nursing education at the University of Iowa saw the School of Nursing with a new head, a new General Hospital, and a new Westlawn dormitory accommodating 414 nurses, including staff and students, in its 245 rooms. In addition, Corder began her twenty-year tenure in conjunction with a new hospitals superintendent, Robert Neff, and a new College of Medicine dean, Henry Houghton.

Conclusion

Mae MacArthur's 1927 resignation highlighted the frustrating ambiguities inherent in nursing and nursing education early in this century. The captive position of nursing education and the nursing service at the University of Iowa, subject to the agendas of University Hospitals' administrators and the dean of the College of Medicine, severely restricted the development of an autonomous profession—that is, one with substantial control over professional education and practice. In 1922, a candidate for the nursing superintendency at the University of Iowa, Effie J. Taylor, who later became dean of the Yale University School of Nursing, pinpointed the weaknesses of the traditional hospital nursing school. In the wake of a campus visit, Taylor described to hospitals Superintendent Arthur J. Lomas her many reservations about the school. Lomas had assured Taylor that the training school was "a recognized department of the University," but Taylor objected that the school was, in the university's own description, "under the administration of the Superintendent of the Hospital" and also under the medical dean's "general direction," a situation that she found incompatible with serious educational objectives.[54]

Closely related to the problem of nursing's continued subordination, indeed a consequence of it, was the wholesale and unrestricted growth in the numbers of graduate nurses in Iowa and nationwide and the difficulty of imposing meaningful standards on professional education and practice. The 1928 report of the Committee on the Grading of Nursing Schools documented the serious problem of the over-production of nursing graduates, a finding at odds with the prevailing sense of a nursing shortage in the 1920s. The committee's twenty-one members, representing the National League of Nursing Education, the American Nurses Association, the National Organization for Public Health Nursing, the American Medical Association, the American College of Surgeons, the American Hospital Association, and the American Public Health Association, noted both the startling growth in numbers of graduate nurses in previous decades and the potentially explosive growth that lay ahead.

In Iowa, the number of graduate nurses per 1,000 population rose from eight in 1900 to 150 in 1920; in comparison, the physician-population ratio declined in the same period from 180 to 148 per 1,000.[55] Nationally, the figures were much the same, with 16 nurses per 1,000 population in 1900 and 141 in 1920; meanwhile, the national physician-population ratio fell from 173 per 1,000 in 1900 to 137 in 1920. More than ninety percent of nursing registries—local agencies matching nurses to nursing positions—reported an oversupply of graduate nurses in hospital nursing, private duty nursing, and public health nursing.[56] Based on such findings, and with the Great Depression just over the horizon, nursing's professional future was, to say the least, a troubled one.

Notes

1. For general descriptions, see James H. Cassedy, "Why Self-Help? Americans Alone with Their Diseases, 1800-1850," in Ronald L. Numbers and Judith Walzer Leavitt, eds., *Medicine Without Doctors: Home Health Care in American History* (New York: Science History Publications/USA, 1977).
2. John M. Toner, "Statistics of Regular Medical Associations and Hospitals of the United States," *Transactions of the American Medical Association* 24 (1873), pp. 329-334.
3. For a fuller chronicle of Mercy Hospital, see Sister Mary Brigid Condon, *From Obscurity to Distinction: The Story of Mercy Hospital, Iowa City, 1873-1993* (Iowa City, IA: Mercy Hospital, 1993).

4. Charles A. Schaeffer, Report to the Board of Regents, 1889, p. 23, University of Iowa Archives.

5. Board of Regents, *Biennial Report, 1899*, p. 12, University of Iowa Archives.

6. See Josephine Dolan, "Nurses in American History: Three Schools— 1873," *American Journal of Nursing* 75 (June 1975), pp. 989-992.

7. Ashley, *Hospitals, Paternalism, and the Role of the Nurse*, p. 21. See also Teresa E. Christy, "The Fateful Decade, 1890-1900," *American Journal of Nursing* 75 (July 1975), pp. 1,163-1,165.

8. The 1880s and 1890s saw burgeoning hospital construction in Iowa, including Mercy Hospitals in several major cities, as well as community and non-denominational hospitals, for example the Jennie Edmundson Memorial Hospital in Council Bluffs and the Cottage Hospital in Creston. Most Iowa hospitals of the era conducted nurse training schools.

9. Account of Ida Hayes, May 1973, Folder 1, Etta Rasmussen Papers, University of Iowa Archives.

10. Nancy Tomes, "'Little World of Our Own': The Pennsylvania Hospital Training School for Nurses, 1895-1907," *Journal of the History of Medicine and Allied Sciences* (October 1978), pp. 507-530.

11. Ann Slater to Lois B. Corder, [no date, but appears to have been c. 1928], MS File, Series I, M-N, School of Nursing-Miscellaneous, University of Iowa Archives.

12. Bertha Kampmeier Box, School of Nursing Papers, University of Iowa Archives.

13. For a detailed view of the discussion and motivation surrounding formation of the society, see Lewenson, *Taking Charge*, pp. 70-82. For first hand testimony, see Isabel A. Hampton, *et al.*, *Nursing of the Sick, 1893* (New York: McGraw-Hill, 1949) and *Papers and Discussions from the International Congress of Charities, Correction, and Philanthropy, Chicago, 1893* (National League of Nursing Education, 1949).

14. See Hine, *Black Women in White*, for a full discussion.

15. From a resolution quoted in Emma C. Wilson, *Historical Outline of the Iowa State Association of Registered Nurses and Related Organizations* (The Association, 1932), p. 10.

16. Mary Lucille Shannon, "Nurses in American History: Our First Four Licensure Laws," *American Journal of Nursing* 75 (August 1975), pp. 1,327-1,329.

17. See Stow Persons, "The Flexner Investigation of the University of Iowa Medical School," *Annals of Iowa* 48 (Summer/Fall 1986), pp. 274-291.

18. Abraham Flexner, "State University of Iowa Medical Department," Box 19-6, GE MacLean Papers, University of Iowa Archives.

19. In 1910, a single Board of Education superseded the previous Boards of Regents that had governed each of the state educational institutions, in-

cluding the state university in Iowa City, the state college in Ames, and the state normal school in Cedar Falls.

20. Unsigned Memorandum, 1916, MS File, Series I, M-N, School of Nursing-Miscellaneous, University of Iowa Archives.

21. University Hospital Annual Reports, 1915-1920, University of Iowa Archives.

22. The plural, University of Iowa Hospitals, appeared in 1919 with the opening of the Children's Hospital on the bluff west of the Iowa River.

23. Lee Wallace Dean to Thomas Macbride, December 19, 1914, Box 1 (1914), Folder 6, Thomas Macbride Papers, University of Iowa Archives.

24. Board of Education Finance Committee Minutes, September 20, 1915, University of Iowa Archives.

25. For a national overview of nursing during World War I, see Philip A. Kalisch and Beatrice J. Kalisch, *The Advance of American Nursing* (Boston, MA: Little, Brown and Company, 1978), pp. 295-325.

26. The Red Cross Nursing Service would not accept Sherburne except under an early release. Haarer notified Red Cross officials in June 1918, that Sherburne would be "released and given diploma as soon as you want her." Penciled notation on letter, A Kerr, Director of Bureau of Enrollment for Red Cross Nursing Service, to M Haarer, June 26, 1918, Record Group 16, Box 1, Folder "Nursing, School of, Historical Sketch," School of Nursing Papers, The University of Iowa Archives.

27. Emma C. Wilson, *Historical Outline of the Iowa State Association of Registered Nurses and Related Organizations*, pp. 97-98.

28. Kalisch and Kalisch, *Advance of American Nursing*, p. 302.

29. "Courses in Red Cross Service," *Bulletin of the State University of Iowa*, June 15, 1917.

30. Kalisch and Kalisch, *Advance of American Nursing*, p. 304.

31. Much of the influenza story related here is taken from MS File, Series I, M-N, School of Nursing Influenza Epidemic Folder, University of Iowa Archives. For a more general perspective, see Alfred W. Crosby, *America's Forgotten Pandemic: The Influenza of 1918* (New York: Cambridge University Press, 1989).

32. See Melosh, *"The Physician's Hand,"* pp. 41-44.

33. Lavinia L. Dock, "What We May Expect from the Law," *American Journal of Nursing* 1 (October 1900), pp. 8-12.

34. See Em Olivia Bevis, "Illuminating the Issues: Probing the Past, A History of Nursing Curriculum Development—The Past Shapes the Present," in Bevis and Jean Watson, eds., *Toward a Caring Curriculum: A New Pedagogy for Nursing* (New York: National League for Nursing Education, 1989), pp. 21-22.

35. Josephine C. Goldmark, *Nursing and Nursing Education in the United States: Report of the Committee for the Study of Nursing Education and Re-*

port of a Survey by Josephine Goldmark (New York: Macmillan Company, 1923).

36. Shortly after Flexner's report, Adelaide Nutting had failed in a prolonged attempt to interest the Carnegie Foundation in conducting a similar survey of nursing education.

37. Richard Olding Beard, "Hospital Economics of the Nursing Situation," *The Modern Hospital* 21 (October 1923), pp. 394-396.

38. Wilson, *Historical Outline*, pp. 20-21.

39. Administration By Laws, 1908-1937, Box 6, Iowa Nurses Association, University of Iowa Women's Archives.

40. The author is not identified, nor is the date; however, internal references suggest that the proposal likely came from Josephine Creelman, perhaps acting in conjunction with one or more of her colleagues, sometime between 1922 and 1925: MS File, Series, I, M-N, School of Nursing-Miscellaneous, University of Iowa Archives.

41. *Bulletin of the State University of Iowa*, New Series, No. 418, August 27, 1927, "Mid-Summer Announcement of the School of Nursing."

42. *Bulletin of the State University of Iowa*, New Series, No. 182, April 1, 1920, "Annual Catalogue of the School of Nursing, 1919-1920."

43. Committee on the Grading of Nursing Schools, *Nurses, Patients, and Pocketbooks*, p. 51.

44. See Rosenberg, *The Care of Strangers*, "Healing Hands: Nursing in the Hospital," pp. 212-236.

45. "Times Have Changed for Nursing Education at UI," *Iowa City Press Citizen*, December 3, 1971.

46. This and much of the following material is taken from Nursing Archive, Student Body of Nurses Minutes, University of Iowa Archives.

47. "House Rules and Information," January 1, 1927, Iowa University School of Nursing, University Hospital, Iowa City, Iowa.

48. Ann Slater to Lois B. Corder, no date (1928), MS File, Series I, M-N, School of Nursing-Miscellaneous, University of Iowa Archives.

49. Quoted in Bonnie K. Smola, "A Study of the Development of Diploma and Baccalaureate Degree Nursing Education Programs in Iowa from 1907-1978," PhD Dissertation, Iowa State University, 1980, p. 110.

50. MS File, Series I, M-N, School of Nursing Curriculum Folder, University of Iowa Archives.

51. For a detailed discussion, see Lee Anderson, "'A Great Victory': Abraham Flexner and the New Medical Campus at the University of Iowa," *Annals of Iowa* 51 (Winter 1992), pp. 231-251.

52. Quoted in "Three Doctors Quit Posts at S.U.I. College," *Des Moines Register*, May 5, 1927.

53. See "Charge Dean Used School for Own Gain," *Des Moines Register*, May 12, 1927; Medical Faculty Minutes, May 17, 1927, University of Iowa Archives.
54. Quoted in Smola, "A Study of the Development of Diploma and Baccalaureate Degree Nursing Education Programs in Iowa from 1907-1978," pp. 241-243.
55. Committee on the Grading of Nursing Schools, *Nurses, Patients, and Pocketbooks*, p. 44.
56. *Ibid.*, p. 80.

Chapter Two

Hard Times and New Directions, 1929-1949

Completion of the new University of Iowa General Hospital and Medical Laboratories in 1928 proved not to be the opening chapter to a new and even more promising era for health sciences education at the university. To the contrary, the November 1928 dedication ceremonies served as a convenient dividing line between, on the one hand, nearly two decades of expansion and reform and, on the other hand, some fifteen years of austerity and uncertainty encompassing the Depression and World War II. For the School of Nursing, as for all the University of Iowa's colleges and departments, the 1930s and early 1940s were difficult years, dominated by shrinking budgets, pay cuts, and staff reductions. However, that extended experience of hardship also shaped nursing's professional development in important ways and, perhaps unexpectedly, opened promising new professional opportunities.

As national unemployment figures exploded from an average of barely more than three percent of the civilian work force in 1929 to twenty-five percent in 1933 and held stubbornly at more than seventeen percent as late as 1939, aggregate personal income in the United States fell from $85.9 billion in 1929 to a low of $47.0 billion in 1933 and recovered only to $72.8 billion in 1939.[1] Meanwhile, the Iowa economy of the 1930s was still predominantly agricultural, and from 1929 into the early and middle 1930s, prices paid Iowa farmers for agricultural produce—both crops and livestock—fell by half to two-thirds. In the 1929 crop year, for example, the average price of corn was eighty cents per bushel; in 1931 and 1932 the price was thirty-two cents. Returns from livestock slumped even more dramatically, as cattle and hog prices fell by two-thirds in the same period. Farm foreclosures and bank failures escalated in the wake of skidding commodity prices, and, as late as

1940, both per capita income and total personal income in Iowa still lagged significantly behind 1929 figures.

In Iowa as elsewhere, economic collapse put enormous pressure on state and local governments and on public institutions of all kinds. Government revenues in Iowa—then derived largely from property taxes at both state and local levels—dwindled, while sky-rocketing unemployment inflated demand for many government services. In 1931, Iowa Governor Dan Turner appointed a six-member Committee on Reduction of Costs of Government to suggest economies in government operations, and through the early 1930s the state legislature instituted substantial funding reductions for the University of Iowa, dropping appropriations twenty-eight percent from 1929 to 1933 and forcing successive salary cuts for university faculty and staff in 1931 and 1932. At the same time, state appropriations for indigent care at the University Hospitals, capped already in the late 1920s at one million dollars annually, slid as well, and patient waiting lists grew at a worrisome pace.

For the University of Iowa in general and for the health sciences campus in particular, World War II brought little relief from the austerity of the 1930s. Nonetheless, the intense war effort from 1942 to 1945 profoundly affected American society and institutions and did so to a significantly greater degree, and with longer lasting effects, than did the wartime experience of 1917-1918. Most immediately, World War II spurred a rapid expansion of nursing education at the University of Iowa and throughout the United States, in part because of special wartime educational programs designed chiefly to produce trained nurses for military service. Beyond that, wartime experience significantly enhanced the professional status of nursing, as it did the professional status of medicine, with major implications for the content and organization of nursing education in the postwar decades.

The Hospital and the Nursing Profession in the Depression

Perhaps surprisingly, the Depression had little obvious effect on the growth of the American hospital system, despite the fact that aggregate personal expenditures for health care goods and services in the United States slumped from nearly three billion dollars in 1929 to less than two billion dollars in 1933.[2] According to American

Medical Association figures, the number of hospital beds in the United States increased from 817,020 in 1920 to 955,869 in 1930, an increase of seventeen percent. In 1935, the total stood at 1,075,139, an increase of 18.5 percent in the five-year period that was in fact the darkest of the Depression. In 1940, the total reached 1,226,245, a further increase of fourteen percent since 1935, some of that owing to Depression-inspired federal subsidies for public construction projects that included hospitals and schools. Hospital utilization also increased in the 1930s; general hospitals' average daily patient census increased from 240 in 1930 to 261 in 1935 and to 325 in 1940.

The United States census recorded 149,000 employed graduate nurses in 1920, 294,000 in 1930, and 377,000 in 1940.[3] The number of nursing schools actually declined from 1,755 to 1,311 between 1920 and 1940, but total nursing enrollments increased considerably during the period, rising from just under 55,000 in 1920 to nearly 79,000 in 1929, slumping to 67,500 in 1935 and then recovering to 85,000 in 1940. More important, the annual production of new graduate nurses rose from some 15,000 in 1920 to nearly 26,000 in 1931 before tailing off to 19,600 in 1935 and rising to 23,600 in 1940.[4] Notwithstanding the growth in America's hospital system, private duty nursing was still the mainstay of professional practice; however, poor economic conditions and the public's increasing reliance on hospital care in time of illness pinched the private duty market and led to serious unemployment and underemployment among graduate nurses. By 1940, private duty nursing in hospitals accounted for as much as eighty percent of all private duty nursing.

As new graduates flooded an already saturated market, nursing leaders and nursing registries in many areas issued public warnings that their local markets could absorb no more job-seekers. A Chicago-based regional placement service instituted in 1931 to serve Illinois, Michigan, Indiana, Wisconsin, and Iowa in fact accomplished very little for Iowa nurses during the 1930s, finding places for only an average of perhaps three dozen nurses each year and as few as eighteen in 1938.[5] A 1934 survey of the University of Iowa School of Nursing's 977 graduates (1900 to 1933) counted just 517 active in nursing, 318 of those in Iowa.[6] During the worst of the Depression, two New Deal programs, the Civil Works Administration (CWA) and, at a later date, the Works Progress Administration (WPA), afforded temporary relief to several thousand unemployed graduate nurses across the United States, nurses who assisted the agencies in various public health endeavors. In one such instance, the University of Iowa Hospitals in early 1934 employed forty-one graduate nurses whose pay was subsidized by the CWA.

The harsh economic conditions of the Depression exacerbated longstanding problems within nursing. As already mentioned, the Depression accelerated the collapse of private duty nursing, a collapse fueled also by consumers' changing health care behaviors and the emergence of the hospital as the central focus of health care. Facing large numbers of graduate nurses unable to earn a living, nursing organizations, including the American Nurses Association and National League of Nursing Education, pressed for the employment of additional nurses in hospitals.[7] The resulting change in nurses' status from independent, if struggling, practitioner to employee was an important moment in the twentieth-century history of nursing. At the same time, continued calls from nursing leaders for higher educational standards and, implicitly at least, a professional hierarchy grounded in academic credentials worsened nursing's internal divisions. Also, and perhaps most importantly, Depression-era pressures made clear that nurse practice acts like Iowa's that reserved the titles "registered nurse" and "graduate nurse" to qualified practitioners but did not define and protect the practice of nursing were of very limited utility in preserving and enhancing the integrity of the nursing profession. Many observers understood that, like physicians or pharmacists, nurses badly needed practice acts barring the untrained from professional practice, while state examining boards badly needed greater powers to inspect nursing schools and to impose stricter regulation on the profession.[8]

Chiefly for reasons of economy, the University of Iowa Hospitals operated below capacity from 1929 to 1945. But stagnant funding levels and diminished operating capacity notwithstanding, patient admissions increased, reflecting the importance of the facilities' indigent care role, the higher incidence of indigency as economic conditions soured, and significant economies in hospital operations. In the five years from 1930 to 1935, admissions rose more than fifty percent, a rate of increase that dropped to just twelve percent from 1935 to 1940, perhaps chiefly reflecting a slight overall improvement in economic conditions. In part, the hospitals accommodated more patients by decreasing the average length of stay, as total patient days increased only twenty-nine percent from 1930 to 1935—well below the rate of increase in patient admissions. From 1935 to 1940, total patient-days at the University Hospitals actually declined three percent.[9]

Early on, the Depression uncovered serious weaknesses in the indigent care system that provided the clinical material essential to both nursing education and medical education at the University of Iowa.[10] Waiting lists for all clinical services grew alarmingly in the early 1930s, and local officials across Iowa employed various strategies to circumvent normal admissions procedures, for example, by direct appeals through political channels and by designating patients as emergency cases. Such problems intensified longstanding political opposition toward the College of Medicine and the University Hospitals and built a temporary coalition in the Iowa legislature to cripple, if not dismantle, the existing indigent care system. That coalition, led by Elbert E. Munger, a Spencer physician, included many members of the state medical society who likewise held grudges, both personal and ideological, against the university. It likewise included hard-pressed farmers who desperately sought property tax cuts and local officials who complained of inequities in the distribution of indigent service among Iowa's ninety-nine counties.

In 1933, the state legislature designated a nine-member task force—led by Munger—to study the indigent care issue and to propose solutions to its major problems. The recommendations in the preliminary task force report, issued April 1, 1933, threatened a significant reduction in the University Hospitals' role in indigent care and also counseled a corresponding reduction in College of Medicine enrollments and, thus, in the hospitals' educational mission.[11] In the summer of 1933, hospitals Superintendent Robert E. Neff, with the approval of the Board of Education, countered with a quota system to apportion indigent admissions among Iowa's counties on the basis of population. Although the quota system did not address the fundamental concerns of critics like Elbert Munger, it effectively fractured the coalition seeking wholesale changes in the indigent care system and ensured the continued flow of indigent patients to the University Hospitals.

Through the Depression years, the University of Iowa Hospitals' nursing service continued to expand, despite attempts early on to reduce staffing levels. In 1929, the hospitals employed forty-five graduate nurses in administrative and supervisory positions, a figure little changed since the early 1920s. However, under the leadership of a new director of nursing, a new hospitals superintendent, and a new medical dean, the hospitals rapidly expanded the ranks of graduates listed in the hospitals' budget as "general duty nurses." The hospitals' budget for 1927-28 listed six general duty positions; in 1929-30, the number grew to twenty; in 1935-36, the total climbed to seventy-four; and, in 1939-40, the total was eighty-eight, echoing the nationwide rise in general duty nurses from 4,000 in 1929 to 27,000 in 1937.[12] The ranks of administrative and supervisory nurses at the University Hospitals grew more slowly, reaching fifty-three in 1935 and sixty-six at the end of the decade, nine of the latter counted as administrative and educational staff, twenty-four as supervisors and thirteen as assistant supervisors in the General Hospital, and ten as supervisors in the Children's Hospital. In addition, the Psychopathic Hospital, which then operated under separate administration, employed twelve graduate nurses.

Faced with added costs of a continually expanding salaried nursing staff, the hospital administration of Robert Neff—ridiculed by some as "Economy" Neff—turned to a variety of cost-cutting strategies. Salary reductions were severe, especially for general duty nurses who saw their annual salaries cut from $1,080 in 1930 to $808 and, ultimately, to $720 by the mid-1930s. Still, the last figure accorded with the average of $756 tabulated in a 1934 survey of graduate nurse salaries at seventy-five hospitals nationwide;[13] moreover, nurses received "maintenance"—room, board, and laundry—in addition to their stated salaries. The State Board of Education in 1933 slashed vacation and holiday benefits in half for all nursing staff and made major reductions in vacation time for students as well. Also, beginning in 1931 and extending through much of the decade, the hospitals' annual budgets included thirty graduate nurses who received only room, board, and laundry for their labors. Those additions boosted the total graduate nursing staff to more than 150 in 1935. Nonetheless, Superintendent Robert Neff complained in September 1936 that conditions "compelled" the hospitals "to accept nurses who in normal times would have been entirely unacceptable."[14] By the late 1930s, annual salaries of administrative and supervisory personnel at the University Hospitals had recovered some lost ground, ranging from $1,000 to $1,300, plus room, board, and laundry. Salaries of general duty nurses rose to $900 plus "maintenance," although the hospitals' annual budgets of the late 1930s listed as many as a dozen nurses, roughly half of them male, who received higher salaries in lieu of maintenance.

The School of Nursing and the Depression

From a total of 240 in 1924-25, enrollments in the University of Iowa School of Nursing rose above 300 briefly in the late 1920s, peaking at 334 students in residence during the 1928-29 academic year. The following year, enrollments dipped slightly to 300, followed by a steep decline in the early 1930s, the total falling to 264 in 1930-31, to 218 in 1931-32, and to 188 in 1932-33. Thereafter, enrollments staged a slow and halting recovery, rising to 201 in 1933-34, to 213 in 1934-35, and to 267 in 1939-40. Those aggregate figures, however, disguised significant variations in enrollment patterns among first-, second-, and third-year classes. In absolute numbers, first-year classes suffered the largest overall decline from the late 1920s to the early 1930s, falling from a high of 151 in 1928-29 to a low of fifty-six in 1931-32. At the same time, second-year classes showed a higher percentage decline, from ninety-seven in 1929-30 to thirty-seven in 1932-33. In contrast, third-year enrollments fell far less dramatically, from a high of 118 in 1928-29 to a low of seventy-four in both 1932-33 and 1933-34.

To some extent, the decline in nursing enrollments reflected hospital administrators' reactions to the Depression. Graduate nurses' slumping salaries in the 1930s and the availability of significant numbers of trained nurses who would work in return for nothing more than room and board fundamentally changed the economic calculus for hospital administrators whose interest lay in maximizing returns on their nursing investments. The decline in nursing enrollments at the University of Iowa, then, reflected in part the University Hospitals' shift from a student nursing staff toward a graduate nursing staff. To some extent, too, declining enrollments reflected the changing economics of nursing education,

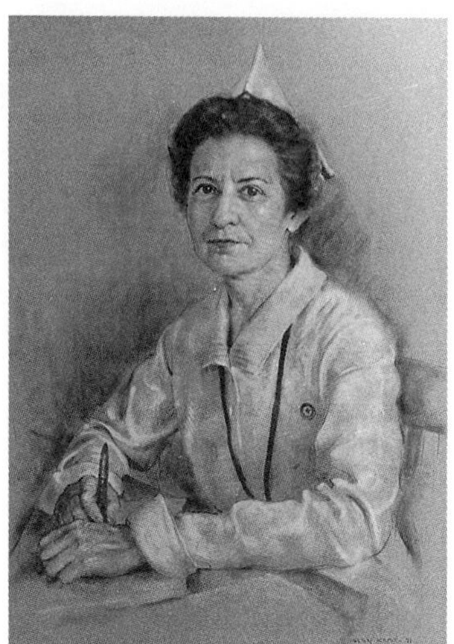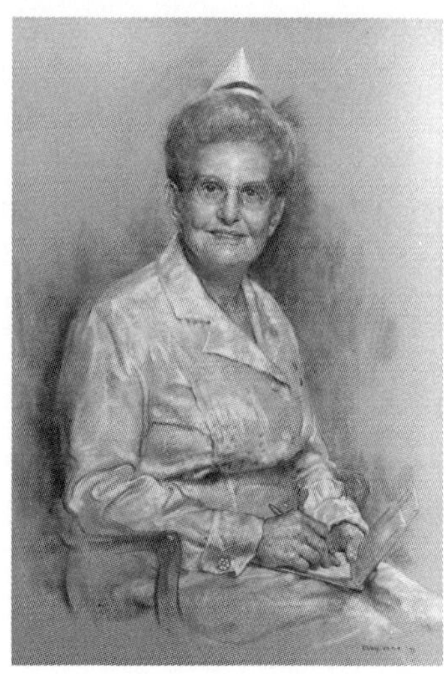

Fig. 2.1. Lois B. Corder, Nursing Director, 1928-47, left, and Lola M. Lindsey, School of Nursing Instructor and Director of Education, 1928-48, right (College of Nursing Collection).

which entailed significant sacrifice in terms of forgone income, a sacrifice that fewer families were willing to shoulder at the depths of the Depression. Moreover, the university, hard-pressed for operating funds, imposed substantial fees—first set at $100 in 1930 and later raised to $165—for first-year students to cover a part of the costs of room, board, instruction, and medical care while the student was not yet engaged in ward duty.

In Iowa and across the nation, the late 1920s and 1930s saw the same lack of standardization in admissions criteria and in curriculum that had plagued nursing education from the turn of the century. A 1930 report counted only five of forty-eight nursing schools in Iowa requiring four years of high school experience for admission; fifteen schools required two years; twenty-six set one year minimums; and two had just an eighth grade requirement.[15] An earlier nationwide survey of 1,500 nursing schools counted just 224 requiring four years of high school for admission, while nineteen required three years, 406 required two years, 813 required one year, and thirty-eight required just an eighth-grade education. At the same time, the latter survey highlighted problems regarding the small size of many sponsoring hospitals and, consequently, the small size of the nursing student body. Nationally, more than a third of hospitals with nursing schools had patient censuses of fewer than fifty per day, and 774 schools—more than half the schools surveyed— enrolled fewer than thirty students.[16] In Iowa, efforts by nursing organizations and the Nurse Examining Board to tighten educational standards, efforts aided by the effects of the Depression, resulted in the closing of several marginal nursing schools during the early 1930s, reducing the Iowa total from fifty-two schools in 1928 to thirty-three in 1933, none of them in hospitals of fewer than fifty beds. In the same period, the total enrollment of student nurses fell from some 2,100 to 1,500.

After eight years' work, the Committee on the Grading of Nursing Schools, in its 1934 final report entitled *Nursing Schools Today and Tomorrow*, offered a discouraging summary of conditions in the nation's nursing schools, highlighting once again the long hours of ward service and the haphazard nature of instruction both on the wards and in the classrooms.[17] Perhaps in part for political reasons, the committee did not disparage the apprenticeship model of training in hospital schools but noted that the high student/teacher ratio made nursing different from earlier apprenticeship programs in professions such as medicine and law. Likewise, the committee noted that head nurses responsible for much of nursing instruction were, on average, just twenty-six years of age and spent less than an hour each day working with students. Meanwhile, the typical student spent more than 7,000 hours on ward duty in the course of the three-year diploma program, compared to the National League of Nursing Education's then recommended 6,252 hours.

The Committee on the Grading of Nursing Schools emphasized the need of an enlarged didactic emphasis to better ground the graduate nurse in the basic sciences and social sciences. However, such a change seemed unlikely when twenty-nine percent of instructors in nursing schools had not themselves completed high school. Overall, the committee's recommendations to address serious and persistent problems in nursing education and in the profession at large—including improving the quality of nursing education and reducing the number of graduate nurses, promoting the use of graduate nurses in hospital care, and achieving autonomy for nursing education—faced seemingly insurmountable fiscal and ideological obstacles. Economic conditions during the Depression only exacerbated obstacles to meaningful professional reforms; meanwhile, most hospital administrators maintained a preference for the more docile student nurses over graduate nurses and scoffed at arguments for greater educational attainments for nurses.[18] Nonetheless, in line with the grading committee's findings, the National League of Nursing Education's revised *Curriculum Guide* of 1937 further reduced total ward hours to 4,800 and increased the recommended classroom hours to 1,200-1,300.

Henry S. Houghton, dean of the University of Iowa College of Medicine and *ex officio* dean of the University of Iowa School of Nursing, delivered a paper in 1931 to the Institute of Nursing Education in Chicago on the central issues and problems in nursing education.[19] Although Houghton was more sympathetic to nurses and their professional aspirations than were many physicians, he nonetheless maintained some skepticism toward nursing elites' arguments in favor of more scientific training for nurses. Admitting that the growth of medical science and technology appeared to have put medicine and nursing on converging paths, Houghton maintained that the two remained "intrinsically different." In his estimation, "The one [medicine] is essentially a matter of erudition," while the other [nursing] involved the "meticulous execution of a plan of action laid down by the physician." Unlike most of his physician colleagues, however, the dean did not discount the need for highly trained nurses for specialized work and for instructional positions, and he proposed replacing the typical hospital nursing school of the day with a two-tiered system of nursing education. The first level in Houghton's system would involve a year of liberal arts education followed by three years' nursing education centered solely on classroom instruction, discounting ward labor as of little or no utility to the student nurse. In the second tier of Houghton's revamped system, promising candidates recruited from the first "purely vocational" training phase would move into a specially designed university degree program offering more concentrated scientific training. For Houghton, economy was one of the virtues of his proposal, noting that salaries for nursing instructors cost the University of Iowa Hospitals some $46,000 annually, money that he thought would be better invested in more graduate nurses to serve patients.

In contrast, Houghton's successor, Ewen Murchison MacEwen, an anatomist who assumed the deanship in 1935, was initially much more traditional in his view of nursing education. In 1936, for example, University of Iowa President Eugene A. Gilmore forwarded to MacEwen a questionnaire prepared by Sister Henrietta Guyot of the Catholic University Department of Nursing Education in Washington, D. C., dealing with standards for nursing schools. MacEwen made plain his view that the primary function of the nursing school was to train bedside nurses, work for which a liberal arts background was superfluous.[20] Setting educational standards too high, MacEwen argued, would result in a drastic reduction in the nursing population and force hospitals to rely on poorly trained practical nurses for patient care. Moreover, MacEwen expressed his preference for the current system of hospital schools, arguing that schools of nursing should be directly connected to hospitals, although not necessarily university hospitals, and that any change in that system would likewise imperil the supply of trained nurses.

Through the 1930s and into the late 1940s, the University of Iowa School of Nursing maintained both the three-year certificate program and the five-year combined program leading to the bachelor's degree and nursing certificate. In addition, students already holding the bachelor's degree could enroll in the School of Nursing in the 1930s and complete the nursing program in two years and three months. The school's published admissions standards for beginning nurses included detailed requirements in several academic areas, ranging from English and mathematics to history and government. The bulk of student nurses' classroom instruction—a total of 755 hours in the mid-1930s—came in the first year, with courses covering a broad spectrum of the basic sciences as well as nursing fundamentals. The second year curriculum included just 240 classroom hours, while "senior ward practice" filled the entire third year until the late 1930s, when the third-year curriculum added two new courses, the first introducing students to a spectrum of professional issues and opportunities and the second providing an introduction to public health nursing.[21]

Nationally, eighty-eight percent of nursing schools surveyed by the Committee on the Grading of Nursing Schools in the early 1930s demanded more than forty-eight hours of student hospital service per week. The University of Iowa Hospitals reduced the working day for students to a maximum of eight hours in 1931, in turn reducing the maximum weekly total to forty-eight hours. It is impossible to document the number of hours actually worked by students, since practice in nursing schools of the era rarely conformed strictly to published criteria. Nonetheless, the University of Iowa's academic program was no doubt more rigorous than most, and published requirements for ward practice in the early 1930s totaled just 3,066 hours: 734 hours during the junior year, 1,404 hours during the senior year, and an additional 992 hours accumulated over the course of two summers.

A 239-page volume entitled *Nursing Procedures*, published in 1930 and outlining the fundamentals of nursing techniques as taught at the University of Iowa, provided insight into the contemporary worlds of scientific health care, nursing, and nursing education.[22] The manual opened with a chapter on hospital housekeeping, instructing students, for example, to "turn all pillows in the same direction" with "open ends away from door" and providing detailed instructions for folding bed linen, making beds, polishing furniture, and caring for appliances and equipment. The second chapter described the patient admission process, including the "admission bath and shampoo," from which the patient emerged in the obligatory hospital robe, gown, and slippers, apparel that came to symbolize the sterile hospital environment and served also to heighten the social distance between patients and caregivers.

The third chapter of *Nursing Procedures* dealt with general care of the patient, focusing chiefly on the issue of patient comfort. Chapter four was entitled simply and straightforwardly "Enemata" and detailed the several kinds and uses of enemas, from purgative, antiseptic, and astringent to carminative, emollient, and nutrient. Chapter five was devoted entirely to "counter-irritation," involving the application of various agents—for example, rubifacients, heat, and cold—"to dilate surface blood vessels" and "to remove inflammation and pain." Chapters six and seven dealt with medications and advanced procedures, the latter including areas such as gastric lavage, lumbar puncture, intravenous infusion, and blood transfusion. Finally, the manual devoted ten chapters to the specialized nursing skills needed in the major clinical specialties, such as internal medicine, surgery, obstetrics, gynecology, orthopædics, and ophthalmology.

Aside from courses in nursing ethics, history, and principles and practice, the School of Nursing relied on outside faculty, chiefly from the College of Medicine, for classroom instruction. Such arrangements were of course common in all departments and colleges of the university and, indeed, constituted one of the virtues of the university system. However, it was also the case that the medical faculty designed the nursing courses they taught; moreover, it was of both symbolic and practical importance that the list of "nursing faculty" in the university catalogues of the time began with the heads of medical and other university departments involved in nursing education. Meanwhile, echoing the uncertain academic status of the nursing school, nurse instructors fell under a secondary category of "administrative and educational nursing staff." Among the administrative staff of the school and the dozens of supervisory nurses with nominal educational responsibilities, just five, not including the school's educational director, held formal university academic status at the level of instructor. Neither Superintendent Lois Corder nor Educational Director Lola Lindsey, both of them graduates of the University of Iowa School of Nursing, held bachelor's degrees. In 1934-35, just three of the school's eight administrative and educational staff possessed bachelor's degrees, as did six of the University Hospitals' fifty-five supervisors, assistant supervisors, and general staff nurses.

In most respects, nursing student life in the 1930s continued much as it had in the 1920s. Students on day duty awakened at 6:00 AM, donned the standard student uniform of blue and white striped dress, white apron, and white hose, and began work on the wards at seven. The day shift, lasting until 4:30 PM, was filled with routine patient care interlaced with instructional activities—for example, demonstrations, classes, and doctors' rounds. School of Nursing rules required students on the night shift (11:00 PM to 7:00 AM) to be in bed by 9:00 AM and to rise at 4:00 PM. Rules likewise required "freshman students to be in their rooms at 8:00 PM for study" Monday through Thursday nights. From the late 1920s to the end of her tenure, disciplinary issues figured prominently in correspondence between Superintendent Corder and the office of the university president. Corder imposed suspensions of varying lengths of time for a variety of infractions, including alcohol con-

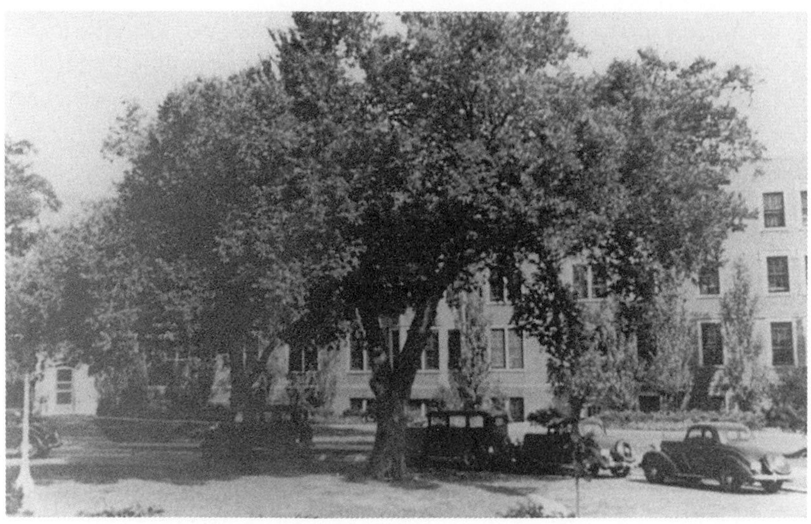

Fig. 2.2. Main Entrance to Westlawn, the nurses' residence and home of the School of Nursing, 1930s.

sumption (apparently the most common of infractions), falling asleep on duty, minor thefts, and improper administration of medications. On the lighter side, school administrators inaugurated a new recreational program in the fall of 1934 aimed at encouraging student interest in hobbies and activities, including music, dancing, writing, bridge, and tennis.

In May 1929, twenty-two School of Nursing students, instructors, and alumnæ organized a local chapter—Gamma chapter—of Sigma Theta Tau, the nursing honor society begun at Indiana University in 1922. In a rite performed every year until 1942, the initiates donned black robes and entered an initiation chamber draped in black to take the oath of membership before an altar equipped with Bible, goblet, and three-branched candelabra. Much of the motivation behind the chapter's formation appears to have come from Superintendent Lois Corder, Director of Nursing Education Lola Lindsey, and Blanche McGurk, Lindsey's first assistant director. Despite hard times and a shrinking membership roll in the early 1930s, Gamma Chapter—organized to foster leadership and scholarship in nursing—played a significant role in national affairs of Sigma Theta Tau. In 1934, Gamma Chapter hosted the national meeting; in addition, Lola Lindsey served as national secretary from

1931 to 1934 and as national vice president from 1934 to 1936. Following in Lindsey's footsteps, Blanche McGurk served for thirteen years, from 1938 to 1951, as national treasurer. Moreover, Lois M. Austin, initiated into Gamma Chapter in 1931, and Rozella M. Schlotfeldt, initiated in 1935, subsequently earned national reputations for their contributions to Sigma Theta Tau and to the larger nursing profession.

The nursing school's alumnæ association, organized in 1911 and a member organization of the Iowa State Association of Registered Nurses, continued its activities, including semiannual—although somewhat irregular—publication of the *Alumnæ Journal.* In 1930, the association's 142 resident members paid $5.00 annual membership fees; the 106 non-resident members paid annual fees of $2.50. In 1936, total membership stood at 325; in 1945, the association claimed 402 dues-paying members. The alumnæ association served a threefold mission: first, it staged a variety of social events to promote professional solidarity among its members; second, it served a charitable function through contributions to the Red Cross and other service organizations, loans to nursing students, and support for sick and needy members; and, third, the association operated an employment registry matching members to both private-duty and institutional jobs.

The Student Nurse Organization (SNO) continued to serve as a social outlet and as an intermediary between students and the school administration, and Superintendent Corder used the organization's meetings on many occasions to raise issues of order and discipline. In January 1929, for example, the group discussed appropriate behavior in the parlors of Westlawn, including "necking, etc.," and, in December 1930, Corder warned students that matrons would "make rounds frequently in parlors" with authority to evict those "not conducting themselves properly."[23] Also at that December 1930 meeting, student members presented a petition containing 239 signatures asking for three days' vacation at Christmas. In their petition, students claimed that the present policy of half-day leaves classed nursing students "with maids, cooks, floor waxers, scrub ladies, and nurse maids," and the *Daily Iowan,* the university's newspaper, reported that many nursing students were prepared to strike over the issue. On that occasion, the students won at least a partial victory, receiving a promise of three days' vacation, although in increments as small as a half-day.[24]

Until World War II, the University of Iowa School of Nursing remained an all-white institution. In one instance preserved in official correspondence, a young African-American woman from Pershing, Iowa, inquired in July 1936 about enrollment in the nursing school. Having arranged an interview with Lois Corder, but having learned also— presumably from Corder—that "no negro [sic] girl" had ever enrolled at the school, the young woman wrote University of Iowa President Eugene Gilmore to ask if school policy precluded her enrollment in either the School of Nursing or the College of Medicine. That letter found its way to College of Medicine Dean Ewen MacEwen, who in turn advised the would-be student to come for her scheduled interview with Corder and noted that any citizen of Iowa meeting academic requirements was eligible for admission to the university. However, as was widely the case at schools of nursing and medicine throughout America, unwritten policy was to discourage such applications. In this instance, Gilmore's secretary advised the president in a penciled note that "Dr. MacEwen said they usually can make these colored girls see that it is unwise for them to enroll."[25] According to a report compiled by Registrar H. C. Dorcas, the entire university enrolled only ninety-nine African-American students, twenty-five of them Iowa residents, and 194 Jewish students, 127 of them Iowans in December 1936.[26]

By the late 1930s, the imprint of more aggressive state licensing boards on nursing education was an increasing concern to University of Iowa officials. In November 1936, in an effort to exercise more stringent oversight of admissions standards, the Iowa Board of Nurse Examiners demanded that nursing schools submit to the board two copies of high school transcripts for all applicants; the board would then approve or disapprove each candidate and return one copy of the transcript to the school. In addition, the board proposed to deny admission to any applicant ranking in the bottom third of her high school class and encouraged schools to admit only those students ranking in the upper half of their graduating classes.[27] The University of Iowa's registrar objected that such policies would deny the university control over its own admissions standards and procedures.[28] College of Medicine Dean Ewen Mac-

Ewen agreed,[29] and the result was an extended series of letters and meetings over that and related issues.

In March 1937, a committee of university officials, including the registrar and the College of Medicine dean, agreed to maintain the university's present admissions policies, at least for the time being.[30] When the Board of Nurse Examiners reiterated its stand in a letter to Corder in April 1937, it was Dean MacEwen who responded to the university president, remarking angrily that the State Board of Education must decide "whether we are running a Nurses' Training School or whether it is being run by a dictator in Des Moines."[31] The question at issue, as outlined by the university attorney in June, was whether or not the Board of Nurse Examiners exceeded its statutory authority in screening admissions.[32] Resting his opinion on interpretations of the Iowa Code, an assistant attorney general in July agreed with university officials that the board had indeed exceeded its mandate in interceding in the admissions process, but the attorney general himself a week later declined to issue a formal ruling on the matter.[33] Finally, in August, Dean MacEwen apprised President Gilmore that negotiations with the nurse examiners had resulted in the board's waiving all the objectionable regulations, explaining that they had been aimed, not at the university, but at the weaker schools in the state.[34]

In another incident, Dean MacEwen notified President Gilmore in August 1938 that the Illinois Board of Nurse Examiners had recently refused registration to graduates of the University of Iowa's combined course, which involved three years' enrollment in liberal arts and two years' enrollment in the School of Nursing. The Illinois board based its ruling on a state law requiring three years' attendance at an approved school of nursing as a prerequisite to licensure. In fact, the Illinois board had announced that change in policy several years before, effective for students admitted after September 1, 1934. In any event, MacEwen claimed complete ignorance of the origins of the University of Iowa's combined course, maintaining—implausibly—that there was "nothing in the records to show how it got into the [university] catalogue." With several students having just completed the third year of liberal arts and preparing to enroll in the School of Nursing, the dean expected "considerable back fire" from this bureaucratic snag. His recommendation was to have the combined program's third-year students register in the School of Nursing and supplement the third-year liberal arts curriculum with ward training. Softening his earlier opposition to liberal arts training for nurses, MacEwen also added that to abolish the combined course would "be a step backward."[35] Moreover, in a subsequent letter to the dean of liberal arts, MacEwen expressed his hope, "before many years," to see a requirement "that all girls entering nursing will pursue at least one year of Liberal Arts courses."[36] In the fall of 1938, the faculty committee of the State Board of Education resolved this conundrum by formally reducing the liberal arts component of the combined program to two years, expanding the nursing component to three years, and using some nursing courses, including physiology, pathology, and bacteriology, to fulfill liberal arts requirements for the bachelor's degree.

Such episodes were symptomatic of broader concerns over standards and accreditation in nursing education, an issue of growing importance in areas beyond nursing as well. In 1938, President Gilmore objected to an inquiry from the National League of Nursing Education regarding the League's accreditation plans for nursing schools. Obviously irritated, Gilmore fired off a letter to Superintendent Lois Corder asking, among other things, "What is the National League of Nursing Education?" His "first impression," he noted, was that the accreditation plan was "a mild form of racket," and he argued that, at some point, "we must look these so-called accrediting bodies squarely in the face."[37] Given the hierarchy of authority in nursing education, Corder responded not to the president but to the dean of the College of Medicine, patiently answering Gilmore's series of questions, outlining the League's history and makeup and the membership of its Committee on Accrediting.[38] Dean MacEwen ventured a cautious endorsement of the League and its goals, although he did, he said, "anticipate a very critical survey" of the nursing school from any visiting League delegation.[39]

In November 1939, Corder reminded MacEwen of the upcoming January 1, 1940, deadline for National League of Nursing Education accreditation applications.[40] Contrary to his earlier more positive response, MacEwen on this occasion was, to say the least, uncharitable. After consulting with hospitals Superintendent Robert Neff during the summer, MacEwen had, he alerted President Gilmore, "told Miss Corder...to inform the League 'to jump in the lake.'" The $250 fee for inspection and $35 annual fee for inclusion in the League's listing of accredited schools rankled the dean; in addition, he saw no reason to accede to the standards of agencies outside Iowa, particularly since most of the nursing school's graduates remained in the state. MacEwen also compared the League's accreditation campaign unfavorably to the American Medical Association and the American Hospital Association, neither of which charged fees for their respective accreditation of medical schools and hospitals.[41] Consistent with his year-earlier response to the issue of accreditation and his ongoing involvement with national groups opposed to the accreditation movement, President Gilmore directed MacEwen not to pay the fees.[42] Not surprisingly, then, the School of Nursing was likewise not a member of the Association of Collegiate Nursing Schools, a group founded in the early 1930s to devise standards and accrediting procedures for university-based schools of nursing.

The School of Nursing and World War II

In July 1940, well before formal American entry into World War II, representatives from a broad range of nursing organizations and agencies—including the American Nurses Association, the National Organization for Public Health Nursing, the National League of Nursing Education, the Army and Navy Nurse Corps, the Veterans Administration, and the United States Public Health Service—created a Nursing Council on National Defense to prepare for the coming emergency. Soon after, Congress significantly broadened the federal role in the provision of health care and specifically in nursing education by passage of the Community Facilities Act, or Lanham Act, of June 1941 providing federal grants to subsidize the operation of health facilities in areas critical to defense production. In July 1941, Congress passed the Labor-Federal Security Appropriations Act specifically providing funds for support of nursing education, the funds to be administered by the Public Health Service. The anticipated demand for military nurses also spurred a federal effort in 1941 to encourage the training of volunteer nurses' aides to assist trained nurses in institutional settings.[43] Already in November 1940, the University of Iowa Hospitals had begun a first-of-its-kind program of instruction for "ward helpers," a program funded by the Works Progress Administration to train women for service in the event of a national emergency. In May 1941, the program enrolled a second class of sixty students.

In December 1941, in the wake of the Pearl Harbor attack, preparedness turned abruptly to mobilization, and through the war years, as the American military effort expanded, so, too, did the recruitment of nurses to military service. The total of military nurses rose from 6,256 in 1941 to 19,025 in 1942, 35,747 in 1943, 48,417 in 1944, and 65,377 in 1945. The 1945 total—54,291 nurses in the Army Nurse Corps, including the Army Air Corps, and 11,086 in the Navy Nurse Corps—was more than triple the maximum of 1918.[44] In December 1943, the University of Iowa School of Nursing *Alumnæ Journal* counted 117 of the school's graduates in military service; overall, American nurses' response to the call for national service was so large and the demand for military nurses was so great that nearly thirty percent of all active graduate nurses were in military service by mid-1945.

Trained nurses contributed to a dramatic reduction in military mortality rates during the war years, as annual death rates among American servicemen fell from 35.5 per 1,000 in World War I to 11.6 in World War II. Notwithstanding their important contributions to the war effort and the admiration routinely expressed by their patients, nurses labored, with only mixed success, to achieve a measure of professional respect in the military, among the most hierarchical and stubbornly patriarchal of all social institutions. Early on, military nurses enjoyed little more than adjunct status, with none of the rank and benefits normally accruing to military personnel. Not until June 1944 did Congress provide Army and Navy nurses temporary rank and privileges for the duration of the war.

The rapid growth of military nursing, greater opportunities in public health nursing and industrial nursing as a result of the war, and the broader range of other opportunities open to young women in the wartime economy quickly reversed the oversupply of graduate nurses that had prevailed through the 1920s and 1930s. The result was a diminished quality of nursing service in American hospitals, the withdrawal of beds from service, and the increasing reliance on a nonprofessional, part-time hospital nursing workforce. At the same time, nursing schools faced increasing difficulty by

1943 in fulfilling expanded enrollment goals. Congress responded with passage of the Bolton Act of June 1943, which created the Cadet Nurse Corps to underwrite the costs of nursing education and to provide monthly stipends to nursing students in return for a commitment to serve in either a military or civilian nursing capacity for the duration of the war. Designed to create graduate nurses in thirty-six months, legislation authorized enrollment of 125,000 nursing students in the Cadet Nurse Corps from June 1943 to June 1945.[45]

The University of Iowa School of Nursing responded to calls from national nursing organizations and from federal government agencies by expanding enrollments in the fall of 1941, welcoming a near-record class of 143 first-year students that pushed total enrollment to 292, the highest since 1930. In November 1941, the university received a $13,675 Public Health Service grant to subsidize the education of twelve students, money paid directly to the University Hospitals. America's formal entry into the war in late 1941 prompted adoption of an accelerated program of instruction in the School of Nursing, as it did in the College of Medicine, and the entering class of 108 in 1942 began work in June instead of September. Despite a smaller first-year class, total enrollments for 1942-43 grew to 307. In the meantime, a $4,000 grant from the W. K. Kellogg Foundation in 1942 funded a trust for student loans in the School of Nursing, funds available to students whose goal was military nursing.[46]

The fall session of 1943 opened with a beginning class of 105 and total enrollment of 278. However, the Public Health Service had already approved the University of Iowa School of Nursing as a Cadet Nurse Corps training site,[47] and the addition of the first group of cadet enlistees in November swelled the school's first-year class to 199 during the 1943-44 winter term. The Cadet Corps curriculum featured a pre-cadet period of nine months, a junior cadet period of twenty-one months, and a senior cadet period of six months, the last taking many students from the University Hospitals for service elsewhere, including military hospitals. In May 1944, 160 cadet nurses, including students enrolled prior to November 1943 who had subsequently enlisted as cadets, marked the end of their pre-cadet training with a formal induction ceremony in the senate chamber of the Old Capitol, a ceremony linked by radio to a companion gathering in Constitution Hall in Washington, DC. In the induction pledge, cadets vowed "to become worthy of the finest traditions of nursing" and pledged "service in essential nursing for the duration of the war."

A second class of 139 cadets enrolled in June 1944 and pushed that year's freshman class to 209, more than a third larger than the previous record of 151 in 1928-29. That June 1944 class included one native American student, an occasion much remarked in the local newspaper and one that appears to have marked the first minority student in the school's history. In the January 1944 winter term, the School of Nursing claimed a total enrollment of 350, and the school counted a total of 550 students in residence at different times from the summer of 1944 through the spring of 1945. The Cadet Nurse program and the attendant enrollment bubble extended also through 1945-46, with a total of 448 students in residence. The training of cadet nurses provided an annual infusion of some $80,000 to the School of Nursing, the federal government paying $430 per student. Moreover, the four groups of cadet nurses enrolled between November 1943 and June 1945—a total of more than 400—affected the school in other ways as well. For example, a $200,000 addition to Westlawn, sixty percent of the cost financed by a Federal Works Administration grant, provided an additional 121 beds for nursing students when completed in 1945.

For the University of Iowa Hospitals, which assumed responsibility for the bulk of nursing instruction, the war years compounded many of the problems left over from the Depression. Meager growth in the hospitals' budget fell well behind the rate of wartime inflation and, among other things, forced significant cutbacks in indigent service. At the same time, vigorous military recruitment efforts diminished the ranks of clinical and teaching staff in both nursing and medicine. By late 1943, College of Medicine Dean Ewen MacEwen grew impatient with the constant pressures from federal agencies to increase enrollments in nursing and medicine and to accelerate the pace of instruction. "Is this a dictatorship?" MacEwen complained in a letter to university President Virgil Hancher.[48]

In 1943, with the nursing shortage growing acute, hospitals Superintendent Robert Neff offered increased salaries to nursing supervisors and later required private duty nurses to serve four weeks each year on the hospitals' general duty staff in return for their hospital privileges.[49] Despite the superintendent's efforts, the number of graduate nurses on duty in the University Hospitals barely held steady in the two years prior to America's entry into the war, and the total fell nearly ten percent to 129 in 1942-43, the lowest total since the early 1930s. By the end of the war, the hospitals administration struggled with a professional nursing staff reduced by some fifty percent from 1939-40. The precipitous decline in graduate nursing staff and the enormous increase in enrollments in the School of Nursing boosted the ratio of students to graduate nurses well beyond levels deemed acceptable in normal circumstances, levels not seen since the 1920s, while national nursing leaders raised concerns regarding the quality of nursing education under wartime conditions.

The University of Iowa School of Nursing and the College of Medicine shared a good many concerns and problems during the war years. For example, both adopted accelerated schedules of instruction as part of the mobilization effort, and both likewise suffered during the war years from severely depleted teaching staffs. In some respects, however, the war affected medical education and nursing education in strikingly different ways. On the one hand, School of Nursing enrollments climbed to historic levels, while, at the same time, a nursing shortage encouraged the addition of marginally trained practical nurses and nurse aides to the University Hospitals' nursing service. On the other hand, the College of Medicine saw a significant decline in student retention and graduation rates during the war, the effects of which lasted until the late 1940s. In some measure, the difference was a simple function of the relative scarcity of men under wartime conditions and, one might add, the College of Medicine's reluctance to admit significantly greater numbers of women—although many other schools of medicine did so. However, the difference in enrollment patterns also reflected the determination of College of Medicine administrators to resist mandatory armed forces placement policies and to match enrollments as closely as possible to diminished teaching resources, a luxury that nursing educators did not enjoy because of the subordination of nursing education to the needs of the University Hospitals. Also unlike physicians, whose standards of professional practice were seldom challenged by wartime experience, nurses were powerless to prevent the dilution of professional practice by the employment of non-professional nursing personnel in the hospital setting.

The Postwar Reorganization of Nursing Education

Wartime experience exerted considerable influence over American nursing and nursing education in the postwar years. Nurses' contributions to the war effort infused the profession with a sense of pride and accomplishment, and, just as important, gave many nurses a new appreciation of large-scale organization and co-operative effort. Moreover, the rapid conversion of university af-filiated nursing schools, like the University of Iowa School of Nurs-ing, to colleges of nursing, a conversion that provided nurses a means to seize control over professional education, was symbolic of nurses' and nursing's newfound status and aspirations in the post-war world. At the same time, the provision of federal aid to nurs-ing education during the war years was itself a major landmark, presaging much greater federal involvement in professional educa-tion in the postwar period.

From 1945 to 1949, nursing enrollments fell from nearly 129,000 to just under 89,000.[50] At the University of Iowa, total en-rollments fell from 363 in the fall of 1945 to a low of 259 in Sep-tember 1948, the latter despite a vigorous recruiting effort in the spring of 1948 that included visits by teams of students and graduate nurses to Iowa high schools. Across Iowa, nursing school enroll-ments fell forty-seven percent from 1945 to 1948 (Figure 2.1), a re-turn to prewar enrollment levels after the termination of the Cadet Nurse Corps program at the University of Iowa and the continued attrition in the number of nursing schools statewide. By 1950, just twenty-nine schools remained in operation in the state.

The slump in nursing enrollments during the late 1940s was deeply troubling because it accompanied yet another wave of con-cern over a nationwide nursing shortage. In a 1949 report, an *ad hoc* Committee on the Function of Nursing organized by the Teachers College of Columbia University estimated the number of active registered nurses in the United States at 280,500 in mid-1948, 167,400 employed in institutions, 22,000 in public health, 52,800 in private duty, 12,700 in industry, and 25,500 in a variety of other positions, including physicians' offices. The committee judged the shortage conservatively at 50,000 nurses.[51] The committee also concluded, as did many other observers, that the shortage of trained nurses was in key respects symptomatic of nursing's broader problems. Those problems, few of them new, ranged from hard work, long hours, tight discipline, and low pay to nurses' ambiguous status in the health care hierarchy and the minimal career expectations of a large majority of nurses.[52] In September 1946, the American Nurses Association, the National League of Nursing Education, and the National Organization for Public Health Nursing had devoted much of a combined meeting to discussion of such fundamental problems in nursing and of strategies for professional development.[53] In Iowa, the fifth district of the Iowa State Nurses Association, in an April 1947 meeting in Cedar Rapids, had compiled a list of recommended personnel practices for area hospitals, focusing in particular on improvements in pay and benefits.[54]

Objectively, postwar conditions for practicing nurses were perhaps no worse than before or during the war; in many respects in fact, conditions in the late 1940s were considerably improved over the 1930s and early 1940s. Graduate nurse pay scales at the University of Iowa Hospitals, for example, although lagging well behind levels in many comparable institutions, more than doubled between 1941 and 1949, increasing from $1,000-1,200 for supervisors and assistant supervisors and $900 for general duty nurses in 1941 to $2,300-2,500 for supervisors and assistant supervisors and $2,000-2,200 for general duty nurses in 1949, all with full mainte-

TABLE 2.1 Total Enrollments in Iowa Nursing Schools, 1941-1949

	First-Year	Second-Year	Third-Year	Total
1941	655	539	545	1,793
1942	1,033	619	584	2,236
1943	1,037	821	632	2,490
1944	1,261	922	765	2,948
1945	1,091	1,041	890	3,022
1946	560	872	980	2,412
1947	499	517	860	1,876
1948	592	465	539	1,596
1949	694	533	453	1,680

Source: *Nursing Needs Resources: Iowa Survey* (1952), p. 33.

nance. Because of the rapid expansion and changing demographics of the graduate nursing staff in the late 1940s, a large majority of nurses received $400-500 in additional salary in lieu of room, board, and laundry. In an effort to entice graduate nurses with children back into the workforce, the University Hospitals opened a free day care unit in 1947. Such measures failed, however, to attract large numbers of women into nursing, perhaps chiefly because women—thanks in part to wartime experience and in part to a vigorous postwar economic expansion—had a broader range of employment and career options, not excluding marriage and childrearing. The perception of a nursing shortage further aggravated nursing's problems by reinforcing hospital administrators' tendencies to augment nursing staffs with practical nurses and untrained aides.

Real or not, the postwar nursing shortage, coupled with the rapid expansion of medical scientific knowledge and health care technologies, prompted renewed attention to some long familiar problems in nursing education. One important result was increased pressures—not just from nursing elites but from more progressive hospital administrators and physicians and many nurses as well—for a more rigorous nursing curriculum to prepare the graduate nurse to supervise the nursing team of practical nurses and aides and to cope with the spiraling technical sophistication of modern health care. In a noted 1948 report, *Nursing for the Future*, Esther Lucille Brown of the Russell Sage Foundation offered her observations on the organization, control, and financing of nursing education, observations that were landmarks in the movement toward collegiate education in nursing. Remarking upon the obvious deficiencies in many of the nation's 1,250 nursing schools, Brown recommended a transition from the hospital school to the nursing college coupled with a meaningful system of institutional accreditation.[55]

Response to the Brown report was less than enthusiastic in some quarters, especially so among hospital nursing schools. The National Organization of Hospital Schools of Nursing, established in opposition to the collegiate plan, played a significant role in the 1949 defeat of legislation in the U. S. House of Representatives that would have provided substantial federal funding for nursing education but would also have given funding preference to collegiate schools. Notwithstanding determined opposition from some quarters, however, the idea of collegiate education in nursing had many backers, especially in higher education circles.

The early postwar decades brought unprecedented growth to the American system of higher education, thanks to the efforts of aggressive university administrators, the rapid growth of federal funding for higher education and for research, and the flood of returning servicemen whose education was subsidized by the "GI Bill." The number of college graduates spiraled rapidly upward in the late 1940s, exceeding 423,000 in 1949-50, compared to 27,400 at the turn of the century and just under 186,000 as recently as 1940-41. As the bubble of wartime veterans subsided, the total of graduates declined to some 300,000 annually by the mid-1950s, a figure still more than fifty percent above prewar totals. To a considerable extent, the postwar boom in higher education was a male phenomenon. Indeed, while the proportion of women among all college graduates had risen from 19.1 percent at the turn of the century to 42.5 percent in 1940-41, it fell to 23.9 percent in 1949-50. As the number of male graduates slumped 44.5 percent from 1949-50 to 1954-55, the proportion of female graduates rose to 36.0 percent in the latter year, although the numbers of female graduates—nearly forty percent of them taking degrees in education—held essentially steady.[56]

Virgil M. Hancher, who served as University of Iowa president from 1940 to 1964, was a determined advocate of a college of nursing. Remembered by many for his demonstrated ambivalence toward innovation, Hancher could be a determined reformer when convinced that existing institutional systems clearly did not work. Such was his response, for example, to the postwar crisis in the College of Medicine over private practice, a crisis that led—more or less by presidential fiat—to institution of the Medical Service Plan, which shared practice revenues among all tenured and tenure-track clinical faculty. Encouraged by the Iowa State Nurses Association, the Nurses' Alumnæ Association, and a good many practicing nurses, Hancher similarly became a champion of reform in nursing education.

During the war years, President Hancher had taken steps to bolster the School of Nursing's lackluster academic image, instituting a system of letter grades (A,B,C,D,F) for nursing students and including nursing in a new course numbering system that assigned to each college and department a distinctive numerical prefix ("96" for nursing courses). However, Hancher saw the existing School of Nursing, with its ambiguous academic standing, as inconsistent with—if not an embarrassment to—the image and mission of the modern university. The university should not, Hancher told one correspondent "conduct merely a training school in nursing."[57] In addition, a baccalaureate program would broaden the geographic and demographic base of nursing education, making it, like the rest of the university, a statewide program with an appeal to young women of all social classes.

Discussion resumed at least as early as May 1945 on the troublesome issue of coordinating the coursework in the combined program so as to satisfy the requirements of both the College of Liberal Arts and state examining boards. The earlier compromise, granting liberal arts credit for designated nursing courses, fell by the wayside after a reorganization of the College of Liberal Arts curriculum implemented in 1945. The dean of liberal arts subsequently rejected an alternative nursing curriculum in January 1946 on the basis that it, too, failed to meet the college's new requirement of ninety semester hours of *bona fide* liberal arts coursework for the bachelor's degree. More important in the long run, the dean offered the opinion that a curriculum leading to the bachelor of science in nursing, rather than in liberal arts, would more appropriately signify a professional nursing education, and he volunteered his college to supply the requisite "scientific and literary subjects" for such a program.[58] For the time being, however, the dean's ruling left no option but to change the five-year collegiate program to a six-year curriculum to provide both three years' work in the liberal arts and three years in nursing. Surely to no one's surprise, the new curriculum instituted in the fall of 1946 resulted in a drastic reduction in enrollments in the combined program, the total falling from fifty-one in 1945-46 to fifteen in 1946-47.

The suggestion from the dean of liberal arts that the solution to the problem with the combined curriculum lay in a baccalaureate nursing program came at a time when President Hancher planned a reorganization of the university administration to create a Division of Health Sciences and Services. Under the direction of Executive Dean Carlyle Jacobsen, the new division would embrace all the health science colleges—medicine, pharmacy, and dentistry—and, perhaps not coincidentally, afford a home for a college of nursing. Furthermore, in April 1947, a special committee of the medical faculty chaired by Phillip Jeans of pediatrics recommended creation of a four-year baccalaureate program in nursing, embracing two and one-half years of didactic work and one and one-half years of work on the hospital wards. The committee also recommended retention of the existing diploma program in view of the nursing shortage but suggested the program's phaseout at the earliest possible date. In presenting the committee's report to Hancher, Dean Ewen MacEwen noted the "tremendous waste of time and money on the three-year girls" under the current system, as dropout rates ran to fifty percent and more, a sharp contrast to the high rate of retention in the combined program.[59]

At an October 1947 meeting of the State Board of Education, President Hancher first discussed his ideas for the implementation of a baccalaureate program. At the board's February 1948 meeting, Hancher raised the issue again, and board members on that occasion advised him to prepare a detailed plan for later consideration. In November 1948, Hancher forwarded to Board of Education members a lengthy memorandum prepared by Dean Carlyle Jacobsen. Jacobsen outlined three levels of nursing education—diploma, baccalaureate, and graduate—and maintained that the university must shoulder greater responsibility for the last two. He also noted that the present administrative arrangement, with the School of Nursing operating as a unit of the College of Medicine, was an obstacle to recruiting capable faculty; the new college, he testified, must enjoy "equal and coordinate status" with the colleges of pharmacy, medicine, and dentistry."[60] In a cover letter, President Hancher also argued for a change in name from "school" to "college," in part to mark a departure from what he called "an indifferent past" in nursing education. In December 1948, the Board of Education, following the recommendation of its faculty committee, gave final approval to creation of a College of Nursing in the university's Division of Health Sciences and Services, contingent upon recruiting "a person with appropriate training, experience, and background to the deanship of the College."

The elevation of nursing education to collegiate status entailed wholesale changes in leadership, since neither Nursing Superintendent Lois Corder nor Education Director Lola Lindsey possessed a college degree. There is first hand testimony that Lindsey, who had been closely involved with Sigma Theta Tau both locally and nationally, was nonetheless strongly supportive of the conversion to baccalaureate status. In contrast, there are few clues to Lois Corder's attitude toward the baccalaureate program and her role in the Board of Education's decision to establish the College of Nursing. Certainly, Corder's relative invisibility in the documentary record is symbolic of her—and her school's—subordinate position in the university hierarchy. On most occasions, after all, and particularly so on important issues, it was the dean of the College of Medicine who spoke for the School of Nursing. Moreover, Corder held dual—and to some extent incompatible—administrative responsibilities embracing both nursing education and the University Hospitals' nursing service. In her role as nursing educator, the superintendent might well applaud reforms in nursing education, but to do so would inevitably mean reduced student hours in the hospitals, which would, in turn, complicate her role as head of the nursing service.

Fairly or not, University of Iowa President Virgil Hancher appears to have identified Lois Corder with nursing education's "indifferent past" at the university. It is certain that Corder had earned a reputation as a stern disciplinarian during her tenure, a trait that generated an increasing volume of complaints from students, from parents, and even from Board of Education members. President Hancher noted in 1944 that he had, in just four years, received numerous complaints "to the effect that Miss Corder's rules are often arbitrary and are enforced in an inflexible manner."[61] However, it should be noted, too, that the archival record contains a good many testimonials to the quality of instruction the School of Nursing provided to some 1,200 graduates under Corder's leadership. One graduate testified that "the discipline, instruction in organization and the assuming of responsibility incorporated in the training at Iowa City have been priceless assets of S.U.I. graduates."[62] Commenting on the "amazing indifference and slovenliness" she had encountered among hospital staff elsewhere since graduation, another was grateful to have been "equipped with a rigid, thorough training."[63] More objectively, the performance of graduates of the University of Iowa School of Nursing on the 1948-49 Nursing State Board Test Pool Exams—standardized, machine-graded exams that were another outgrowth of World War II—put the school at the top of the state's twenty-nine nursing schools.

In any case, as momentum built toward establishment of a baccalaureate program, Corder resigned effective February 1, 1947, having accepted a position as superintendent of nurses at the Santa Fe Coastal Lines Hospital in Los Angeles. President Hancher responded with thanks for her "loyal and efficient service," and Corder offered the president her "heartiest good wishes for your continued success and faith in your future plans"—the latter perhaps *prima facie* evidence of her support for the baccalaureate program then in the planning stage.[64] College of Medicine Dean Ewen MacEwen and new University Hospitals Superintendent Gerhard Hartman concurred on the interim choice of Lola Lindsey as acting director of the School of Nursing and Maureen Marble, previously first assistant director of nursing, as acting director of nursing in the University Hospitals. Both the dean and the superintendent also concurred on plans to see the School of Nursing "set up in a manner similar to the other schools of the University [i.e., on a collegiate basis],"[65] a move that would inevitably limit Lindsey's tenure. Barely two months later, Marble resigned and was replaced as director of nursing by Gelia Clyde, a 1932 graduate of the Iowa State Teachers College, a veteran of the Army Nurse Corps, and holder of a master's degree in nursing from Western Reserve University.[66] Clyde in turn resigned in November 1948, replaced by Marie Tener as acting director. Lola Lindsey, meanwhile, resigned her position as director of nursing education effective January 1, 1949, just after the Board of Education gave final approval to the baccalaureate program.

As one observer later recalled, those transitional years constituted "a time of great uncertainty."[67] However, university officials received a reassuring flow of correspondence in support of the baccalaureate plan. In August 1947, the Iowa State Nurses Association forwarded a lengthy resolution endorsing creation of a college of nursing "in order to further nursing education, both on the undergraduate and graduate level, in Iowa."[68] In September, the University of Iowa Nurses' Alumnæ Association presented a shortened version of the same resolution.[69] In November, a similar appeal arrived from the president and secretary of the Iowa State League of Nursing Education.[70] Letters from individual nurses, most of them alumnæ, stressed several advantages to a baccalaureate program, including the opportunity to provide nurses with an education comparable to that enjoyed by other professionals, to prepare nursing leaders for the postwar world, and to establish formal graduate courses.[71] Typically, one nurse wrote that she and her colleagues were "deeply concerned about the lack of progress of the School of Nursing in recent years" and wanted to see the university pursue the many "possibilities for improvement."[72]

Having won the State Board of Education's approval for the new college, the most important concern for university officials in late 1948 and early 1949 was the hiring of faculty and the selection of a dean, or, more properly, a dean-elect who would assume the existing title of director of nursing education during the interim period before formal inauguration of the college. Executive Dean Carlyle Jacobsen was already hard at work on those problems by the end of 1948, and in January 1949 the Board of Education approved the appointments of Amy Frances Brown as an assistant professor and Evelyn T. Crary as an associate, a step just below assistant professor. Both were promised annual salaries of $4,200. With the concurrence of University Hospitals Superintendent Hartman, Jacobsen recommended Myrtle E. Kitchell for the deanship in February 1949.[73]

Myrtle Kitchell was born in Iowa and graduated from high school in Minnesota. After receiving her BSN from the University of Minnesota School of Nursing in 1939 and spending three years in hospital nursing, Kitchell served three years as assistant chief nurse with the 26th General Army Hospital in England, Africa, and Italy and eight months with the 52nd station hospital in Italy. Returning to the University of Minnesota late in 1945, she became an instructor in the School of Nursing and received a master's degree in education in 1947. At the time of her discussions with University of Iowa officials, Kitchell was a doctoral student in the University of Minnesota College of Education and was, by her own recollection, initially not much interested in the position in Iowa City. When Dean Jacobsen and Superintendent Hartman interviewed Kitchell in Minneapolis in January 1949, their would-be dean took a hard line regarding her requirements for the new college, but the two men seemed undeterred. Moreover, testimony from other officials at the University of Minnesota, the Department of the Army, and the Public Health Service reassured them that Kitchell "was held in high regard by nursing leaders." Kitchell subsequently visited the University of Iowa campus on February 11 and 12, and the State Board of Education approved her appointment as dean-elect in May 1949, effective September 1 or as soon as the new dean could terminate her responsibilities in Minnesota.

During the summer of 1949, Myrtle Kitchell was already at work on the organization of the new college. In July, Kitchell submitted to Dean Jacobsen the first of a series of recommendations from the nascent nursing faculty, suggesting that the university set tuition at $65 per semester for resident and non-resident nursing students, impose charges for room and board during the two years of non-clinical studies, and vest responsibility for admissions decisions in the nursing faculty. Kitchell also noted that the faculty was set to begin work on a new curriculum, focusing initially on the first two, non-clinical years.[74] By the end of September, Kitchell had also drafted a faculty manual for the college.[75] The manual defined two classes of faculty: first, those employed full-time in nursing education and designated with academic ranks from assistant instructor to full professor and, second, those with appointments in the University Hospitals but actively engaged in nursing education and designated by clinical rank. Only faculty with academic appointments in the College of Nursing would enjoy the right to vote on faculty matters. In contrast to the struggles over the distribution of authority then taking place in the College of Medicine, the nursing manual was a remarkably democratic document, ceding to the faculty the right to consult with the dean on matters of policy, to participate on an executive committee of the college and on standing and special committees, to elect a faculty secretary, to hear reports from the dean at regular faculty meetings, and to call special faculty meetings by petition.

The faculty manual also addressed curricular philosophy and objectives, pledging to offer "a broad education for professional nursing" and to do so "without discrimination as to race, color, or creed." While continuing "for the present" the three-year diploma program, concern clearly centered on the baccalaureate program, which would blend liberal arts and professional instruction in a curriculum extending over four calendar years—the equivalent of five academic years. The manual promised to train nurses able to function "in any field of nursing," with an emphasis on "the individualization of care and the development of judgment in planning to meet the patient's needs"—a subtle reminder of nursing education's newfound independence and the potential ramifications of that independence for nurses' on-the-job responsibilities. Graduates of the program would receive the bachelor of science in nursing and the certificate of graduate nurse.

The actual design of such a curriculum and the setting of standards for student performance were difficult and time consuming chores, involving considerable debate and soul-searching on the part of curriculum committee members. At the outset, the committee rejected most elements of the existing academic curriculum which, in the committee's estimation, consisted of "many short unrelated courses," reflecting chiefly what medical faculty members thought nurses ought to know. The committee was no more enthusiastic about the practical component of the curriculum, reflecting chiefly the needs and priorities of the University Hospitals. In addition, the overlap of old and new programs compounded the committee's difficulties, particularly with the capabilities of existing students "open to considerable question."[76]

In early December 1949, Dean Kitchell presented the committee's finished work covering the first two years of both the three-year diploma and four-year baccalaureate programs.[77] The freshman year of the four-year program, totaling forty semester hours spanning the standard academic year and summer session, contained eight semester hours of chemistry, eight hours of communications skills, eight hours of history, and four hours of psychology, along with personal hygiene, physical education, mathematics, and an orientation to nursing. The sophomore year, totaling forty-four semester hours, brought a greater focus on the sciences and the basic elements of nursing, including four hours of microbiology, eight hours of anatomy and physiology, eight hours of sociology, and nine hours of the foundations of nursing, along with dietetics, child development, and a more advanced course in the care of adults and children. Meanwhile, the revised three-year program received a greater emphasis on classroom instruction, with considerable overlap in coursework with the four-year program. The details of clinical instruction for both three- and four-year programs remained uncertain; however, one important issue had been resolved in September 1949 with Marie Tener's permanent appointment as director of nursing services in the University Hospitals, a position of vital importance, Kitchell noted, "if the School of Nursing is to go forward" and one that Tener was to hold for sixteen years.[78]

Declaring their "belief in democratic values" and in the "inherent dignity of the individual," Kitchell and her colleagues also promulgated rules governing student deportment and responsibilities that were, in many respects, more lenient than previous codes. Kitchell and her colleagues counseled students that nursing was a "service profession" involving "certain personal sacrifices," yet they were also adamant that nursing students should be drawn into the larger university community. In keeping with that goal, they designed a curriculum that gave students the opportunity to participate in extracurricular activities and to experience the full range of university and family life.[79] New rules also allowed senior nursing students to live outside Westlawn for the final six months of their training.[80]

Conclusion

On December 6, 1948, the University of Iowa School of Nursing marked its fiftieth anniversary with a golden jubilee banquet at the Iowa Memorial Union. The school's acting director, Lola I. Lindsey, was the guest of honor, receiving an opal ring and a gold engraved jewelry box from students and colleagues as a token of appreciation for her twenty-seven years of service to the school. Surely, the banquet was, for Lindsey and for many others, a bittersweet occasion, since the transition from a school of nursing to a college of nursing was well underway and Lindsey had just announced her resignation. Barely one year later, on December 3, 1949, the university held yet another celebration, this one a reception and dinner marking the birth of the College of Nursing and honoring the new dean and faculty, an event that, from a historical perspective, overshadowed the golden anniversary of the previous year.

Inspired by changes in nursing education and practice during the 1930s and World War II as well as by the promised emergence of the research university, the postwar movement toward baccalaureate programs marked a major turning point in the professional development of American nursing. Likewise, the establishment of the University of Iowa College of Nursing was a critical moment in the local history of nursing education. The College of Nursing for the first time afforded academic nurses the opportunity to define professional education in their own terms and to create a curriculum and set standards of evaluation and performance apart from the immediate interests of the College of Medicine and the service needs of the University Hospitals. Just as important for the long term, colleges of nursing like that at the University of Iowa afforded nurses a largely self-directed institutional niche within which to elaborate an independent knowledge base, a central element in the making of a profession.

Historians contend that graduates of hospital diploma schools by and large resisted the transition to baccalaureate programs, fearing, not unreasonably, that the inception of the bachelor of science in nursing degree would depreciate the graduate nurse's training and skills in the marketplace.[81] However, the evidence from Iowa suggests strong support among diploma nurses, especially among graduates of the University of Iowa School of Nursing, for a fundamental reorganization of nursing education. The nurses who wrote to President Virgil Hancher and other university officials in support of the collegiate idea often explicitly recognized the shortcomings in their own educational experiences, including the marginalization of nursing students within the university community, and they understood, too, the limits those shortcomings placed on their professional aspirations. Moreover, most of them emphasized that creation of the College of Nursing carried with it opportunities for specialized graduate training, opportunities currently unavailable to Iowa nurses.

Nursing alumnæ, the nursing faculty and dean, university officials, and a range of other interested observers held high expectations for the new College of Nursing. Yet many unanswered questions remained in 1949, for the college was, after all, barely more than a skeleton, its future contingent upon an array of internal and external factors, some of which were obvious and some not. Among the most important unknowns were, first, the future relationship between the College of Nursing and the College of Medicine and the relationship between the College of Nursing and the University Hospitals; second, the nursing dean's ability to recruit and retain qualified faculty, especially in light of the small numbers of nurses possessing bachelor's and graduate degrees; and, third, the dean's ability to attract sufficient financial resources to accommodate the expected growth in undergraduate enrollments and to implement the much anticipated graduate offerings.

Notes

1. *Historical Statistics of the United States*, Part 1 (Washington, DC: U. S. Department of Commerce, 1975), pp. 126, 241.
2. *Ibid.*, pp. 319.
3. *Ibid.*, pp. 78, 80, 140.
4. *Ibid.*, p. 76.
5. "Statistical Data Relating to Nurses from Iowa Registered Nurse Placement Service," Box 69, Folder INA: Membership Nurse Placement Service, 1940-45.
6. "Annual Report of the University Hospitals, State University of Iowa, for the year ending June 30, 1934," *Bulletin of the State University of Iowa* New Series 771 (December 22, 1934). The survey also showed that the 953 graduates still living in 1933 were evenly divided between married [476] and unmarried [477], but it did not include numbers of married and unmarried graduates among the population still active in nursing.
7. Reverby, *Ordered to Care*, pp. 186-191.
8. See George V. Fleckenstein, "Nurse Practice Acts," *American Journal of Nursing* 36 (March 1936), pp. 230-234.
9. See Samuel Levey, *et al.*, *The Rise of a University Teaching Hospital*, A *Leadership Perspective: The University of Iowa Hospitals and Clinics* (Chicago: Health Administration Press, 1997), p. 148.
10. For a fuller account of the indigent care controversy, *Ibid*, pp. 147-158.
11. "Preliminary Report of the Committee Acting Under Joint Resolution No. 7," *Journal of the House of Representatives* (Des Moines, IA: State of Iowa, 1933), pp. 1130-1136.
12. Barbara Melosh, "The Physician's Hand,'" p. 168.
13. "Graduate Staff Nursing," *American Journal of Nursing* 36 (June 1936), pp. 591-596.
14. RE Neff to EA Gilmore, September 18, 1936, Folder 57, 1936-37, EA Gilmore Papers, University of Iowa Archives.
15. "State Registration Requirements for Entrance to Nursing Schools," *American Journal of Nursing* 30 (May 1930), pp. 618-619.
16. "Some Problems in Grading Our Schools of Nursing," *Trained Nurse and Hospital Review* 77 (November 1926), pp. 507-509.

17. Committee on the Grading of Nursing Schools, *Final Report of the Committee on the Grading of Nursing Schools* (New York: The Committee, 1934).

18. For a discussion of the comparative advantages and disadvantages of graduate and student nurses to the hospital administrator, see Malcolm MacEachern, "Which Shall We Choose—Graduate or Student Service?" *Modern Hospital* 38 (June 1932), pp. 97-98, 102-104.

19. Houghton summarized his arguments in HS Houghton to WA Jessup, February 23, 1931, Box 79-87A, Folder 82, 1930-31, WA Jessup Papers, University of Iowa Archives.

20. EA Gilmore to H Guyot, September 1, 1936, Folder 82, 1936-37, EA Gilmore Papers, University of Iowa Archives.

21. Public health nursing opportunities with the public schools and local health agencies in Iowa were severely limited. A 1938 survey of Iowa's public health resources concluded that the powers and responsibilities vested by statute in local government agencies were "largely neglected" and that, as a result, average per capita expenditure on public health programs of all kinds came to just 5.5 cents. See Iowa State Planning Board, *Public Health Resources in Iowa* (Des Moines, IA: Iowa State Planning Board, 1938).

22. *Nursing Procedures* (Iowa City, IA: State University of Iowa, 1930).

23. Minutes of Student Organization of Nurses, January 1929 and December 1930, School of Nursing, University of Iowa Archives.

24. *Daily Iowan*, December 9, 1930.

25. Gertrude M. Ferguson to EA Gilmore, July 1936; EM MacEwen to GM Ferguson, July 24, 1936, Folder 82, EA Gilmore Papers, 1936-37, University of Iowa Archives.

26. HC Dorcas to EA Gilmore, December 1, 1936, Folder 100, 1936-37, EA Gilmore Papers, University of Iowa Archives.

27. Iowa Board of Nurse Examiners to LB Corder, November 28, 1936, Folder 82, EA Gilmore Papers, 1936-37, University of Iowa Archives.

28. HC Dorcas to LB Corder, December 4, 1936, Folder 82, 1936-37, EA Gilmore Papers, University of Iowa Archives.

29. EM MacEwen to EA Gilmore, December 2, 1936, Folder 82, 1936-37, EA Gilmore Papers, University of Iowa Archives.

30. HC Dorcas to EA Gilmore, March 26, 1937, Folder 82, 1936-37, EA Gilmore Papers, University of Iowa Archives.

31. EM MacEwen to EA Gilmore, May 6, 1937, Folder 82, 1936-37, EA Gilmore Papers, University of Iowa Archives.

32. CM Updegraff to EA Gilmore, June 16, 1937, Folder 82, 1936-37, EA Gilmore Papers, University of Iowa Archives.

33. P Freeburn (Office of the Attorney General) to MR Pierson (State Board of Education), July 14, 1937; MR Pierson to EA Gilmore, July 21,

1937, Folder 82, 1936-37, EA Gilmore Papers, University of Iowa Archives.

34. EM MacEwen to EA Gilmore, August 13, 1937, Folder 82, 1936-37, EA Gilmore Papers, University of Iowa Archives.

35. EM MacEwen to EA Gilmore, August 6, 1938, Record Group 16, Box 1, Liberal Arts and Nursing Folder, 1947-48, School of Nursing Papers, University of Iowa Archives.

36. EM MacEwen to George Kay, August 17, 1938, Record Group 16, Box 1, Liberal Arts and Nursing Folder, 1947-48, School of Nursing Papers, University of Iowa Archives.

37. EA Gilmore to LB Corder, February 23, 1938, Folder 82, 1937-38, EA Gilmore Papers, University of Iowa Archives.

38. LB Corder to EM MacEwen, March 1, 1938, Folder 82, 1937-38, EA Gilmore Papers, University of Iowa Archives.

39. EM MacEwen to EA Gilmore, March 4, 1938, Folder 82, 1937-38, EA Gilmore Papers, University of Iowa Archives.

40. LB Corder to EM MacEwen, November 7, 1939, Folder 82, 1939-40, EA Gilmore Papers, University of Iowa Archives.

41. EM MacEwen to EA Gilmore, November 9, 1939, Folder 82, 1939-40, EA Gilmore Papers, University of Iowa Archives.

42. See, for example, Jonathan J. Tigert, "Objectionable Practices of Accrediting Agencies," a paper circulated in April 1939 by the Joint Committee on Accrediting of the Association of Land Grant Colleges and Universities and the National Association of State Universities, found in Folder 82, 1938-39, EA Gilmore Papers, University of Iowa Archives. See, also, subsequent correspondence from Tigert to Gilmore, December 11, 1939, and April 5, 1940, Box 82, 1939-40, EA Gilmore Papers, University of Iowa Archives.

43. For fuller discussion, see Kalisch and Kalisch, *Advance of American Nursing*, pp. 447-450.

44. *Ibid.*, p. 485.

45. For more historical background on the Cadet Nurse Corps, see Federal Security Agency, *The United States Cadet Nurse Corps and Other Federal Nurse Training Programs* (Washington, DC: US Government Printing Office, 1950).

46. VM Hancher to Kellogg Foundation, June 18, 1942, Folder 113, 1941-42, VM Hancher Papers, University of Iowa Archives.

47. See Board of Education Minutes, September 14, 1943, University of Iowa Archives.

48. EM MacEwen to VM Hancher, December 17, 1943, Folder 113, 1943-44, VM Hancher Papers, University of Iowa Archives.

49. RE Neff to VM Hancher, January 12, 1943, Folder 57, 1942-43; RE Neff to BB Hickenlooper, February 16, 1944, Folder 57, 1943-44, VM Hancher Papers, University of Iowa Archives.

50. *Historical Statistics of the United States*, p. 76.

51. The Committee on the Function of Nursing, *A Program for the Nursing Profession* (New York: The Macmillan Company, 1949), pp. 12, 33.

52. Kalisch and Kalisch, *Advance of American Nursing*, pp. 493-496.

53. See "The Biennial," *American Journal of Nursing* 46 (November 1946), pp. 728-783.

54. "Desired Working Conditions Outlined by Nurse Association," *Iowa City Press Citizen* April 26, 1947.

55. Esther Lucille Brown, *Nursing for the Future* (New York: Russell Sage Foundation, 1948).

56. Figures are from the United States Office of Education, quoted in *Information Please Almanac, 1957*, pp. 287-88.

57. VM Hancher to Vera Sage, October 22, 1947, Folder 116, 1947-48, VM Hancher Papers, University of Iowa Archives.

58. HK Newburn to VM Hancher, January 18, 1946, Records Group 16, Box 1, Folder Liberal Arts and Nursing, 1947-48, School of Nursing Papers, University of Iowa Archives.

59. CE Jacobsen to VM Hancher, April 9, 1947, Folder 115, 1946-47, VM Hancher Papers, University of Iowa Archives.

60. VM Hancher and CE Jacobsen to state board of education, November 1948, Folder 120, 1948-49, VM Hancher Papers, University of Iowa Archives.

61. VM Hancher to EM MacEwen, August 18, 1944, Folder 115, 1944-45, VM Hancher Papers, University of Iowa Archives.

62. Ellen Bergman to LB Corder, February 25, 1945, Folder 115, 1944-45, VM Hancher Papers, University of Iowa Archives.

63. Evelyn Watson Good to LB Corder, November 4, 1946, Folder 115, 1946-47, VM Hancher Papers, University of Iowa Archives.

64. LB Corder to EM MacEwen, December 23, 1946, Folder 58, 1946-47; VM Hancher to Corder, January 8, 1947; Corder to Hancher, January 10, 1947, Folder 115, 1946-47, VM Hancher Papers, University of Iowa Archives.

65. Allin W. Dakin to VM Hancher, January 24, 1947, Folder 115, 1946-47, VM Hancher Papers, University of Iowa Archives.

66. G Hartman to Administrative Department Heads, March 28, 1947, Folder 58, 1946-47, VM Hancher Papers, University of Iowa Archives.

67. Etta Rasmussen to Earl Rogers, February 28, 1980, Record Group 16, Box 1, Folder Nursing-History, School of Nursing Papers, University of Iowa Archives.

68.   Iowa State Nurses Association to VM Hancher, August 29, 1947, Folder 116, 1947-48, VM Hancher Papers, University of Iowa Archives.
69.   Nurses' Alumnæ Association to VM Hancher, September 11, 1947, Folder 116, 1947-48, VM Hancher Papers, University of Iowa Archives.
70.   Mona Jackson and Helen Cromwell to VM Hancher, November 10, 1947, Folder 116, 1947-48, VM Hancher Papers, University of Iowa Archives.
71.   See, for example, Lillian Roper [class of 1927] to VM Hancher, September 6, 1947, Folder 116, 1947-48, VM Hancher Papers, University of Iowa Archives.
72.   Mrs. RC Lommasson to VM Hancher, December 5, 1948, Folder 120, 1948-49, VM Hancher Papers, University of Iowa Archives.
73.   CE Jacobsen to VM Hancher, February 25, 1949, Folder 120, 1948-49, VM Hancher Papers, University of Iowa Archives.
74.   ME Kitchell to CE Jacobsen, July 19, 1949, Folder 118, 1949-50, VM Hancher Papers, University of Iowa Archives.
75.   Folder 118, 1949-50, VM Hancher Papers, University of Iowa Archives.
76.   Curriculum Committee minutes, October 11 and 13, 1949, Records Group 16, Box 1, Information-Nursing, Folder Committee on Curriculum, 1949-50, School of Nursing Papers, University of Iowa Archives.
77.   ME Kitchell to CE Jacobsen, RI Tidrick, and G Hartman, December 6, 1949, Box 9, Folder Dean Jacobsen correspondence, College of Nursing Papers, University of Iowa Archives.
78.   ME Kitchell to CE Jacobsen, September 16, 1949, College of Nursing Papers, Box 9, Folder Dean Jacobsen correspondence, University of Iowa Archives.
79.   "Basis for Judgment Concerning Absence from Class and Adjustments in Hours of Practice," November 21, 1949, Records Group 16, Box 1, Information-Nursing, Folder Committee on Curriculum, 1949-50, University of Iowa Archives.
80.   ME Kitchell to CE Jacobsen, September 10, 1949, Box 9, Folder Dean Jacobsen correspondence, College of Nursing Papers, University of Iowa Archives.
81.   The most thorough discussion of internal divisions is perhaps Barbara Melosh, "A Charge to Keep," in *The Physician's Hand*, pp. 37-76.

Chapter Three

Building a College of Nursing, 1950-1964

To the surprise of most Americans, their memories scarred by the recent Depression, the first two postwar decades brought sustained economic expansion unlike anything since the surge of industrialization and westward migration in the nineteenth century. In the two decades from 1946 to 1965, the gross national product grew at an annual rate of 3.7 percent, rising from $208 billion to $685 billion.[1] In Iowa, median family income tripled from $3,000 to $9,000 in the same period. In turn, economic prosperity fed government expenditures at all levels, a trend with profound implications for American society in general and for American health care in particular. Federal government expenditures rose from a postwar low of $36.5 billion in 1948 to $118 billion in 1965, while state and local government expenditures increased from just $14 billion in 1946 to more than $86 billion in 1965.

Behind those aggregate figures lay important trends for health care, both in Iowa and in America at large. Included in growing federal and state budgets were enormous increases in appropriations for education, including education in the health care professions, for medical scientific research, and for health care goods and services. Total public expenditures for education rose from $4 billion in 1946 to $30 billion in 1965; total spending for higher education rose from just over $1 billion to more than $8 billion over the same period. Similarly, federal expenditures for medical scientific research rose from $90 million in 1948 to $1.5 billion in 1965. Moreover, as annual per capita spending on health care goods and services rose from $68 to $187, a remarkable series of scientific and technological advances invested the health care professions with new prestige and, at the same time, raised the expectations of health care consumers.

The early postwar period was also one of extraordinary growth in American hospitals, growth nurtured by the general economic expansion, by the spread of private health insurance,[2] and by the Hill-Burton Hospital Survey and Construction Act of 1946, which ultimately funneled billions of dollars into hospital construction. In the 1950s, the American hospital became home to an expanding array of sophisticated health care technologies—their use, to a considerable extent, organized and supervised by more and better trained registered nurses.

Against that backdrop of economic prosperity and expanded investments in education, medical scientific research, and health care, the late 1940s and 1950s saw more and more colleges and universities adopt baccalaureate programs in nursing. After decades of frustration, nursing school accreditation also had a perceptible effect in the 1950s, thanks in part to federal regulations requiring that nurses seeking employment in government agencies and institutions present credentials from accredited educational institutions. Colleges of nursing also began—slowly at first but at an accelerating pace in the 1960s—to establish graduate training programs at the master's level and a few at the doctoral level, offering advanced education to prepare nurses for more specialized roles in administration, clinical practice, teaching, and research. At the same time, practical nursing programs, conducted often under the adult education umbrella in the public schools, and associate degree programs, conducted in expanding networks of community colleges, grew rapidly.

In many ways, then, the period from 1950 to 1964 was a formative one for modern American nursing, certainly so for nursing education. During the 1950s and early 1960s, nursing care, especially in the hospital setting, became more intensive in nature and more technology-oriented, while registered nurses, particularly those with baccalaureate training, assumed increasing supervisory responsibilities, passing on to subordinates many of the routine care functions that had comprised the bulk of instruction at prewar hospital diploma schools. The emphasis on educational credentials in nursing benefited the new colleges of nursing, which profited, albeit at a later date and in lesser degree than did colleges of medicine, from the unprecedented postwar infusion of public and private funds into education and research in the health sciences.

A Sketch of Postwar American Nursing

The Korean War opened the 1950s and introduced American society to a harsh new set of geopolitical realities. For Americans in general and for American nurses in particular, the "forgotten war" of 1950-53 was the third major wartime experience of the century. In the summer of 1950, the Joint Committee on Nursing in National Security, including representation from six major nursing organizations, devised a detailed plan for the mobilization of nurses to meet the nursing needs of the military services while minimizing disruption of domestic nursing staffs. In fact, the war entailed an abbreviated mobilization of nursing personnel, and the combined strength of Army and Navy nurse corps peaked at roughly 8,800, less than fifteen percent of the World War II maximum. Nonetheless, the extremes of climate and terrain, as well as the often brutal nature of the conflict, made nursing during the Korean War especially demanding. Moreover, nurses played important roles in the success of several innovations in the delivery of health care to combatants, including the new Mobile Army Surgical Hospital units (MASH units) designed to provide front-line medical and nursing care. Overall, such innovations held battle and non-battle death rates during the war significantly below World War II levels.[3]

The Korean War may not have affected American nursing so profoundly as did World War II; nonetheless, wartime advances in medical, surgical, and nursing care signaled an emergent revolution in the foundations of American health care. Accelerating through the 1950s and 1960s, that revolution brought much-publicized advances in several areas, from cancer therapy and kidney dialysis to cardiac catheterization, open heart surgery, and synthetic "wonder drugs," including antibiotics, antihistamines, tranquilizers, and antihypertensives. Just as important, that revolution also saw the wholesale reconstruction of America's hospital system.[4] From 1946 to 1965, the number of short-term general hospitals in America increased 29.1 percent, from 4,400 to 5,700, and the number of hospital beds rose even more steeply, jumping 56.7 percent from 473,000 to more than 741,000. In the same period, the average daily patient census in American hospitals grew from 341 to 563, and *per diem* hospital costs increased 374 percent, from an average of $9.39 to $44.48. The Hill-Burton Hospital Survey and Construction Act of

1946 (Public Law 79-75) was important in recasting America's hospitals; in the quarter century after 1946, the US Public Health Service disbursed $3.7 billion in Hill-Burton construction funds. During the same period, Congress also appropriated hundreds of millions of dollars for an ambitious expansion of the Veterans Administration hospital system.

In part because of the twin revolutions in technologies and facilities, the number of active graduate nurses in the United States increased from some 375,000 to over 613,000 from 1950 to 1965, with hospital nurses making up roughly sixty percent of the total. However, the increase in graduate nurses employed in hospitals did not keep pace with the expansion in hospital beds and the increased staffing levels necessitated by the growing intensity of nursing care. Hospitals, then, relied to an ever greater extent on auxiliary nursing personnel—for example, practical nurses and aides—for the delivery of nursing services.

By the early 1960s, the complexion of American nursing was substantially changed from the immediate postwar years and earlier. A 1962 American Nurses Association survey counted 848,000 licensed professional nurses (registered nurses) in the United States—a sixty-eight percent increase over the 504,000 in the 1949 inventory.[5] The 532,000 active nurses in 1962 exceeded the 299,000 of 1949 by seventy-eight percent. In Iowa, active nurses made up fifty-five percent of the 15,592 registered nurses, compared to sixty-three percent nationally. Across the United States, males accounted for just under one percent of the total of active nurses in 1962.

According to the 1962 ANA survey, more than sixty percent of active nurses, or 335,000, were employed in hospitals or other institutions; twelve percent, or 64,100, were engaged in private duty nursing; eight percent, or 44,000, were employed as office nurses by physicians and dentists; nearly five percent, or 24,000, were in public health nursing; and three percent, or 16,000, were in nursing education. In Iowa, the figures were sixty-one percent in hospitals, nine percent in private duty, eleven percent in doctor's and dentist's offices, two percent in public health, and four percent in education. Of the 335,000 nurses employed nationwide in hospitals and other institutions, fifty-nine percent, or 199,000, were general duty or staff nurses. As might be expected, private duty nurses were, on average, significantly older—median age 49 years—than their colleagues in other fields.

Marriage and child-rearing were major factors in nurses' career patterns. Eighty-two percent of all inactive nurses in the United States and eighty-five percent of inactive nurses in Iowa were married in 1962, compared to the sixty-one percent of active nurses nationwide and sixty-three percent in Iowa who were married. Moreover, while nearly half of all active nurses nationwide were under forty years of age, the proportion of active nurses among age groups 20-29 and 30-39 showed substantial variation, suggesting the impress of marriage and child-rearing responsibilities on nurses' career patterns. Just thirty percent of the under-thirty group were inactive, compared to forty-three percent of the 30-39 group, a cohort especially apt to be burdened by child-rearing duties. In Iowa, thirty-five percent of the 20-29 age group were inactive, compared to fifty-three percent in the 30-39 group. In contrast, the proportion of inactive nurses in the 40-49 age group fell to thirty-two percent nationwide and to forty-two percent in Iowa.

There was also a slow but significant change in registered nurses' educational backgrounds. In 1952, only 27,039 of 374,584 registered nurses, just over seven percent, held bachelor's degrees, and 3,806, or one percent, held master's degrees.[6] Barely a handful of nurses held PhDs at the time; a count in 1950 found just twenty-two, with a further fifty nurses—among them the University of Iowa College of Nursing's new Dean Myrtle Kitchell—then enrolled in doctoral programs.[7] In comparison, the 1962 ANA survey included an inventory of the educational qualifications of more than 130,000 nurses in fifteen states, not including Iowa, indicating that eighty percent of active nurses in those states were graduates of hospital diploma programs, while twelve percent were graduates of bachelor's programs. In addition, the 1962 count included 1,649 active nurses holding master's degrees in nursing and 600 holding master's degrees in other areas, 104 active nurses holding PhDs in nursing and thirty-eight holding PhDs in other areas.[8]

The University of Iowa College of Nursing circulated the results of a survey of its own in 1962, this one identifying career patterns of more than 3,000 graduates of the college and its predecessors, the Nurse Training School and the School of Nursing.[9] The college reported that forty-two percent of the 1,296 respondents still lived in Iowa, and ninety-eight percent had worked as nurses at one time or another after graduation. Different graduate cohorts, however, showed significantly different patterns of work. More than fifty-seven percent among the 1907-1935 cohort had worked in nursing at least ten years, but the figure dropped to fewer than fifty percent of 1936-1940 graduates and fell even further to thirty-four percent for the World War II cohort of 1941-1945 graduates. Barely more than twenty-one percent of 1946-1950 graduates had been actively engaged in nursing for ten years or more.

Unlike the ANA report, the University of Iowa study argued that marriage itself had little impact on nursing careers but agreed that child-rearing, in contrast, had a significant effect. Countering that claim, however, more than eighty percent of unmarried respondents graduating between 1931 and 1955 remained active in nursing in 1961; yet, among married women with no children in that group, only 50.9 percent remained active. Among all married graduates in the 1931-1951 classes, those with children and those without, just 27.2 percent were active in nursing at the time of the survey. At the same time, survey results suggested that holders of bachelor's degrees were more likely to pursue graduate education than were diploma school graduates. Among the 779 diploma graduates responding to the survey, just thirteen had acquired master's degrees by 1961; in comparison, thirty-three of the 517 respondents who were graduates from the combined program and its baccalaureate successor possessed master's degrees in 1961.

The 1950s brought a significant reorganization of professional nursing organizations. Early in the decade, after several years of study, the American Nurses Association merged with the National Association of Colored Graduate Nurses, and the ANA also established special interest sections to address the needs of nurses in a variety of specialized fields.[10] Also, the National League of Nursing Education, the National Organization of Public Health Nurses, and the Association of Collegiate Schools of Nursing merged to form the National League for Nursing.[11] Meanwhile, membership in nursing organizations remained low, a reflection of the limited career aims of many nurses and perhaps their equally limited professional esteem. In 1960, the Iowa Nurses Association (successor to the Iowa State Association of Registered Nurses and the Iowa State Nurses Association) claimed 2,551 members, representing thirty-six percent of the association's potential membership. By that time, too, the INA had instituted a range of special interest sections: general duty nursing, head nursing, occupational health nursing, office nursing, private duty nursing, and public health nursing.

Several important studies projecting the future of American nursing surfaced in the 1950s and early 1960s, underlining nursing trends, pointing to the strengths and weaknesses of existing educational programs, and projecting future nursing needs. *Nursing for a Growing Nation*, published by the National League for Nursing in 1957, counted 430,000 active professional nurses in 1956 and calculated a national ratio of 258 nurses per 100,000 population—254 per 100,000 in the midwestern states. In line with expected population growth and desirable increases in the nurse/population ratio to the range of 300-350 per 100,000, the report projected a demand for 600-700,000 active nurses in 1970, requiring the training of 380,000 diploma nurses and 180,000 baccalaureate nurses in the period from 1957 to 1970.[12] A second study, compiled by the US Surgeon General's Consultant Group on Nursing and published in 1963 under the title *Toward Quality in Nursing: Needs and Goals*, contained a broad-ranging call for federal aid for nursing education.[13] Under present circumstances, the report's authors warned, far too many nursing schools were providing inadequate education, while nursing as a whole was not recruiting its share of promising students, perhaps because of nursing's low status as measured both in public esteem and in monetary terms. Perhaps the most important points raised in the report were, first, the need for more nurses with graduate degrees and, second, the need for federal aid to spur the general expansion of nursing education at all levels, from practical nursing to doctoral programs.

Federal funding of basic nursing education was an outgrowth of such reports and studies, bolstered also by the intensive lobbying efforts of major nursing organizations. Passage of the Health Professions Educational Assistance Act of 1963 (PL 88-129), like most health "manpower" legislation of the era, was motivated chiefly by concerns over declining medical school applications and a looming "physician shortage." Nonetheless, that act was the first to provide direct federal aid—in the form of student loans and grants—to undergraduate education in the health professions and to provide federal subsidies for the construction of new educational facilities.[14]

Close on the heels of the 1963 act, the Nurse Training Act of 1964 (PL 88-581) specifically provided basic nursing education a combination of student loans, graduate traineeship programs, special projects and planning grants, and funding for the construction of educational facilities.

As noted in the previous chapter, the immediate post-World War II years saw a precipitate enrollment decline in nursing education programs nationwide. High student attrition rates worsened the enrollment decline; one national study reported attrition in the graduating class of 1949—the entering class of 1946—at thirty-one percent, with "matrimony" far and away the most common cause of withdrawal (thirty-four percent) followed by "failure in classwork" (eighteen percent).[15] Myrtle Kitchell estimated the attrition rate at thirty percent in the entering class of 1946 at the University of Iowa School of Nursing.[16] By 1950, however, nursing enrollments had begun to recover, and the student body had also become more diverse. In 1951, the 1,170 nursing programs, both diploma and baccalaureate, were twenty percent fewer in number than two decades earlier, but total enrollments were higher at 102,509. The total student population embraced 2,971 African-Americans in 236 schools, 1,023 men in 117 schools, and 12,301 diploma nurses enrolled in baccalaureate programs. In 1951, Iowa nursing schools enrolled 2,180 students, 1,950 of them Iowa residents. More than 700 Iowans were enrolled in nursing schools out of state in that year.[17]

From the mid-1950s, three long-term trends were especially prominent in American nursing education (Table 3.1). The first was the explosive growth in practical nursing programs and the ap-

TABLE 3.1. Nursing Programs and Graduates, 1948-49 to 1964-65

	Practical Nursing		Diploma Nursing		Baccalaureate Degree		Associate Degree	
	Programs	Graduates	Programs	Graduates	Programs	Graduates	Programs	Graduates
1948-49	71[a]	1,500[a]	n/a	21,379	n/a	1,294	n/a	n/a
1954-55	395	9,694	963	25,873	154	2,601	19	199
1959-60	661	16,491	908	25,288	172	4,136	57	789
1964-65	984	24,331	821	26,795	198	5,381	174	2,510

[a]1948 estimates.

Sources: *Nursing Outlook* and *American Journal of Nursing*

pearance, at least by 1964-65, of significant numbers of associate degree programs. The second major trend was the continuing decline in the number of diploma schools, a decline that reflected ongoing pressures on marginal programs. The third trend was the slow increase in the numbers of baccalaureate programs through the 1950s, following the explosive growth of the late 1940s and early 1950s and preceding a second growth surge in the early 1960s. Throughout the period, graduates of baccalaureate programs made up a small, but slowly increasing, minority of all new registered nurses—six percent in 1949, rising to some sixteen percent in 1965.

Federal subsidies appropriated under the National Vocational Education Acts fueled the rapid growth in practical nursing programs. Practical nursing programs were attractive not only because of their relatively short duration and low tuition, they were also more democratic vehicles for nurse recruitment than the older diploma programs or the newer baccalaureate programs. In 1954, twenty-eight percent of the more than 12,000 students enrolled in practical nursing programs were non-white and nearly four percent were men.

Building a College of Nursing: Faculty

From 1950 to 1964, three deans led the University of Iowa College of Nursing, fulfilling essential administrative roles, performing important formal and informal political functions within the university and beyond, and setting standards that guided other faculty and students. The first, introduced in the previous chapter, was Myrtle Kitchell, who came to the University of Iowa as a doctoral candidate and received her PhD in educational administration and educational psychology from the University of Minnesota in 1955. Just thirty-two years of age when she arrived in Iowa City, Kitchell was widely recognized as a promising young leader in American nursing.

President Virgil Hancher keenly appreciated Kitchell's importance to the college and the university. When former University of Iowa Executive Dean Carlyle Jacobsen, who had played a principal role in bringing Kitchell to the new college in 1949, wrote in 1951 from his new post as executive dean for medical education at the State University of New York in Albany to inform Hancher of his interest in Kitchell for an as yet undefined position on his campus, the president responded that the loss of the nursing dean "would cripple us a great deal."[18] In early 1953, Hancher worried over Kitchell's recent visit to Western Reserve to explore the deanship at that school, warning University of Iowa Provost Harvey Davis that Kitchell had expressed some reservations about the future of the College of Nursing, concerns grounded in ongoing problems with a handful of physicians in the College of Medicine. Hancher himself noted that the newly appointed dean of the College of Medicine, Norman Nelson, was said to hold "traditional" attitudes toward nurses and nursing.[19] Notwithstanding Hancher's repeated concerns, however, Kitchell remained in office until the end of the 1956-1957 academic year, when she began a brief hiatus from academia in order to raise her two children.

Before Kitchell's departure from the deanship, Provost Davis polled the nursing faculty regarding the selection of a new dean, asking for news of developments in nursing education and their implications for the college, ideal qualities in a dean, and suggested candidates.[20] In November 1956, Kitchell herself submitted to Davis a list of prospective candidates, a list that included Helen Nahm of the National League for Nursing, Agnes Love of the University of Michigan, and Rozella Schlotfeldt—the last a graduate of the University of Iowa School of Nursing and later dean at Western Reserve University.[21] Subsequently, the dean appointed a committee of three to evaluate likely candidates.[22] In spring 1957, President Hancher appointed a three-member executive committee, chaired for the first month by Mary M. Lohr and thereafter by Etta Rasmussen, to take charge of the College of Nursing during the interim period.[23] However, the search for a new College of Nursing dean dragged on beyond expectations, and from fall 1958 Rasmussen served as acting dean.

Myrtle Kitchell's eventual successor, Mary Kelly Mullane, visited the University of Iowa campus December 8-10, 1958. Mullane was a New York City native and had received a nursing diploma from Holy Name Hospital School of Nursing in Teaneck, New Jersey, in 1931, a bachelor of science degree with a major in teaching in schools of nursing from Teachers College of Columbia University in 1936, a master of arts degree in administration in nursing schools from Teachers College in 1942, and a PhD from the University of Chicago in administration in higher education in 1957.

Mullane had considerable experience both in nursing service and nursing education, including a twelve-year stint as associate professor and assistant to the dean at the Wayne State University College of Nursing. A longtime associate at Wayne State applauded in particular Mullane's open-mindedness and her social skills and assured University of Iowa President Virgil Hancher that she "showed evidence of real scholarship" and would insist on high standards for faculty and students.[24] Early in 1959, Mullane published *Education for Nursing Service Administration: An Experience in Program Development by Fourteen Universities*, a retrospective description and analysis of a W. K. Kellogg Foundation project to fund graduate programs in nursing service administration—a project in which the University of Iowa College of Nursing had participated.[25] At the time of her Iowa City interview, Mullane was also a member of the National League for Nursing's subcommittee on practical nurse education. The Iowa State Board of Regents (successor to the State Board of Education) announced her appointment in January 1959, effective July 1, 1959.[26]

While Mary Mullane's tenure in the deanship was relatively short, just three years, she presided over a landmark curriculum revision and transition—described in detail below—resulting in adoption of the long-awaited four academic-year curriculum in the fall of 1961 and the phaseout of student nursing service in the University Hospitals. In spring 1962, President Hancher received word of University of Illinois President David Henry's interest in appointing Mullane dean of his university's nursing school in Chicago.[27] Not only did that position fit with Mullane's big city background; it also owed much to a long professional association between Henry and Mullane, an association begun at Wayne State University. In her formal letter of resignation in July 1962, Mullane expressed confidence in the future of the college, commended President Virgil Hancher, Provost Harvey Davis, and the College of Nursing faculty for their support, and noted that she had accepted the Chicago position because of the challenge it presented and because of her personal friendship with Henry.[28]

In September 1962, a five-member search committee reported to President Hancher that it had finished another survey of faculty opinion on the future of the college and on desired qualifications in a new dean and had also considered possible candidates.[29] Among the goals of the college, the committee listed the integration of the general nursing program into the basic baccalaureate program, accreditation of the master's program and reinstitution of the nursing administration program, inauguration of a doctoral program in cooperation with other Big Ten schools by 1972, development of faculty research, and continued provision of nursing leadership to the state of Iowa.

Contrary to the urgings of many parties, including the State Board of Nurse Examiners, the search committee proceeded slowly, and during the ensuing interregnum a series of acting deans—most prominently, Florence Sherbon—guided the college.[30] As had been the case in 1957-58, the primary cause of delay appears to have been the lack of suitable candidates, especially candidates holding the PhD. In response to an inquiry from the Board of Nurse Examiners in the summer of 1963, a member of the university's central administration explained simply that "there are not many nurse educators with a PhD."[31]

Mullane's successor and the third dean of the College of Nursing, Laura Corbin Dustan, visited the college in the fall of 1963, and the Board of Regents approved her appointment in January 1964, effective in September of that year. A Vermont native, Laura Dustan graduated from the University of Vermont in 1940 with a degree in home economics, having been, as she later remembered it, "roped into" home economics in place of the general science major that she had first envisioned.[32] After applying to both Yale and Western Reserve for graduate study in nursing, Dustan attended Western Reserve from 1940 to 1943, earning her master's degree in nursing. Following a teaching stint at Western Reserve during the war years, she completed a course in nurse midwifery in 1946 and became maternity nursing supervisor at a New York City teaching hospital. In the 1950s, after three years in public health nursing in New York, Dustan returned to the University of Vermont as an assistant professor—later associate professor—in public health nursing, also completing work in 1956 for a master's degree in public health nursing curriculum and teaching from Columbia University's Teachers College.

Recognizing the importance of a PhD for access to the higher levels of nursing administration, Dustan enrolled in the doctoral program of the school of education at the University of California, Berkeley, in 1960, attracted to the Bay area in part by the proximity of Helen Nahm, one of the most important figures in American nursing at the time. Dustan received her PhD in 1963 and took a position with the National League for Nursing's Board of Review for Accrediting of Baccalaureate Programs, which, she later recalled, constituted a central experience of her career, an experience that impressed her with the potential of baccalaureate education in nursing, while, at the same time, affording a first-hand view of the generally inadequate facilities that burdened most baccalaureate programs. Coming to the University of Iowa in 1964, Dustan was impressed by the fact that, in the new four academic year curriculum, the College of Nursing's students were "real students" for all four years. Like each of her predecessors, Dustan, too, saw the College of Nursing through an important transition, in her case the planning and construction of the present College of Nursing Building in the late 1960s and early 1970s.

For Myrtle Kitchell, Mary Mullane, and Laura Dustan, one of the dean's most important responsibilities lay in faculty recruitment, a vexing problem for nursing educators nationwide, especially in the new baccalaureate programs. In 1952, the National League for Nursing counted 10,406 nurses directly involved in professional nursing education programs of all kinds. Of that total, 4,559, or 43.8 percent, held bachelor's degrees, 1,140, or 11.0 percent, held master's degrees, and nearly all the remainder, more than 4,700, held hospital diplomas.[33] With more than 100 new colleges of nursing seeking faculty members in the early 1950s, the pool of potential faculty, especially faculty with advanced degrees, was comparatively small, and competition in their recruitment was correspondingly intense. Furthermore, rising expectations through the 1950s and into the 1960s regarding faculty credentials coupled to the slow expansion of graduate programs meant that demand for faculty continued to run well ahead of supply.

Early in her tenure, Myrtle Kitchell reflected on the factors at work in faculty selection and organization.[34] First, Kitchell noted that a baccalaureate program placed far greater demands on faculty than did the older apprenticeship mode of training. Much the same was true, she noted, of the strengthening movement toward accreditation of nursing schools. In addition, she argued that the manifold changes in nursing practice meant that faculty members must master an ever larger body of knowledge and experience in order to perform their educational functions. Finally, just as important as the specifics of faculty selection was the creation of an organizational structure in the college that would combine functions and personnel in efficient ways while encouraging and rewarding the participation of each faculty member.

When Myrtle Kitchell arrived in Iowa City in the summer of 1949, she was, as noted in the previous chapter, the third member of the new College of Nursing faculty. By the fall of 1951, that skeleton group had expanded to include, in addition to Kitchell, one associate professor, six assistant professors, four associates, and six instructors. The college's instructional staff also included various members of the University Hospitals nursing service as well as personnel from area public health agencies and visiting nurse associations. In 1954, the faculty numbered five associate professors, five assistant professors, seven associates, and eight instructors. In comparison, Dean Kitchell reported to Provost Harvey Davis in March 1956, that the nursing faculty at the University of Minnesota included two professors, two associate professors, six assistant professors, and 22 instructors, and both Ohio State University and the University of Michigan reported similar numbers.[35]

In the last half of the 1950s and the early 1960s, College of Nursing faculty numbers increased at a more rapid pace, especially in the instructor ranks. In 1959, during the transition between Deans Myrtle Kitchell and Mary Mullane, the faculty consisted of Acting Dean Etta Rasmussen, who was also an assistant professor, one full professor, two associate professors, six assistant professors in addition to Rasmussen, two associates, and twenty-four instructors. By the fall of 1964, the faculty included Laura Dustan, professor and dean, one professor emeritus, seven associate professors, sixteen assistant professors, and twenty-nine instructors—the associate category having disappeared. By and large, the major expansion in faculty numbers from the mid-1950s to the mid-1960s reflected rising accreditation criteria, the demands of an expanded graduate program, and the college's increasing responsibility for clinical instruction—or, perhaps more accurately, the conversion of hospital work into formal clinical instruction.

Problems in identifying and recruiting faculty only worsened over time as demand—fueled by faculty growth at nursing schools across the nation, by rising expectations regarding faculty credentials, and by the fact that too few nurses, for whatever reasons, sought graduate training—increased far faster than did the supply of candidates. As a result, faculty recruitment absorbed a disproportionate share of the deans' and department heads' time and effort. Although complete data are lacking, a third or more of the faculty recruited to the University of Iowa College of Nursing between 1949 and 1964, especially at the associate or instructor level, came to the college with only bachelor's degrees. Many of those subsequently earned master's degrees, either from the University of Iowa or elsewhere. By the same token, many of those who resigned faculty positions in the 1950s and 1960s did so to pursue advanced degrees. In 1954-55, ten of the eleven faculty members in the ranks of assistant professor and above held master's degrees, five of those from Columbia University, and one held a doctorate in education from Stanford University. Of the fifteen associates and instructors, just three held advanced degrees. The situation was much the same at other Big Ten schools, where the faculty at Ohio State University, for example, included one doctoral degree, fifteen master's degrees, and seventeen bachelor's degrees—fifteen of the latter at the level of instructor.[36]

Despite long-standing problems in faculty recruitment and to some extent in faculty retention, Dean Mary Mullane reported in September 1961 that the college had made significant progress in responding to criticisms lodged in 1959 by the Collegiate Board of Review of the National League for Nursing that too few faculty possessed training and experience to match their areas of teaching responsibility.[37] A combination of intense recruitment efforts and concerted efforts at faculty development, including university support for faculty attendance at professional meetings and faculty leave for further education, had, Mullane reported, done much to correct the problem. In the dean's count, just nine of thirty-six faculty members had graduate training specific to their areas of teaching responsibility in the fall of 1959, while three had training in a related area. In the fall of 1961, in contrast, twenty-three of forty faculty members had the requisite training in their major areas of responsibility, and five more had training in related areas.

Nonetheless, the unceasing search for new faculty continued into the early 1960s as the college struggled to maintain adequate faculty numbers. Having resolved in July 1962 not to reappoint any current staff holding bachelor's degrees and hoping also to avoid hiring any new instructors at the bachelor's level, college faculty nonetheless welcomed twelve new instructors with bachelor's degrees in September 1963, but did so with the caveat that each must enroll in at least one graduate course per semester.[38] Early in 1964, the faculty reaffirmed the graduate enrollment requirement, advising department chairs to assign correspondingly lighter workloads to affected faculty members.[39] In the fall of 1964, two of the twenty-five College of Nursing faculty at the rank of assistant professor and above held doctorates, twenty held master's degrees, and one held a bachelor's degree, leaving one unaccounted for in official records. Nine of twenty-nine instructors held master's degrees, while the remaining twenty held bachelor's degrees. At the same time, Dean Laura Dustan notified Willard Boyd, the university's dean of faculties, of the need to recruit additional faculty, in part to replace under-qualified members.[40]

At times, particularly by the early 1960s, faculty salaries were an impediment to faculty recruitment. In the summer of 1957, the College of Nursing executive committee received a report on faculty salaries, noting a range from $10,000 for full professors, $7,400-8,200 for associate professors, $7,000-7,800 for assistant professors, $6,000-$7,400 for associates, and $4,000-$6,000 for instructors.[41] Figures at the lower levels were comparable to pay scales for supervising nurses at the University Hospitals, while figures at the higher levels were somewhat below the figures applying in other University of Iowa colleges and were well below base salaries in the College of Medicine's clinical departments, where faculty also augmented their base salaries substantially from practice revenues distributed through the college's Medical Service Plan. Nursing faculty salaries increased slowly through the late 1950s and into the early 1960s, and the college judged in May 1963 that the existing scale placed the University of Iowa in "a good position" compared to competing schools. Still, Dean Dustan asked just over a year later to increase entry-level assistant salaries to $8,000, an increase mandated, she argued, by the highly competitive job market.[42]

Problems in the setting of promotion policies echoed the general problems in faculty recruitment. University of Iowa policy regarding promotion ostensibly blended four elements: academic credentials, teaching ability, service record, and research productivity. The university faculty handbook of the late 1950s specified "the doctorate or its equivalent" and a "record of scholarly investigations supported by publications or the equivalent in terms of assistance in the direction of doctoral dissertations" as prerequisites for appointment at the assistant professor level. Also, the handbook specified that appointments at the rank of assistant professor "ordinarily do not exceed a total of seven years." For promotion to the tenured ranks of associate or full professor, institutional standards were correspondingly higher. In all cases, the handbook noted that "length of service" was not "of itself a qualification" for promotion.

The College of Nursing could not hope to meet those criteria, and Provost Harvey Davis afforded the college considerable leeway in interpreting and applying general university standards. In 1957, the College of Nursing faculty established guidelines setting the master's degree as the threshold for promotion to full professor, mandating "creative performance in nursing practice" and "contribution[s] to the literature" for promotion to associate professor, and requiring active participation in professional organizations, "creative teaching," and service to the college, the university, and the state for promotion to assistant professor.[43] The college also buttressed its promotion policies with detailed guidelines for merit pay increases within rank. In 1963, aiming to increase research productivity, the college adopted the further requirement that "faculty of professorial rank should be encouraged, if not required, to write at least one scholarly paper annually which would be publishable."[44]

As that faculty addendum recognized, nursing research was an essential factor in faculty growth and in faculty evaluation for the long term. Nursing research and the elaboration of a body of nursing knowledge apart from medicine were also crucial to the professional autonomy of nursing. In the period from 1950 to 1964, however, most College of Nursing faculty engaged in little or no research, a pattern reproduced generally at colleges of nursing nationwide. One problem, as one observer has noted, was that few faculty had sufficient backgrounds "either to do research adequately or to educate students to do it."[45] A second problem was the lack of funding, public or private, for nursing research. By the early 1960s, then, as funded research and scholarly publication rapidly became the *sine qua non* of academic life in most University of Iowa departments and colleges, including the health sciences colleges, the College of Nursing lagged badly behind, with few faculty members possessed of research training and with little available research funding.

In describing the slow growth of research in nursing, Myrtle Kitchell Aydelotte noted in a 1995 interview that she and other *Nursing Research* editorial board members were "hard pressed to find something to publish" in the journal's inaugural 1952 issue. A limited research program begun in 1950 by the American Nurses Association led—thanks in part to a $100,000 ANA donation—to creation in 1955 of the American Nurses' Foundation, which provided one of the first significant funding sources for nursing research. Still, for nursing, as for other fields, federal funds held the key to the expansion of research efforts, and it was not until fiscal year 1956 that the US Public Health Service Division of Nursing Resources received its first congressional appropriation of $625,000 for the support of nursing research.

The University of Iowa's Myrtle Kitchell and Marie Tener, the latter head of the nursing service in the University Hospitals, were among the initial recipients of USPHS research funds. In 1957, Kitchell and Tener won a $100,000 award for a study designed to test the assumption that more intensive nursing care—achieved either through increased staffing levels or through better training— would enhance patient welfare.[46] Published in 1960 under the title *An Investigation of the Relation Between Nursing Activity and Patient Welfare*, the authors concluded that neither increased staffing levels nor intense in-service training programs had a significant effect on patient welfare. Disappointing though its conclusions may have been, the Kitchell-Tener study, the College of Nursing's first major externally funded research project, was an important milestone.

Faculty involvement in the university and in broader nursing communities at local, state, and national levels was also a goal of the

College of Nursing. Acting through formal and informal channels, Myrtle Kitchell went to great lengths to earn a place for herself—and, thus, for her college—within the university structure. Much the same was true of Kitchell's successors, and, with some exceptions, their efforts were rewarded. However, as Kitchell recognized early on, nurses' reception within the broader university hinged on solid academic credentials and their demands, based upon those credentials, to be taken seriously. Likewise, in part as a matter of necessity and in part as a matter of choice, College of Nursing faculty worked extensively with administrators and staff of the University Hospitals nursing service, collaborating on educational and research problems, and also with medical faculty, especially in the basic science areas.

Myrtle Kitchell also initiated a pattern of interaction with broader professional communities. At a national level, Kitchell held a variety of offices and committee assignments in the 1950s; she was, for example, a member of the National League for Nursing Collegiate Board of Review and the American Nurses Association finance committee as well as national president of Sigma Theta Tau. In Kitchell's view, her involvement in national nursing circles provided continuing education in current concerns and issues that was a benefit to the college, while her participation also enhanced the college's national visibility. That pattern continued in the late 1950s and early 1960s, as the college routinely supported faculty travel to national conferences and professional meetings. Likewise, in 1963, the American Nurses Association invited the college to host a national workshop for its general duty and head nurse sections, and registrations for the August sessions totaled over 500. Throughout the period, Kitchell and her successors in the dean's office also received numerous requests from schools across the nation seeking information on curriculum and instructional methods and on possible faculty candidates.

In much the same way, the College of Nursing nurtured connections with the community of Iowa nurses, chiefly through activity in professional associations and through an expanding array of continuing education programs. By 1961, the college had one faculty member devoted full-time to the coordination of continuing education programs, and programs both on and off campus enrolled 327 nurses in the 1961-62 academic year. The college's 1963-64 report on continuing education included off-campus conferences for nursing home administrators and cooperative ventures with several organizations, including the Iowa Nurses Association, Iowa Heart Association, and American Cancer Society. All told, seven conferences drew a total attendance of 634, with nurses from nine states represented.[47]

Nursing Students at the University of Iowa

The University of Iowa as a whole grew rapidly in the early postwar years. In 1950, at the peak of the postwar enrollment surge, the university counted 10,386 students, compared to 6,667 a decade earlier and fewer than 3,200 at the depths of World War II. In the College of Nursing, baccalaureate enrollments rose rapidly in the early 1950s (Table 3.2), and the college also enrolled the first male nursing students, although the percentage of males in the student body never reached as high as two percent during the fifteen-year period to 1964. In the fluid educational and practice environ-

TABLE 3.2. University of Iowa College of Nursing Undergraduate Enrollments and Degrees, 1948-1965

	Total	Male	Female	Degrees
1949-50	263[a]	0	263	0
1950-51	345	4	341	0
1951-52	311	4	307	2
1952-53	426	5	421	38
1953-54	511	7	504	58
1954-55	532	6	526	68
1955-56	524	4	520	80
1956-57	515	4	511	111
1957-58	502	4	498	111
1958-59	463	2	461	91
1959-60	455	3	452	106
1960-61	370	3	367	92
1961-62	388	4	384	80
1962-63	414	2	412	78
1963-64	429	1	428	90
1964-65	428	7	421	96

[a]Three-year diploma program enrollments plus nineteen freshmen in baccalaureate program.
Sources: University of Iowa *Catalogues;* Comparative Enrollment Reports, Office of the Registrar; University of Iowa College of Nursing

ments of the early 1950s, the total of bachelor's degrees awarded rose at a more gradual pace than did enrollments, coming into line with senior enrollments (not shown in the table) only in the middle of the decade. Toward the end of the 1950s, perhaps reflecting the combined effects of economic recession and changes in leadership in the college, enrollments slumped mildly. However, enrollments recovered in the early 1960s, a recovery partially disguised by the fact that freshmen students were no longer counted among the nursing student body.[48] In fact, as early as 1960, the college capped admissions because of space and personnel limitations; moreover, the pending influx of postwar "baby-boomers" prompted projected enrollment of as many as 300 freshmen by 1970.

From 1951, total enrollment figures included both students in the basic program for first-time nursing students and the so-called general program catering to students already holding hospital school diplomas. Indeed, the college offered two programs for diploma nurses. The general program consisted chiefly of the liberal arts components of the basic program, plus the more specialized College of Nursing offerings, including courses in public health nursing and hospital nursing administration. The second option for diploma holders, open until 1958, was an undergraduate program in psychiatric nursing supported by US Public Health Service grants provided by the National Institute of Mental Health under the National Mental Health Act of 1946, a program that was part of an extraordinary postwar expansion in federal and state facilities and programs for the care of the mentally ill and the training of mental health professionals. In place of the comprehensive junior and senior year nursing courses, students in the psychiatric nursing program enrolled in a series of courses in psychology (seven semester hours) and psychiatric nursing theory and practice (fourteen semester hours).

Enrollments in the general program rose from twenty-four in 1952 to forty-six in 1956, with an additional fifteen students in the psychiatric nursing option in the latter year. By 1960, with the psychiatric nursing option having disappeared, the single general program enrolled forty-two students. However, in 1959-60, the program saw major changes, most important a reduction from sixty to thirty-five semester hours in the maximum transfer credit, a reduction resulting from criticisms from the university's central administration and from National League for Nursing accreditation officials. Under the new structure, the general program added several new courses, including courses in public health nursing and nutrition, Comprehensive Nursing I and II, and an increase in the natural science requirement from three to sixteen semester hours.

In the early 1950s, the College of Nursing maintained the older diploma nursing program, chiefly in response to the much-noted nursing shortage of the period and to appease critics in the College of Medicine and in the University Hospitals administration who opposed the transition to a baccalaureate program. However, College of Nursing officials drew a sharp distinction between the baccalaureate and diploma programs. The former, they advised, was "to prepare students broadly by the integration of professional study and the study of the liberalizing subjects so essential to the practice of a profession" in order to prepare students for the full range of career opportunities in hospital and public health nursing. In contrast, the diploma program was simply "for students interested in preparing for bedside nursing in hospitals."[49] The college admitted no new students into the diploma program after 1952, awarding a total of 358 certificates through 1956 when the final class graduated.

The College of Nursing also played a major role in the development of practical nursing in Iowa. At the instigation of the Iowa State Nurses Association, the state legislature revised the Iowa Nurse Practice Act in 1949, including in the statutes for the first time a functional definition of practical nursing and also providing for licensure of practical nurses. Responding to continued criticism from the College of Medicine and the University Hospitals regarding the need for nurses "having less education than the professional nurse," faculty of the University of Iowa College of Nursing prepared a plan for a practical nursing program,[50] a program inaugurated in January 1953 to coincide with the termination of the college's diploma program. The college recruited Etta Rasmussen, then head of both nursing education and nursing service at St. Luke's Hospital in Cedar Rapids, to organize and direct the program, which operated initially with an annual budget of some $20,000 and which enrolled an average of 20-25 students each year.

From the first, the practical nursing program was a source of contention. Despite its popularity among physicians and hospital administrators, many nursing faculty opposed the program on grounds that it was not properly part of the college's mission. In December 1959, Dean Mary Mullane conceded the need for practical as well as professional nurses; however, Mullane maintained that the purpose of the university was to educate professionals. Thus, in her view, the practical nursing program lay outside the college's purview, although it could be justified as a laboratory for the development of curriculum and teaching strategies for use in other such programs. On that basis, nursing faculty voted in January 1960 to continue the program for an indefinite period.[51]

While holding responsibility for the University of Iowa practical nursing program, Etta Rasmussen served also in an advisory capacity at other practical nursing programs around the state, and she served on a six-member committee appointed by the National League for Nursing and the US Office of Education in 1960 to conduct regional conferences for instructors in schools of practical nursing. By 1963, Rasmussen was state supervisor of practical nursing programs, and ten Iowa programs—one at the university, three in area adult education programs, three in vocational-technical schools, and three in junior colleges—employed thirty-seven instructors and shared nearly $200,000 in federal, state, and local funds.[52]

University of Iowa President Virgil Hancher shared concerns over the propriety of the university's practical nursing program, and his administration conducted a 1964 survey on the question.[53] To no one's surprise, University Hospitals officials, adamant about the need for well-trained practical nurses, were pleased with the program. University Vice President of Medical Services Robert Hardin expressed his approval, but added that he preferred not to "tell the College of Nursing what it should do." In the end, Hancher's administration recommended continuation of the practical nursing program at a reduced level, thus lessening the burden on faculty members in nursing and in basic science areas and also lessening the drain on university resources. Subsequently, the College of Nursing faculty voted once again to continue the program on a demonstration basis.

Building a College of Nursing: The Baccalaureate Program

An overriding concern of deans and faculty in the College of Nursing was to create—for nurses and for the public—an image of nursing as a profession. In a 1995 interview, Myrtle Kitchell remembered having been told by the university registrar soon after her arrival on campus that previous practice had been to send to the School of Nursing those female students judged unsuited to the liberal arts. Whether or not it was true, the registrar's remark more or less accurately captured the School of Nursing's image and its standing within the university, and was probably not far off the mark as an assessment of the academic potential of nursing students. In March 1950, the curriculum committee reported, for example, that nineteen of sixty-eight seniors carried grade point averages below 2.0, as did twenty-five juniors.[54] Spurred by such gloomy reports, Dean Kitchell and her successors sought to attract more promising students to nursing and to raise admissions standards, relying upon a variety of screening methods including personal interviews, letters of reference, and a roster of standardized examinations. By the early 1960s, class grade point averages had risen to respectable levels, standing at 2.75 for seniors and 2.72 for sophomores and juniors.[55] In the early 1960s, the college also sought to reward academic achievement by establishing a dean's list for outstanding students.

In addition to upgrading the academic environment, Myrtle Kitchell was also determined that, to the extent possible, students in the new baccalaureate program should enjoy the full range of university student life. For the short term, that meant entertaining students in her private home and broadening nursing students' access to the diverse array of university activities and services, from sporting events and student health to campus organizations and dormitories. For the long term, it meant the elimination of student nurses' service obligations in the University Hospitals and their liberation from Westlawn, the old nurses' dormitory. By integrating nursing students into the university at large, Kitchell aimed to impress upon them that nursing, like the liberal arts or business, belonged to a community of higher education and, just as important, that the baccalaureate nurse was as much a professional as was the engineer or pharmacist.

The nature of student life tended to create solidarity among nursing students. All students belonged to the Student Nurse Organization that operated with activity funds allocated by the university and with a faculty advisor chosen by the dean from a list of candidates nominated by the students. In the early 1950s, the college created a faculty committee on student welfare and also employed a guidance counselor, who became an administrative assistant to the dean, in order to provide additional attention to students' needs and problems, to foster students' involvement in university affairs, and to boost students' professional identification through activities such as the annual capping ritual. Beyond that and unlike students in other professional schools on campus, nursing students shared not only classes and laboratories as they moved in blocks through the curriculum; juniors and seniors also continued to share living quarters in Westlawn until the early 1960s.

While nursing students' wider exposure to university life no doubt contributed to a better rounded educational experience, it also, for better or worse, eventually diminished students' direct identification with other nursing students, with the College of Nursing, and with the nursing profession. A 1961 report of the Iowa Board of Nurse Examiners observed that student interest in professional affairs, specifically the activities of the Student Nurse Association of Iowa "does not appear to be great."[56] Likewise, a group of senior students at the University of Iowa College of Nursing complained in 1963 of the lack of "professional dignity and standards" displayed by younger students, citing the prevalence of bobby socks and tennis shoes, short skirts, and brightly painted fingernails.[57] The students also charged that some nursing faculty were poor role models in that regard and asked that "the younger members of the College of Nursing be instilled with the same code of standards, feeling of pride, and professional dignity...that was taught to us." In much the same vein, the faculty expressed its concern in early 1964 over freshmen pre-nursing students' apparent lack of interest in the Student Nurse Organization.[58] Over the long term, then, the goal of integrating students—and faculty as well—into the university, by housing freshman and sophomore students in the women's dormitories and encouraging their participation in university activities, was at odds with the goal of creating a common professional identity. However, some degree of discordance and disorder may have been the price, gladly paid by some, of breaking with the rigid and intellectually limited diploma school atmosphere of the past.

In the 1950s and early 1960s, nursing educators faced many serious problems in defining and implementing an academic curriculum appropriate to the professional nurse. Nurse educators in hospital diploma schools had, after all, traditionally exerted little control over the nursing curriculum; thus, pioneers like the University of Iowa's Myrtle Kitchell inherited educational systems largely devoid of emphasis in the humanities and social sciences and featuring, at best, a patchwork of courses in the physical and biological sciences. The new breed of nurse educators also faced the problem of gauging and then achieving an effective balance between academic and clinical components of the curriculum, an especially sensitive problem because of the traditional focus on clinical experience in nursing education and the continued dependence of many hospital nursing services on student labor.

In the years from 1950 to 1964, the University of Iowa College of Nursing faculty conducted near constant curricular reviews and revisions. An original curriculum committee, organized in 1949, struggled first and foremost to achieve recognition of nursing as an academic discipline. Gathering input from nursing faculty and from faculty in other colleges and departments, including internal medicine, surgery, pharmacology, pathology, psychology, and sociology, the full committee and its specialty subcommittees devised a series of new and redesigned basic science and clinical courses for the four-year curriculum. In some respects, the basic science courses posed the most serious problems because of competing demands, chiefly from the College of Medicine, for teaching faculty and space and because of deep-seated bias on the part of some medical faculty against women in the "hard" sciences.

By the fall of 1952, the college settled on a basic curriculum blending liberal arts, basic sciences, and early clinical experience in the first two years, including the summer following the sophomore year, with clinical courses and experience in medical-surgical nursing, maternal and infant nursing, psychiatric nursing, and public health nursing dominating the junior and senior years, including summers. Also in 1952, the college set the curriculum for the general program for graduate nurses and for the specialized track in psychiatric nursing. The basic curriculum, but not the general curriculum, won NLN accreditation in 1952. The curriculum committee then continued to work on several fronts, addressing the duplication of content among courses, the integration of basic science concepts and clinical practice in the student's overall learning experience, and the strengthening of both the general program and the public health nursing component of the basic curriculum (Figure 3.1).

Initially, many baccalaureate nursing programs retained parts of their hospital diploma school backgrounds, shifting the primary emphasis toward academic work but maintaining, for the time being, the tradition of student hospital labor. Such was the case at the University of Iowa, where, during her campus interview in early 1949, Myrtle Kitchell saw the hospitals' clinical chiefs and the hospitals' administration as cautious at best in their responses to baccalaureate education in nursing. Although generally anxious to see improvements in nursing education, both physicians and hospital administrators understood that the conversion to a baccalaureate program meant the certain surrender of their long-standing control

Fig. 3.1. College of Nursing Basic Curriculum, 1954-55

Freshman Year	Semester Hours
Communication Skills	8
Physical Education Skills	2
Mathematics Skills	4
Introduction to Chemistry	8
Orientation to Nursing	3
Elementary Nutrition	3
Western Civilization	4

Sophomore Year [Inc. Summer Session]	Semester Hours
Western Civilization	4
Introduction to Psychology	4
Anatomy	4
Foundations of Nursing	12
Introduction to Sociology	3
Microbiology for Nurses	4
Physiology for Nurses	4
Well Child Development	3
Medical and Surgical Nursing	3

Junior Year [Inc. Summer Session]	Semester Hours
The Family	3
Community Hygiene	3
Nursing of Mothers & Infants	3
Medical and Surgical Nursing of Children and Adults	4
Medical and Surgical Nursing	4
Fundamentals of Community Health	3
Clinical Experience	20

Senior Year [Inc. Summer Session]	Semester Hours
Nursing in the Social Order	2
The Urban Community	3
Psychiatric Nursing	3
Surgical Nursing	1
Surgical Nursing	2
Literature	8
Clinical Experience	20

over the nursing curriculum and, just as important, threatened the eventual loss of student labor in the hospitals.[59]

A special committee appointed by hospitals Superintendent Gerhard Hartman in the fall of 1950, noted bluntly that the advent of the baccalaureate program "threatens the diploma program and hence our future supply of graduate nurses and the amount of service from student nurses."[60] Much of the current shortage of nursing personnel, the committee charged, reflected nursing leaders' intent to raise educational standards in nursing at the expense "of providing patient care [i.e., through student apprenticeship]." Moreover, the committee complained that not only did nursing faculty seek to reduce student service hours; they had also arranged clinical experience in such a way that "ward teaching and classes" disrupted students' "practical work." Finally, committee members lamented the fact that no College of Medicine clinical faculty held places on the College of Nursing curriculum committee and recommended the appointment of a special committee made up of nurses and physicians "to review the curricula for both the three and four year programs." Thus, perhaps the most difficult of all curriculum goals in the 1950s was that of reducing and finally eliminating the hospitals' claim on student time and the clinical medical faculty's claim on the nursing curriculum.

Substantial expansion in University Hospitals operations in the late 1940s and 1950s exacerbated staffing problems and helped to fuel the debate over student nursing service. From 1945-46 to 1960-61, the last year prior to the implementation of a four academic-year curriculum in nursing, total patient admissions at the hospitals rose from 17,133 to 24,796, an increase of nearly forty-five percent. During the same period, the staff-to-patient ratio rose as well, and the hospitals administration scrambled to fill its nursing needs, even hiring medical and dental students as part-time aides. High turnover rates among full-time nurses aggravated staffing problems, the rate reaching thirty-nine percent among supervisors and head nurses and eighty-five percent among general duty nurses in 1951. In 1954, Nursing Director Marie Tener reported that the most important reason cited by nurses for leaving was "family responsibilities," the most common of which was the husband's graduation from the university.[61] The second largest group were nurses who professed only to have sought temporary employment, a group that likely included many nurses hired to staff polio wards. The third largest group cited "desire for new experience," which Tener surmised was often a euphemism for job dissatisfaction. Meanwhile, with private patients making up only twenty-one percent of admissions in 1945-46 and just twenty-five percent in 1960-61, the University Hospitals remained largely an indigent care institution, overwhelmingly dependent upon relatively inflexible state appropriations for operating revenues. That, too, heightened the administration's concern over maintaining the student nurse labor force.

In the end, the gradual withdrawal of nursing students from the nursing service was a significant factor in University Hospitals' increase in permanent nursing staff in the last half of the 1950s, as the number of general duty nurses, for example, rose from 142 in 1954 to 207 in 1959.[62] However, turnover rates among nurses remained high, hovering at seventy-four percent in 1958. [63] Whatever their shortcomings, then, nursing students, especially junior and senior students, represented a reliable work force, one that physicians and hospital administrators surrendered only reluctantly.

In February 1950, a College of Nursing faculty committee reported that junior students spent an average of 35.5 hours per week in the hospitals; seniors spent thirty-six hours.[64] In April 1951, Dean Myrtle Kitchell estimated that her students would provide more than 263,000 hours of hospital service, worth some $250,000, from summer 1951 through spring 1952.[65] While conceding the necessity of continued student labor, Kitchell and the nursing faculty immediately embarked upon a series of long-term steps aiming, first, to win control over student hours and work assignments in the hospitals, second, to achieve incremental reductions in students' hospital workload, and, ultimately, to end the student work obligation altogether.

Several collateral issues entered into the discussion of nursing students' hospital service. In March 1950, Dean Kitchell noted that under existing arrangements the college incurred significant expenses—including maintenance and operation of Westlawn, student laundry, and clerical expenses associated with student hospital service—that were rightly chargeable not to the college but to the hospitals.[66] More important, Kitchell and others questioned "the quality as well as quantity of nursing care" afforded by the University Hospitals, and Kitchell in particular offered detailed suggestions for improvement of the nursing service.[67] Likewise, the quality and degree of student supervision in the hospitals was an issue. Few nursing service personnel directly involved in student supervision possessed either advanced degrees or training in education, and a 1951 College of Nursing executive committee report based on a study of the student nursing service in October and November of 1950 charged that as many as ten percent of students were on duty without supervision by a registered nurse and that students accrued significant overtime hours.[68] Closely related to the problem of supervision were the troublesome issues of assigning academic credit to ward service and evaluating student performance. Marie Tener, as head of the University Hospitals' nursing service, was generally supportive of the College of Nursing's goals, despite the negative implications for her service. Also, many College of Medicine faculty were supportive, especially those who worked closely with the College of Nursing in providing instruction in the basic sciences and in clinical areas.

Nonetheless, the effort to diminish student nurses' work obligation provoked a strong reaction from some quarters in the College of Medicine and from the hospitals administration. In a June 1951 report to university President Virgil Hancher, a special committee headed by University Hospitals Assistant Director Glen Clasen leveled a series of complaints at the College of Nursing. Overall, the college's educational goals were not, the committee charged, "in keeping with the needs for improving the nursing service of the University Hospitals." Nursing faculty had put in place a curriculum "without advice or active participation by the medical faculty and the hospital administration," and, in the committee's judgment, baccalaureate training "indoctrinates the student with the importance of college degrees and minimizes the importance of patient care." To avert "a crisis which threatens to disturb if not to disrupt the operation of the University Hospitals," the committee recommended representation of the medical faculty and the hospital administration "on all policy-forming committees in the College of Nursing." Furthermore, the committee recommended that the medical faculty be empowered to declare a nursing emergency when conditions warranted, allowing the nursing service director to assign students as necessary. Should such measures fail to correct existing problems, the committee proposed re-establishment of the hospital diploma school.[69]

In the face of such extraordinarily intrusive aims, President Hancher remained a staunch ally of the College of Nursing, and he responded to the committee's lengthy indictment in a characteristically blunt message to the secretary of the medical faculty. While conceding that establishment of the College of Nursing had sparked "certain problems," Hancher contended that "even more problems would have been created without it." In fact, Hancher reminded his correspondents, "one of the reasons for the creation of the College of Nursing was the way in which the School of Nursing had languished while it was under the supervision of the Dean and the faculty of the College of Medicine." The school, he noted, had sunk so low that "it either had to be abolished or substantially reorganized."[70] Hancher, then, made plain to the medical faculty and the hospitals' administrators that they had little choice but to work with the College of Nursing.

The issue of student nursing reached a critical stage in 1952, with the initial junior class finishing its first year of ward service. Perhaps with the idea of minimizing frictions between the college and the hospitals, President Hancher proposed in 1952 to make Myrtle Kitchell director of University Hospitals nursing services as well as dean; however, Kitchell refused, arguing that such a dual role would be unworkable under current conditions and thinking, too, that it would undermine the college's hard won autonomy. With President Hancher intervening once again to force acceptance from the Hospital Advisory Committee, the College of Nursing at that time set new policies reducing junior and senior nursing students' hours to thirty-two per week, effective during the spring semester of 1953, with a further reduction to thirty hours effective in the fall semester. Simultaneously, the college instituted two other major changes, both of them discussed earlier, discontinuing the carryover diploma program and approving the practical nursing program. Dean Kitchell also reported to President Hancher that the nursing faculty preferred a major reorganization of the basic curriculum "so that it will cover a period of four academic years," a reorganization that would entirely eliminate the traditional hospital service.[71] In preparing for a series of meetings with College of Medicine Dean Norman Nelson in 1954, Kitchell reiterated in her notes that "the [nursing] faculty does not support the belief that a nursing service should be dependent upon services rendered by students."[72]

By the end of the decade, junior and senior students' hospital obligations had fallen to 28 hours per week. More important, on October 7, 1955, the nursing faculty had given formal notice of their intention to move forward with the four academic year curriculum shorn of hospital service.[73] However, that step was long delayed by political considerations and by the many thorny issues of content and organization involved in such a thorough curricular revision. The curriculum committee's subcommittee on the basic sciences, for example, wrestled inconclusively with the problem of identifying the basic science principles involved in clinical nursing and, after two subcommittee members spent several hours in a fruitless effort to define the science of the enema, finally dismissed the project as "unrealistic."[74] Likewise, the curriculum committee faced the forbidding task of redesigning, in collaboration with the hospitals administration and medical faculty, the clinical training components of the curriculum, deciding when and where to assign students to the major clinical areas and settling upon nursing faculty assignments for clinical supervision. Not until February 1957, after consultation with all affected university colleges and departments, did the nursing faculty approve an outline of the proposed curriculum, tentatively setting the fall of 1958 for its implementation.[75]

At that point, many details remained unfinished, not least the problem of gaining approval from the university administration and the State Board of Regents. While the curriculum committee continued through 1957 and 1958 to fine tune its earlier curriculum draft, continued grumbling from the College of Medicine and from the University Hospitals was only one of several factors that delayed the process.[76] The interregnum in the dean's office from May 1957 to July 1959 was another major obstacle. In the university setting in general and perhaps especially in the health sciences, the lack of a dean tends to bring important matters to a standstill, a reflection not so much of the competence or incompetence of interim deans and committees as of the insecurities of outside parties, including public and private funding agencies, the central university administration, and the university's governing body. Yet another significant obstacle in the way of the new nursing curriculum was the economic recession of the late 1950s that led the state legislature to look askance at new spending proposals—in this instance, significantly more funding for nursing faculty and as much as $300,000 for additional nursing personnel in the hospitals.[77]

After Mary Mullane assumed the deanship in July 1959, momentum began to build once again behind the curriculum change, driven by the convictions of the dean herself and also by the recommendation contained in the April 1959 National League for Nursing accreditation report that—in accord with guidelines in the NLN "Self-Evaluation Guide for Collegiate Schools of Nursing"—the college take steps to ensure that "service expectations of University Hospitals in no way interfere with the freedom of the faculty in developing and implementing the curriculum."[78] As work progressed on the new curriculum, Dean Mullane reminded the nine-member curriculum committee, which included two student members, that the College of Nursing existed within a university and that the great majority of nursing students were juniors and seniors; therefore, the dean advised, the nursing curriculum should be intellectually challenging.[79] In March 1960, the committee received reports on the latest curriculum proposals from each of the college's departments, and in April decided upon a series of final recommendations to the faculty as a whole, asking the faculty also to reaffirm its commitment to the four academic year format and its faith in the quality of the graduates from such a program.[80] Finally, on December 9, 1960, the State Board of Regents, acting upon the recommendation of university President Virgil Hancher, approved the change to the four academic year curriculum in September 1961, with "nursing practice limited to the amount and type necessary for the education of those enrolled in the program."[81] However, since students were not admitted to the College of Nursing until the sophomore year, the change effectively began with the sophomore class enrolled in the fall of 1962 (See Figure 3.2).

With that victory in hand, the curriculum committee continued its work in several areas. Most immediately, the college faced the embarrassing lack of accreditation for its general baccalaureate program for diploma nurses, particularly its public health nursing component, which had been a subject of continuing discussion and negotiation with National League for Nursing accreditation authorities since the mid-1950s. By the late 1950s and early 1960s, the University of Minnesota's accredited program had, at the request of the Iowa Department of Public Health, conducted extension courses for public health nurses in several Iowa locations. However, Mary Mullane reported to President Hancher in March 1961 that Minnesota officials had informed her that the university "would not much longer be able to do these things."[82] At the same time, Iowa State University had for some years offered a variety of extension courses in non-nursing areas such as child development, nutrition, and sociology for the benefit of Iowa's practicing diploma nurses; in addition, and even more galling to Mullane, an Iowa State University professor of engineering conducted an extension course in nursing management.

Fig. 3.2. College of Nursing Basic Curriculum, 1964-65

Freshman Year	Semester Hours
Rhetoric	8
Historical-Cultural	8
Mathematics	4
Elementary Human Anatomy	4
Orientation to Nursing I	1
Orientation to Nursing	0
Electives	0-8

Sophomore Year	Semester Hours
Introduction to Psychology	4
Introduction to Sociology	3
Nutrition	3
Microbiology	4
Human Physiology	4
Foundations of Nursing	6
Practicum—Found. of Nursing	4
Human Growth and Dev.	4
Electives	0-4

Junior Year	Semester Hours
Literature	4
Sociology	3
Medical-Surgical Nursing	6
Practicum—Medical Nursing	3
Practicum—Surgical Nursing	3
Maternity Nursing	3
Practicum—Maternity Nursing	3
Nursing Care of Children	3
Practicum—Care of Children	3
Fundamentals of Management and Teaching in Nursing	3

Senior Year	Semester Hours
Literature	4
Fundamentals of Community Health	2
Psychiatric Nursing	3
Practicum—Psych. Nursing	3
Public Health Nursing	3
Practicum—Public Health	3
Practicum—Management and Teaching	3
Nursing in the Social Order	2
Senior Nursing	4
Practicum—Senior Nursing	3

The University of Iowa College of Nursing, the dean maintained, should take over such educational responsibilities, and she promised to pursue that objective with an aggressive combination of accreditation initiatives and community outreach efforts. In its 1959 review, the NLN Collegiate Board of Review had denied accreditation to the general curriculum and the associated public health program because of reservations about content, principally basic science content, as well as questions concerning the supervision of public health field training. In June 1960, after the college had provided further information, the NLN again denied accreditation, citing the same objections.[83] However, in May 1961, partly in response to prodding from Mullane and her public health faculty and partly as a result of curriculum adjustments, the NLN Board of review granted approval of the baccalaureate general program, including public health.[84]

Building a College of Nursing: Graduate Education

For a variety of reasons, graduate education in nursing developed slowly through the 1950s. Some of the problems were institutional in nature, including the lack of resources to support graduate education and the reluctance of many within the broader university community to recognize the legitimacy of graduate education in nursing. Likewise, some of the problems had to do with the peculiar history of nursing education. Among those the most important were, first, the lack of qualified nursing faculty, particularly faculty with research backgrounds and preferably with doctoral degrees, and, second, the protracted debate within nursing over a standardized baccalaureate curriculum shorn of elements of specialization. In short, the development of graduate programs awaited the drawing of distinct lines between undergraduate and graduate education.

National data on enrollments in master's and doctoral programs in nursing are scanty through the 1950s. The late 1950s and early 1960s, however, saw the implementation of firm guidelines for standard master's programs, and, by 1960, the National League for Nursing published detailed annual reviews of graduate education. The NLN's 1960-61 report counted 2,175 nurses enrolled in master's degree programs, 1,424 of those, or 65.5 percent, enrolled on a full-time basis. By 1964-65, not only had the population of master's degree students grown to 2,836, an increase of nearly a third, but the proportion of full-time students had risen to 74.0 percent. Meanwhile, doctoral programs in nursing in those years were far more modest in number and expanded at a considerably slower pace. NLN data showed just 132 nurse PhD candidates in 1960-61, sixty-nine of those full-time students;, and the total for 1964-65 rose only to 157 students, ninety-four of them full-time. The number of nurses receiving PhDs was correspondingly low, just eleven in 1960-61 and only twenty-five in 1964-65.

Planning for graduate education began early at the University of Iowa College of Nursing. During her time as dean and in the forty years since, Myrtle Kitchell Aydelotte has been adamant on the subject of graduate education for nurses, arguing that academic credentials are crucial to the elevation of nurses' professional status in the health care hierarchy, especially vis-à-vis physicians. As early as June 1950, just one year into her tenure as dean, Kitchell sent to university President Virgil Hancher a detailed proposal for a graduate training program in nursing service administration.[85] Noting the lack of such programs in the midwest region, the dean cited the "tremendous growth in hospitals, the rapid changes in medical care, the increased emphasis upon positive health, [and] the changing character of nursing itself" as justification for a program that would promote intensive research in the area of nursing service administration while also preparing well-trained administrative personnel, both of which would allow the more efficient utilization of scarce nursing resources.

"Very selective" admissions criteria contained in the proposal went beyond the standards set by the university's Graduate College. In addition to a bachelor's degree from "any college or university recognized in good standing" by either the Association of American Universities or regional accrediting agencies, the college would assess candidates on the basis of personal background, academic record and experience, as well as performance on the Graduate Record Exam and other standardized tests. As first proposed and as later implemented, the curriculum—conducted with the cooperation of the College of Commerce, the College of Liberal Arts, and the Graduate Program in Hospital Administration—encompassed one academic year and one summer session and included courses in psychology, statistics, and administration as well as field experience in the study of specific problems in nursing administration. The program did not require a thesis, but did propose oral and written comprehensive examinations.

By late 1950, Kitchell and other University of Iowa officials were directly involved in planning a W. K. Kellogg Foundation program to sponsor graduate programs in nursing service administration in selected colleges and universities around the country.[86] In November 1950, several University of Iowa staff, including Kitchell, nursing director Marie Tener, and representatives from political science and education as well as the central university administration, attended a preliminary Kellogg Foundation planning conference. Also in attendance were representatives from other educational institutions, the American Red Cross, the US Public Health Service, and the Army, Navy, and Air Force Nurse Corps. In December, Herman Finer, director of the Nursing Service Administration Research Project at the University of Chicago, visited the University of Iowa campus to discuss the proposed graduate program with university personnel, and Kitchell attended a month-long curriculum development workshop in early 1951 sponsored jointly by the Kellogg Foundation and the University of Chicago.

The University of Iowa was one of fourteen colleges and universities eventually chosen to participate in the Kellogg program, each institution receiving a five-year grant with the understanding that the host institutions would take increasing fiscal responsibility for the programs during the grant period and assume full funding at the end of the five years.[87] Funded at $77,000 for five years and directed by Louise M. Schmitt, the Iowa program welcomed its first class of students in September 1951, after considerable discussion and negotiation over course content and objectives with participating faculty from other colleges and departments. The first five students received their Master of Science in Nursing Service Administration degrees in August 1952.

Intended to integrate "specialized study" with "study in other areas essential to successful management of nursing service," the program's curriculum aimed to provide students with "knowledge of administration," "knowledge of functions of nursing and current nursing practice," "knowledge and understanding of the significance of good human relations," "awareness of the implications of social and cultural change [on patient health and nursing practice]," and the "ability to apply processes essential to carrying out the function of nursing service."[88] Through 1955, thirteen students completed the program. In 1956-57, as the program continued on a one-year grant extension funded by unexpended balances from previous years, enrollment stood at seven, with six of those students also supported by US Public Health Service Professional Nurse Training Grants authorized by the Health Amendments Act of 1956 (PL 84-911).[89]

The Kellogg Foundation's objectives to foster the study of problems in nursing service administration and to provide instruction to nurses already employed in administrative positions were important elements in the University of Iowa program. Program graduates produced some two dozen theses addressing a broad variety of research issues in administration. In addition, at least thirty non-degree students enrolled at various times in one or more courses in the nursing service administration program. Moreover, the college offered "an inservice program for graduate nurses on-the-job in hospitals throughout the region."[90] In April 1952, the college conducted the first of four scheduled continuing education conferences for directors and assistant directors of hospital nursing services, attracting a total of thirty-eight nurses from twenty-five hospitals in nineteen Iowa counties. The second of the scheduled conferences, held in July 1952, attracted forty-one participants. For the duration of the Kellogg grant, the college continued a variety of educational out-reach programs.

In a 1956 report on the nursing service administration program, the college noted that the chief obstacles facing prospective students were, first, the difficulties in arranging full-time leave from existing employment and, second, the lack of student financial aid, apart from the limited research assistantships available to the college.[91] On the positive side, the report claimed increasing numbers of inquiries from employers seeking "qualified nursing service directors," with several hospital administrators visiting the campus to meet with faculty and to interview students.

From the mid-1950s, interest in nursing administration programs declined substantially nationwide, and nursing education at both undergraduate and graduate levels turned toward the development of clinical specialties. At the University of Iowa College of Nursing, the graduate curriculum committee began work on a new curriculum in late 1955 and early 1956. The committee first grappled with basic questions, beginning with whether or not graduate education in fact prepared the nurse to perform activities beyond those assigned to the baccalaureate nurse.[92] The committee also discussed the differences between functional and content specialization, the former designed to prepare nurses for careers in one of four functional areas, research, teaching, practice, or administration, and the latter meant to provide specialty training in recognized clinical areas, such as medical-surgical nursing, pediatric nursing, psychiatric nursing, or public health nursing. Finally, the committee compiled a list of the basic concepts of nursing practice, pointing to the nurse's "closeness to the patient," the nurse's role in "management of care," and a range of ancillary functions, including teaching and counseling. Overall, the committee expressed its preference for a graduate program oriented toward development of "an increasingly high level of competence in a field of clinical nursing" grounded in "a comprehensive and creative understanding of the theory relevant to a specialized function."

In March 1958, the committee submitted a four-semester curriculum culminating in the master of arts. The stated aim of the program, the heart of which was a series of courses in advanced nursing skills and techniques, was "to enhance and broaden professional nurses' knowledge and competency in a specialized area of clinical training"—with initial offerings limited to medical-surgical and psychiatric nursing—and to prepare nurses for "positions of responsibility in hospitals, other health agencies and education programs." Implemented in September 1958 with an enrollment of nine students, eight of them funded by US Public Health Service traineeships, the new program was a three-semester sequence—with an optional fourth semester—requiring a total of thirty-six semester hours credit with thesis or forty-five semester hours without thesis. The thesis option was designed for students who might wish to pursue further education, while the non-thesis option was a terminal degree.[93] Enrollments in September 1959 stood at fifteen, and thirteen students received their master's degrees in 1959-60. Thereafter, enrollments plummeted to just four in 1960-61.

However, the graduate faculty had begun a review of the master's program in 1959, discussing a range of basic questions, including questions raised in a recent National League for Nursing conference on graduate education.[94] In April 1959, an outside consultant urged faculty to consider the graduate program in light of anticipated demand for graduate education, both state and regional, and to keep in mind the two basic types of students drawn to graduate programs: experienced nurses, who often supplemented a diploma education with baccalaureate and master's degrees, and "the young graduate [baccalaureate] who can be prepared for research and creative teaching."[95] The profession depended upon the first "to build good teaching and to open doors for students," the consultant noted, "but we cannot expect that she will enhance or add to the knowledge of nursing." In the consultant's assessment, the future of nursing lay in the hands of a new generation of properly trained academic nurses for whom the master's program was a crucial first step toward more thorough academic preparation and careers in research and teaching.

The subsequent reorganization of the graduate program, much of that accomplished during the 1960-61 academic year, appears to have been motivated chiefly by the desire to win NLN accreditation at a time when fewer than seventy percent of master's programs nationwide enjoyed NLN accreditation.[96] Reiterating the nationwide emphasis on specialization at the master's level in nursing, the redesigned program would train nurses "for positions as teachers and supervisors" in medical-surgical, pediatric, and psychiatric nursing and "provide a foundation on which post-masters and doctoral programs in nursing and related areas may be built." The result was a three-semester program offering concentrations in the three stated clinical areas, with medical-surgical nursing first offered in the fall of 1961 and pediatric and psychiatric nursing added the following year, the last supported by a grant from the National Institute of Mental Health. The new program incorporated the same options of thirty-six semester hours with thesis or forty-five semester hours without thesis as had the previous program. Also like the previous program, the new offerings in the clinical specialties offered a fourth semester to students "who may contemplate further educational preparation beyond the master's level." Finally, in addition to the choice of a clinical concentration, the program required that students also select a minor concentration in either administration or teaching. For the first time, the College of Nursing master's program won NLN accreditation in 1962.

At the same time, nursing service administration found a new champion in Dean Mary Mullane. In April 1960, less than a year after assuming the deanship, Dean Mullane wrote university President Virgil Hancher regarding the defunct administration program. Having invested considerable time and energy in the original Kellogg program, Mullane was a staunch advocate of the administration concept, a subject she raised again in May 1961. A graduate program in nursing service administration, the dean noted, was "sorely needed by Iowa's hospitals, nursing homes, and public health agencies," even though she conceded that the college lacked the resources at the present time to revive the program and the project would have to wait "until funds are available."[97] A year later, in June 1962, the dean recruited Eva Erickson to revive the nursing service administration program,[98] a plan that encountered stiff resistance from her own faculty, many of whom argued for clinical specialization over functional specialization in graduate education. As a consequence of faculty resistance and Mullane's unexpected resignation of the deanship, nursing service administration remained in limbo until 1966.

Conclusion

For nurse educators at the University of Iowa and elsewhere, the chief challenge of the 1950s and early 1960s lay in defining what a college of nursing should be and what nursing education should accomplish and in winning institutional and public support for those goals. According to an outline sketched by Myrtle Kitchell in 1954, the College of Nursing's essential functions were to develop collegiate programs for basic nursing students and for diploma nurses, to develop graduate education and continuing education programs, and to serve as a site for experimentation and demonstration in nursing instruction and practice.[99] From 1950 to 1964, thanks to the dedication of its deans and faculty and to the support from the university's central administration, the College of Nursing made significant strides on all those fronts, expanding student enrollments and faculty numbers, implementing substantial revisions of the curriculum, achieving accreditation in all major program areas, and nurturing connections to the wider nursing profession. Moreover, the college stood as the flagship of nursing in the state of

Iowa, recognized as such not only by its deans and faculty but also by the Iowa Board of Nurse Examiners and by a wide cross section of Iowa's practicing nurses, increasing numbers of whom were graduates of the college.

Notwithstanding such successes, the aspirations of nurse educators at the national level and at the University of Iowa outpaced achievements, leaving significant issues and problems unresolved. At the University of Iowa, the College of Nursing's makeshift physical facilities in the basement of Westlawn—the half-century-old dormitory for nursing students and graduate nurses—perhaps best symbolized the plight of nursing education. Consisting largely of converted dormitory rooms recently abandoned by students who had fled to alternative housing, those quarters were cramped and ill-equipped and, even more important, projected a poor image of the college. Moreover, the University Hospitals, desperate to accommodate its rapidly expanding operations, also had designs on space that the college occupied. One important challenge facing the college in the middle and late 1960s, then, was to seize a place for nursing education in what proved to be an ambitious reconstruction of the University of Iowa campus.

Facilities were only one element in nursing's still marginal place within the community of higher education. A second, equally important, concern was the lagging academic credentials and research productivity of nursing faculty. Despite the marked expansion of graduate education in nursing in the late 1950s and early 1960s, the College of Nursing's search for qualified nursing faculty was unending and in some degree disappointing, with serious ramifications for the future of nursing education. Similarly troubling were the lack of a viable, independent research culture in nursing and the halting and uncertain growth of a base of specialized nursing knowledge, problems exacerbated by the lack of local facilities for nursing research and by the fact that federal funding of training and research programs in nursing failed to keep pace with funding levels in many other disciplines and professions.

Notes

1. Economic statistics from *Historical Statistics of the United States: Colonial Times to 1970.*

2. Wartime wage and price controls contributed significantly to the spread of private health insurance, encouraging labor unions to include such non-wage benefits in their collective bargaining packages. That wartime pattern and the longstanding American aversion to "big government" and "socialized medicine" combined, for better or worse, to link health insurance firmly to employment in postwar America.

3. For a more detailed description of nursing during the Korean War, see Kalisch and Kalisch, *The Advance of American Nursing*, pp. 538-546.

4. *Ibid.*

5. American Nurses Association, *The Nation's Nurses: The 1962 Inventory of Professional Registered Nurses* (ANA, 1965).

6. Eugene Levine, "How Many Nurses Have College Degrees," *Nursing Outlook* 2 (January 1954), p. 23.

7. "Doctoral Degrees," *American Journal of Nursing* 50 (June 1950), pp. 377-78. The count was based upon a survey of 113 institutions offering doctoral degree programs.

8. ANA, *The Nation's Nurses.* Because it did not include any southern states, the 1962 ANA count likely overstated the proportion of bachelor's degree nurses; however, it did suggest a significant ten-year increase in the number of nurses holding graduate degrees, particularly since the fifteen-state total did not include several populous northern states such as New York, Pennsylvania, and Ohio.

9. State University of Iowa College of Nursing, "Alumnæ Newsletter #2," Spring 1962, Folder 71, VM Hancher Papers, The University of Iowa Archives.

10. See Committee on the Structure of National Nursing Organizations, *New Horizons in Nursing* (New York: Macmillan Company, 1950).

11. For background to the reorganization, *Ibid.*

12. National League for Nursing, *Nurses for a Growing Nation* (New York: The League, 1957).

13. US Surgeon General's Consultant Group on Nursing, *Toward Quality in Nursing: Needs and Goals* (Washington, DC: US Public Health Service, 1963).

14. Prior to the early 1960s, the American Medical Association, while enthusiastically supporting federal aid for hospital construction and grudgingly tolerant of federal funding of medical scientific research, was adamantly opposed to direct federal involvement in medical education,

opposition that effectively blocked aid not only to medical education but to education in the other health professions as well.

15. "Withdrawal of Students," *American Journal of Nursing* 50 (March 1950), pp. 184-185.

16. ME Kitchell to HH Davis, July 3, 1952, Folder 114, 1952-53, VM Hancher Papers, The University of Iowa Archives.

17. "Student Enrollment—1951," *American Journal of Nursing* 51 (July 1951), pp. 470-473; "Graduate Nurses Enrolled in Colleges and Universities," *American Journal of Nursing* 51 (August 1951), pp. 528-529.

18. CE Jacobsen to VM Hancher, July 20, 1951, and Hancher to Jacobsen, July 26, 1951, Folder 116, 1951-52, VM Hancher Papers, The University of Iowa Archives.

19. VM Hancher to HH Davis, March 19, 1953, Folder 114, 1952-53, VM Hancher Papers, The University of Iowa Archives.

20. Faculty Meeting Minutes, October 19, 1956, Box 9, College of Nursing Papers, The University of Iowa Archives.

21. ME Kitchell to HH Davis, November 13, 1956, Box 9, "Correspondence with Dr. Harvey Davis, September 1956 through August 1957," College of Nursing Papers, The University of Iowa Archives.

22. ME Kitchell to Faculty, January 29, 1957, Box 9, "Kitchell's Communications to the Faculty and Staff Groups," College of Nursing Papers, The University of Iowa Archives.

23. VM Hancher to E Rasmussen, M Lohr, and M Lyford, April 16, 1957, and Rasmussen to Hancher, April 30, 1957, Folder 71, 1956-57, VM Hancher Papers, The University of Iowa Archives.

24. Gordon H. Scott to VM Hancher, January 13, 1959, Folder 71, 1958-59, VM Hancher Papers, The University of Iowa Archives.

25. Mary K. Mullane, *Education for Nursing Service Administration: An Experience in Program Development by Fourteen Universities* (Battle Creek, MI: WK Kellogg Foundation, 1959).

26. University officials made the decision to recommend Mullane to the regents immediately after her campus visit. See HH Davis to MK Mullane, December 19, 1958, Folder 71, 1958-59, VM Hancher Papers, The University of Iowa Archives.

27. VM Hancher to Allin Dakin, May 9, 1962, Folder 71, 1961-62, VM Hancher Papers, The University of Iowa Archives.

28. MK Mullane to VM Hancher, July 16, 1962, Folder 71, 1962-63, VM Hancher Papers, The University of Iowa Archives.

29. Minutes of Committee for Selection of Dean, September 15, 1962, Folder 71, 1962-63, VM Hancher Papers, The University of Iowa Archives.

30. Vera Sage of the board urged Virgil Hancher to see to the replacement of Mullane as quickly as possible, emphasizing the importance of the col-

lege's place in nursing education in Iowa; Hancher noted on the margins of Sage's letter, "We are proceeding—How fast, God knows—I hope the committee keeps moving." Sage to VM Hancher, July 26, 1962, Folder 71, 1962-63, VM Hancher Papers, The University of Iowa Archives.

31.   Allin Dakin to Vera Sage, July 24, 1963, Folder 71, 1963-64, VM Hancher Papers, The University of Iowa Archives.

32.   A delightful raconteur, Laura Dustan provided a wealth of information and insight in a telephone interview with the authors on September 5, 1995.

33.   Levine, "How Many Nurses Have College Degrees," p. 23.

34.   Myrtle E. Kitchell, "Organizing a Faculty," *The American Journal of Nursing* 51 (December 1951), pp. 740-742.

35.   ME Kitchell to HH Davis, March 7, 1956, Box 9, "Correspondence with Dr. Harvey Davis, September 1955 through August 1956," College of Nursing Papers, The University of Iowa Archives.

36.   ME Kitchell to HH Davis, March 7, 1956, Box 9, "Correspondence with Dr. Harvey Davis, September 1955 through August 1956," College of Nursing Papers, The University of Iowa Archives.

37.   "Progress Report of the College of Nursing of the State University of Iowa to the Collegiate Board of Review National League for Nursing, September 1961," Folder 71, VM Hancher Papers, The University of Iowa Archives.

38.   Box 3, Folder "Administrative Staff Minutes, 1962-63," December 6, 1962, and August 15, 1963, College of Nursing Papers, The University of Iowa Archives.

39.   Box 3, Folder "Administrative Staff Minutes, 1963-64," February 10, 1964, College of Nursing Papers, The University of Iowa Archives.

40.   Laura Dustan to WL Boyd, September 8, 1964, Box 9, Folder "Dean Boyd—General, 1964-66," College of Nursing Papers, The University of Iowa Archives.

41.   Memorandum from Lila Wagner to Etta Rasmussen, July 18, 1957, Box 3, Executive Committee Budget, 1957-58, College of Nursing Papers, The University of Iowa Archives.

42.   Box 3, Folder "Administrative Staff Minutes, 1962-63," May 23, 1963, and Box 9, Folder "Dean Boyd—General," Laura Dustan to WL Boyd, September 24, 1964, College of Nursing Papers, The University of Iowa Archives.

43.   Minutes of Special Faculty Meeting, April 12, 1957, Box 9, Folder "Kitchell's Communications to the Faculty and Staff Groups," College of Nursing Papers, The University of Iowa Archives.

44. Box 3, Folder "Administrative Staff Minutes, 1962-63," March 14, 1963, College of Nursing Papers, The University of Iowa Archives.

45. Janie M. Brown, "Master's Education in Nursing, 1945-1969," in M. Louise Fitzpatrick, ed., *Historical Studies in Nursing* (New York: Teachers College Press, 1978), p. 119.

46. Ronald Scantlebury [NIH] to MK Aydelotte, March 1, 1957, Folder 71, 1956-57, VM Hancher Papers, The University of Iowa Archives.

47. Fifth Annual Report on Continuing Education, 1963-64, Box 2, Folder "Annual Reports 1964," College of Nursing Papers, The University of Iowa Archives.

48. The spring semester of 1961, for example, found 197 prenursing, freshman students enrolled in the college of liberal arts.

49. State University of Iowa *Catalogue, 1950-51*, pp. 216-217.

50. ME Kitchell, August 4, 1952, Box 15, Folder "Nursing Service Administration Program," College of Nursing Papers, The University of Iowa Archives.

51. Faculty Minutes, December 4, 1959, and January 15, 1960, Box 5, Folder "College of Nursing Faculty Minutes, 1953-62," College of Nursing Papers, The University of Iowa Archives.

52. Box 3, Administrative Staff Minutes, 1963-64, September 26, 1963, College of Nursing Papers, The University of Iowa Archives; see also folder marked "Iowa Department of Public Instruction, Division of Vocational Education, Practical Nurse Education Section."

53. R Heffner to F Sherbon, June 10, 1964, Folder 71, 1963-64, VM Hancher Papers, The University of Iowa Archives.

54. Curriculum Committee Minutes, March 6, 1950, Box 3, Folder "Committee on Curriculum Minutes, 1949 through April 1953," College of Nursing Papers, The University of Iowa Archives.

55. Administrative Staff Minutes, October 25, 1962, Box 3, Folder "Administrative Staff Minutes, 1962-63," College of Nursing Papers, The University of Iowa Archives.

56. Iowa Board of Nurse Examiners, "Report of Survey of State University of Iowa, College of Nursing, April 10-13, 1962," Folder 71, 1962-63, VM Hancher Papers, The University of Iowa Archives.

57. Memorandum from Florence Sherbon to administrative faculty, November 26, 1963, Box 3, Administrative Staff Minutes, 1963-64, College of Nursing Papers, The University of Iowa Archives.

58. College of Nursing Faculty Minutes, January 10, 1964, Folder 71, 1963-64, VM Hancher Papers, The University of Iowa Archives.

59. Myrtle Kitchell Aydelotte shared her memories of this period in an August 18, 1995 interview.

60. Report of the Special Committee for the Study of Nursing Service, University Hospitals; see also ME Kitchell to HH Davis, November 27, 1950, Box 15, Folder "Nursing Service at University Hospital (Marie Te-

ner) 1949-55," College of Nursing Papers, The University of Iowa Archives.

61. Marie Tener, *Report of Department of Nursing Service, 1/1/53-1/1/54*, University of Iowa Hospitals.

62. Box 2, Folder "Annual Report to the Iowa Board of Nurse Examiners Basic Program, 1954-59," College of Nursing Papers, The University of Iowa Archives.

63. "Report of the Activities of the Nursing Service Department in State University of Iowa Hospitals, January 1, 1958-December 31, 1958," University of Iowa Graduate Program in Hospital and Health Administration Collection.

64. Box 3, Folder "Executive Committee Minutes, 1949-51, February 15, 1951," College of Nursing Papers, The University of Iowa Archives.

65. "Prediction of Hours of Nursing Service Provided by Students in College of Nursing July 1, 1951-June 30, 1952, Incl.," Box 15, Folder "Nursing Service at University Hospital (Marie Tener) 1949-55," College of Nursing Papers, The University of Iowa Archives.

66. ME Kitchell to CF Jacobsen, March 23, 1950, Box 9, Folder "Dean Jacobsen Correspondence," College of Nursing Papers, The University of Iowa Archives.

67. ME Kitchell to RL Jackson, April 14, 1951, Box 7, Folder "Hospital Advisory Committee 1950-55," College of Nursing Papers, The University of Iowa Archives.

68. Box 3, Folder "Executive Committee Minutes, 1949-51," February 15, 1951, College of Nursing Papers, The University of Iowa Archives.

69. Gerhard Hartman to HH Davis, June 13, 1952, and "Progress Report of the Special Committee for the Study of Nursing Education and Nursing Service," June 5, 1951, Folder 114, 1952-53, VM Hancher Papers, The University of Iowa Archives.

70. VM Hancher to Paul Huston, June 22, 1951, Folder 108, 1950-51, VM Hancher Papers, The University of Iowa Archives.

71. ME Kitchell to VM Hancher and HH Davis, November 12, 1952, Box 9, Folder "Unlabelled," College of Nursing Papers, The University of Iowa Archives.

72. "Brief Prepared for Series of Conferences with Dean Norman Nelson, March 1954," Folder 118, 1953-54, VM Hancher Papers, The University of Iowa Archives.

73. ME Kitchell to HH Davis, December 30, 1955, Box 9, Folder "Correspondence with Dr. Harvey Davis, September 1955 through August 1956," College of Nursing Papers, The University of Iowa Archives.

74. Box 9, Folder "Kitchell's Communications to the Curriculum Committee," Curriculum Committee Minutes, March 8, 1957, College of Nursing Papers, The University of Iowa Archives.

75. ME Kitchell to HH Davis, February 20, 1957, Box 9, Folder "Correspondence with Dr. Harvey Davis, September 1956 through August 1957," College of Nursing Papers, The University of Iowa Archives.

76. For "grumbling," see NB Nelson, G Hartman, and G Clasen to HH Davis, May 1, 1958, Folder 41, 1957-58, VM Hancher Papers, The University of Iowa Archives.

77. MK Mullane to HH Davis, November 21, 1960, Folder 71, 1960-61, VM Hancher Papers, The University of Iowa Archives.

78. NLN Collegiate Board of Review, "Comments and Recommendations," Report of Visit for Accreditation Purposes, February 16-21, 1959," University of Iowa College of Nursing.

79. Curriculum Committee Minutes, December 11, 1959, Box 3, College of Nursing Papers, The University of Iowa Archives.

80. Curriculum Committee Minutes, April 8, 1960, Box 3, College of Nursing Papers, The University of Iowa Archives.

81. State Board of Regents Minutes, December 9, 1960, The University of Iowa Archives.

82. MK Mullane to VM Hancher, March 27, 1961, Folder 71, 1960-61, VM Hancher Papers, The University of Iowa Archives.

83. Mary Quarmby to MK Mullane, June 2, 1960, Folder 71, 1960-61, VM Hancher Papers, The University of Iowa Archives.

84. Mary Quarmby [NLN] to MK Mullane, May 19, 1961, Folder 71, 1960-61, VM Hancher Papers, The University of Iowa Archives.

85. ME Kitchell, "The Development of Programs for Nursing Service Administration," June 30, 1950, Folder 118, 1949-50, VM Hancher Papers, The University of Iowa Archives.

86. The university already had links to the Kellogg Foundation, which had recently provided a $50,000 grant to subsidize establishment of the new graduate program in hospital administration.

87. Mildred Tuttle to ME Kitchell, July 25, 1951, Folder 116, 1951-52, VM Hancher Papers, The University of Iowa Archives.

88. From a retrospective review and summary of objectives, October 1956, Box 6, Folder "Graduate Faculty Meetings 1956-57," College of Nursing Papers, The University of Iowa Archives.

89. Both the American Nurses Association and the National League for Nursing actively promoted the nurse traineeship program. From 1957 to 1959, the US Public Health Service awarded professional nurse training grants to more than 3,800 recipients, disbursing a total of $11 million.

90. "Annual Report—Program in Nursing Service Administration," Folder 114, 1952-53, VM Hancher Papers, The University of Iowa Archives.

91. Report of Five-Year Review of Nursing Service Administration Project, Box 6, Folder "Graduate Faculty Meetings 1956-57," College of Nursing Papers, The University of Iowa Archives.

92. Review of work accomplished, October 10, 1957, Box 6, Folder "Graduate Faculty Meeting Minutes September 1957-August 1958," College of Nursing Papers, The University of Iowa Archives.

93. E Rasmussen to W Loehwing, Dean of the Graduate College, September 9, 1958, Box 9 "Correspondence with Walter Loehwing, September 1958 to June 1959," and State University of Iowa College of Nursing, Master's Degree, March 1958, Box "Nursing Information," Folder "Nursing, School of, Miscellaneous," College of Nursing Papers, The University of Iowa Archives.

94. National League for Nursing Department of Baccalaureate and Higher Degree Programs Work Conference on Graduate Education in Nursing, March 16, 17, 18, 1959, Box 6, Folder "Graduate Faculty Committee Minutes September 1958-September 1959," College of Nursing Papers, The University of Iowa Archives.

95. Graduate Faculty Committee Minutes, April 22, 1959, Box 6, Folder "Graduate Faculty Committee Minutes September 1958-September 1959," College of Nursing Papers, The University of Iowa Archives.

96. "Nursing Education Today: On Accreditation," *American Journal of Nursing* 60 (October 1960), pp. 1,475-1,478.

97. MK Mullane to VM Hancher, May 1, 1961, Folder 71, 1960-61, VM Hancher Papers, The University of Iowa Archives.

98. Eva Erickson provided her recollections in a telephone interview with the authors on September 14, 1995. This account draws heavily upon testimony from Erickson, Etta Rasmussen, and Myrtle Adylotte.

99. ME Kitchell, "Brief Prepared for Series of Conferences with Dean Norman Nelson, March 1954," Folder 118, 1953-54, VM Hancher Papers, The University of Iowa Archives.

Chapter Four

Forging a New Professionalism, 1965-1980

The 1950s and early 1960s were important years for the University of Iowa College of Nursing, years dominated by efforts to define a professional curriculum, recruit qualified faculty, and, slowly but definitively, distance nursing students from the University Hospitals. In all that, the college had much in common with the growing number of collegiate schools of nursing nationwide. However, at the University of Iowa and elsewhere, the first two postwar decades had also left many fundamental questions about the future of nursing and nursing education unanswered, an especially troublesome concern at a time when the health care system placed increasingly heavy demands—in terms of both education and job performance— upon the health care professions in general and upon nursing in particular.

Through the 1960s and 1970s, the texture of American health care changed in dramatic ways. First, health care became more accessible, thanks to the spread of private health insurance, the provision of health care benefits to the elderly and indigent through Medicare and Medicaid, and the continued expansion of hospitals and supporting facilities. Second, the ongoing technological revolution in health care intensified, bringing scores of new drugs and new technologies into the health care marketplace and accelerating the pace of specialization in the health care professions. Third, aggregate health care costs spiraled upward at an alarming rate, fostering initial efforts at cost containment that, while themselves largely ineffective, set the stage for more stringent efforts in the 1980s and 1990s.

For the nursing profession, the health care system's dynamism raised several concerns. One of those was the nurse's role and authority in the area of patient care, a question closely tied to the issue of the nurse's educational qualifications and professional status and also to the legal definitions of nursing in state licensing statutes. Another concern was the definition and certification of emerging clinical specialties in nursing. Still another concern was nurses' ambiguous place within the rapidly evolving health care reimbursement system, a system shaped to an ever greater extent by third-party payers. Altogether, the challenges of the 1960s and 1970s nurtured a new, more activist bent among nurses, an activism embracing both collective bargaining and political action.

Nurse-educators shared many of the concerns of the profession at large, and they faced a range of special problems as well. Responding to repeated calls for larger nursing enrollments, the University of Iowa College of Nursing in the mid-1960s laid plans for an ambitious expansion in both undergraduate and graduate education programs, plans that envisioned a doubling of undergraduate enrollments and a tripling of graduate enrollments by the mid-1970s. Federal funding, derived chiefly from the Nurse Training Act of 1964 and its successor acts, was a major element in College of Nursing plans, playing a major part in the realization of a new nursing building and providing capitation funds, scholarship and loan funds, and training grants in support of undergraduate and graduate education. Likewise, federal funds subsidized several other initiatives at the college, including continuing education programs and a thorough revision of the undergraduate curriculum.

At the same time, rising expectations in nursing education brought to a flash point long-smoldering questions surrounding nurse educators' academic credentials and research productivity. As early as 1970, a report by the National Commission for the Study of Nursing and Nursing Education, a project organized by the National League for Nursing and the American Nurses Association, underlined the need for improved educational programs in nursing and increased attention to nursing research, especially research into "the impact of nursing practice on the quality, effectiveness, and economy of health care."[1] At the University of Iowa College of Nursing, efforts to bolster graduate education and faculty research, in tandem with the university administration's insistence that the college bring its promotion and tenure practices into line with university policy, led to a late 1970s crisis in the college. Painful though it was, that crisis was ultimately the precursor to significant reforms in the 1980s that catapulted the college into the front rank of American nursing schools.

The Demographics of Nursing, 1966-1980

As had been true throughout the postwar years, the single most striking influence on the professional development of American nursing in the late 1960s and 1970s was the continued expansion of America's hospitals, the aggressive growth in specialized care services, and the consolidation of the hospital's position at the center of the health care system. Several factors fueled hospital growth, including the combination of federal, state, and local support for hospital construction, the expanded coverage of private health insurance plans, the accelerating revolution in health care technologies, the ongoing—indeed, intensified—emphasis on acute care, and passage of Medicare and Medicaid legislation in 1965, legislation that ultimately pumped hundreds of billions of dollars into the health care economy.

Perhaps surprisingly, the number of hospitals actually declined slightly nationwide in the late 1960s and 1970s, slipping from 7,127 in 1964 to 7,015 in 1978. The number of hospital beds declined as well, falling 18.6 percent from 1,696,039 to 1,380,645 in the same period. In Iowa, both the number of hospitals and total beds remained virtually unchanged over that period, with 138 hospitals and 21,613 total beds in 1964 and 141 hospitals and 21,847 beds in 1978. Hospital admissions, on the other hand, rose 32.1 percent nationwide from 28,266,239 to 37,243,182 between 1964 to 1978. In Iowa, hospital admissions rose 29.0 percent, reaching 576,577 in 1978.[2] Meanwhile, total expenditures for hospital care in America rose from $14.0 billion in 1965 to more than $101 billion in 1980, an astonishing and, for many observers, unsettling 621 percent increase.[3] In Iowa, per capita hospital expenditures increased from $68 to $307 from 1966 to 1978.[4]

The number of practicing registered nurses grew from 504,000 in 1960 to 700,000 in 1970 and to 1,119,000 in 1980. Similarly, the number of registered nurses per 100,000 population increased from 282 to 506 in those two decades, chiefly reflecting increased staffing levels in America's hospitals. In 1964, American hospitals employed some 382,300 registered nurses; in 1980, hospitals employed more than 957,000 nursing personnel, 775,000 of them registered nurses.[5] In Iowa, the total of 8,555 active registered nurses in 1962 grew to 15,083 in 1978; of the latter, 9,765 or 64.7 percent were employed either full- or part-time in hospitals, a figure almost identical to the national rate of 64.9 percent.

As in earlier years, large numbers of registered nurses were not a part of the nursing workforce in the late 1960s and 1970s, either unemployed or employed in areas outside nursing. In Iowa in 1978, for example, there were over 20,000 employed registered nurses, but just the 15,083 noted above reported employment in nursing. In 1980, the American Nurses Association estimated that more than 388,000 nurses in the United States held jobs outside nursing. Such figures may have under-reported part-time employment in nursing; still, it appears that many women continued to withdraw from the nursing workforce at least during childrearing years and that there remained serious job dissatisfaction within the nursing profession. Indeed, the theme of job dissatisfaction among nurses was a staple in the professional literature of the 1970s.

In a 1975 study of nursing turnover at thirteen Chicago and San Francisco hospitals, Joanne Comi McCloskey, who later joined the University of Iowa nursing faculty, reported that the most frequently mentioned complaints of nurses who had recently changed jobs dealt with educational issues, the lack of career advancement, and the lack of recognition of nurses' contributions to patient care.[6] In McCloskey's study, salary ranked only fifth on nurses' lists of job enrichment concerns, despite the fact that as late as 1980 median salaries of head nurses in hospitals of 500 beds or more ranged only from $14,700 to $19,600,[7] a salary range perhaps comparable to that of resident physicians and significantly below that, for example, of community pharmacists.

For some nurses at least, collective bargaining was a means toward greater professional autonomy and, thus, greater job satisfaction.[8] The Taft-Hartley Act of 1947 had exempted nonprofit hospitals from collective bargaining requirements, but, after decades of protest from nurses and other hospital workers, Congress overturned that exemption in 1974, by which time the American Nurses Association had long been on record in favor of collective bargaining as an acceptable job strategy for nurses. Indeed, the ANA and its state affiliates had registered as labor organizations under provisions of the Landrum-Griffin Act of 1959. In addition to pay and benefits, collective bargaining afforded nurses the tools to negotiate a variety of professional issues, such as work rules and standards of care.[9]

The 1974 victory left two important issues unresolved: first, the status of many supervisory nurses remained in limbo, since the Taft-Hartley Act excluded supervisory personnel from participation in collective bargaining units with rank-and-file workers, and, second, the 1974 act did not address the question whether nurses were professionals and therefore entitled to separate bargaining units. In 1975, the National Labor Relations Board decided both issues in favor of nurses, ruling in a California case that nurses were professionals under the law and ruling in a Massachusetts case that head nurses—whose primary responsibility lay in overseeing patient care rather than in supervising other nurses—were not supervisory personnel as defined in Taft-Hartley.

The wider adoption of systems of clinical nursing specialties helped to some extent to ease problems of job satisfaction and nurse retention. At the University of Iowa Hospitals, Myrtle Kitchell Aydelotte became director of nursing in 1968 and immediately began a reorganization of the nursing service, a reorganization supported by the hospitals and clinics administration and one that led to increased staffing levels, significant changes in administrative structures, and the organization of the nursing service around a series of clinical nursing specialties. Ironically, Aydelotte was recruited to the position as nursing director by hospitals' Associate Director Gene Clasen, with whom Aydelotte had often been at odds during her years as dean of the College of Nursing. Nonetheless, with health care becoming increasingly complex and the University Hospitals moving increasingly toward a tertiary care role, Clasen conceded to Aydelotte significant powers, including control over the nursing budget.[10] One concomitant of Aydelotte's reorganization of the nursing service was a significant change in the educational background of the University Hospitals' nursing staff, with new emphasis on the baccalaureate degree as the entry level credential in the nursing service and with the recruitment of master's level nurses as administrators and as clinical nurse specialists.

As nursing became more technical and more specialized and as sentiment for an expanded health care role for nurses intensified, questions of continuing education and specialty certification in nursing grew in importance. In January 1974, the American Nurses Association issued its first standards for continuing education programs, and the ANA's Council on Continuing Education began implementing a system of continuing education accreditation in 1975. Meanwhile, the continuing education offerings of the University of Iowa College of Nursing expanded apace throughout the 1960s and 1970s, especially so after the institution of state-mandated continuing education for the health professions in the late 1970s. The ANA also took a leading role in the area of specialty certification, awarding the first certificates in 1975 and, by the end of that year, offering certification in five defined areas: pediatric ambulatory nursing, geriatric nursing, psychiatric and mental health nursing, medical-surgical nursing, and maternal-child health nursing.

Behind a long list of major new initiatives in nursing stood the question of nurses' professional autonomy, an increasingly important and at times contentious issue, one linked in important ways to the emergence of the women's movement and also to the general tone of unrest in American society. The 1971 Nurse Training Act authorized funding for development of nurse practitioner programs, and a 1972 Department of Health, Education and Welfare study entitled *Extending the Scope of Nursing Practice* recommended greater utilization of advanced-practice nurses in a range of primary care functions. However, the advent of advanced-practice nurses was not without controversy within the profession. In a dialogue published in the seventy-fifth anniversary edition of the *American Journal of Nursing* in 1975,[11] one author charged that the nurse practitioner was nothing more than a barely disguised physician assistant, a condition that reduced nursing to a subordinate and watered-down version of medicine. A second author, in contrast, while conceding that the nurse practitioner and the physician assistant were alike in some superficial aspects, described fundamental differences between the two, particularly the nurse practitioner's claim to a much broader professional jurisdiction and her status as an independent professional practitioner.

Notwithstanding the nurse practitioner debate, the vast majority of nurses still practiced in more or less traditional settings, primarily in hospitals, throughout the 1960s and 1970s. Most nurses, then, practiced in institutions dominated by physicians who jealously guarded their prerogatives regarding access to patients; moreover, nurses labored within the confines of reimbursement systems that ignored nursing as a distinct element of patient care. At a time when some form of national health insurance seemed imminent, most observers saw little promise of significant improvement in the situation of practicing nurses.[12] Still, most nursing leaders entertained hopes that improved educational credentials could aid in nurses' quest for professional recognition. As a result, the 1960s and 1970s brought the steady expansion of graduate programs at master's and doctoral levels, as well as establishment of the American Academy of Nursing in 1973 to recognize the contributions of nursing leaders.[13]

Finally, the 1970s brought important changes in state laws governing the practice of nursing. In Iowa, state law in the 1960s defined the role of the registered nurse in very narrow terms, focusing on "the observation of symptoms" and "the accurate recording of facts and carrying out of treatments and medication prescribed by licensed physicians." In short, Iowa law in 1962 defined nursing chiefly in relation to the practice of medicine. However, a series of statutory changes followed in the 1970s. In 1974, the state legislature expanded the Board of Nursing from five members to seven with the addition of two public members; for the first time, the law also specified board representation for baccalaureate programs, diploma programs, associate degree programs, nurse practitioners, and practical nurses. A 1976 statute (H.F. 1503) set nursing apart from medicine and vested nurses with a degree of professional autonomy, empowering the registered nurse to "[F]ormulate nursing diagnosis and conduct nursing treatment of human responses to actual or potential health problems through services, such as case finding, referral, health teaching, health counseling, and care provision which is supportive to or restorative of life and well-being." Of course, the registered nurse could also, as under the previous statute, "[E]xecute the regimen prescribed by a physician." In 1977, as part of a comprehensive reform of the general statutes governing the professions (S.F. 312), the state legislature mandated that all state licensing boards formulate continuing education requirements. Importantly, the 1977 legislation also augmented licensing boards' investigative and disciplinary authority, including the creation of peer review committees and the power to command physical and mental examinations of licensees. In subsequent years, professional licensing boards in Iowa assumed much more aggressive leadership roles, continually testing the bounds of professional jurisdiction and, in doing so, jostling with the jurisdictional claims of other professional groups.

Nursing Students and Programs

The major story in basic nursing education from 1965-66 to 1979-80 (Table 4.1) was the expansion of baccalaureate and associate degree programs and the steady decline in the number of diploma programs. In that fourteen-year period, the number of baccalaureate programs nationwide rose from 210 to 385, an increase of 83.3 percent; the number of associate degree programs rose from 218 to 707, a 224 percent increase; and the number of diploma programs fell from 797 to 311, or 61.0 percent. In Iowa between 1970 and 1979, the number of diploma programs fell by half, from eighteen

TABLE 4.1. US Nursing Enrollments and Graduates, 1965-66 to 1979-80

	Associate Degree		Diploma Nursing		Baccalaureate Degree		Practical Nursing[a]	
	Enroll-ments	Graduates	Enroll-ments	Graduates	Enroll-ments	Graduates	Enroll-ments	Graduates
1965-66	11,564	3,349	93,760	26,278	30,378	5,498	36,729	25,688
1966-67	15,338	4,654	90,651	27,452	33,081	6,131	41,077	27,644
1967-68	20,936	6,218	84,413	28,197	36,599	7,145	44,292	30,833
1968-69	27,471	8,701	77,776	25,114	40,341	8,381	48,342	34,864
1969-70	34,537	11,678	72,798	22,856	43,460	9,105	53,080	37,128
1970-71	44,593	14,754	71,055	22,334	48,897	9,913	57,890	38,556
1971-72	56,300	19,165	71,466	21,592	59,785	11,027	58,186	44,446
1972-73	67,543	24,850	71,694	21,445	73,890	13,132	57,085	46,456
1973-74	78,673	29,299	68,760	21,280	85,156	17,049	58,872	46,863
1974-75	85,452	32,622	64,083	21,673	94,951	20,241	59,453	46,080
1975-76	89,492	35,094	60,213	19,861	100,680	22,678	59,370	48,081
1976-77	92,404	36,815	56,091	18,014	101,046	23,632	58,003	47,297
1977-78	92,387	37,069	52,858	17,131	102,494	24,497	55,620	45,991
1978-79	92,961	36,763	48,059	15,820	101,239	25,349	53,241	45,066
1979-80	93,485	36,509	43,651	14,495	100,444	25,411	53,874	42,536

[a]Through 1969-70, the figures are for the full academic year; thereafter, the figures are for fall admissions.

Source: National League for Nursing

to nine; conversely, the number of associate degree programs rose from eight to eighteen; and the number of baccalaureate programs grew from four to seven. Moreover, behind those numbers in Iowa and across the nation lay matching trends in student admissions, total enrollments, and graduates.

The reasons for the large-scale demographic trends in nursing education were many. Certainly, rising costs were an important factor in the decline of diploma schools, a result of rising expectations in nursing education and the resistance of third party payers to the cost-shifting that subsidized nursing education in hospitals. Certainly, too, federal funding played a major role in the expansion of baccalaureate education in nursing.[14] At the same time, the enlarged pool of student recruits reflected a wide range of factors, including the increasing financial rewards in nursing, the more aggressive professional posture of nursing, and a diminished market for elementary and secondary teachers linked to declining numbers of school-age children.[15] As in many other states, the rapid expansion of the community college system in Iowa fueled the rapid growth in associate degree programs and enrollments. In October 1964, Iowa counted just thirty-five students enrolled in associate degree programs; by October 1979, the count had grown to 1,348. Finally, the health care marketplace began in the 1970s to confer significant advantages upon baccalaureate degree holders. By the end of the 1970s, nurses with baccalaureate and graduate degrees claimed disproportionate representation in supervisory positions and in newly emergent clinical specialties; conversely, disproportionate numbers of diploma nurses held employment as general duty or staff nurses.

Federal funding was particularly important in the steady growth of baccalaureate programs. In 1968, Congress extended the five-year Nurse Training Act of 1964 for an additional two years, providing $260 million to the US Public Health Service Division of Nursing for construction grants, student assistance, and special projects through 1971. The Nurse Training Act of 1971 once again extended those programs, in 1974 alone distributing nearly $26 million in loans to 37,000 students and more than $21 million in scholarships to 21,500 students at 1,265 participating schools of nursing. The 1971 act also provided capitation grants distributing funds directly to schools of nursing on the basis of student enrollments; in

1972, the University of Iowa College of Nursing received more than $150,000 from that source.

Behind the scenes, however, the Nixon administration expressed strong opposition to federal support for nursing education, an opposition echoed in the Ford administration. President Ford refused in late 1974 to approve a three-year $650 million Nurse Training Act, arguing that the federal government could ill afford such expenditures at a time of serious budget problems and that, in any event, the nation already faced an "oversupply" of nurses.[16] In July 1975, both House and Senate overrode a second presidential veto and enacted a combined Nurse Training, Health Revenue Sharing, and Health Services Act that authorized $553 million for nursing education through 1978. Nonetheless, appropriations under the 1975 act and successors fell well short of the sums authorized, falling from a peak of $156.5 million in 1973 to just $42.3 million in 1984.[17]

At the University of Iowa College of Nursing, the level and reliability of federal and state funding was an ongoing concern in the 1970s, particularly so as growing enrollments commanded greater faculty numbers and enlarged instructional facilities. According to a December 1971 report from the university's vice president for health affairs, the College of Nursing's count of federal funds rose from some $64,000 or 15.3 percent of the college budget in the 1961-62 fiscal year to just over $492,000 or 38.9 percent of the college budget in 1970-71.[18] During the same period, College of Nursing allocations from the university's general fund—made up of state appropriations, tuition receipts, and federal grant overhead—grew from $313,000 to $749,000, but fell from 74.6 percent to 59.2 percent of the overall college budget. The latter figure represented just 1.7 percent of total university allocations, compared, for example, to the College of Medicine's 14.8 percent share. Meanwhile, federal loan programs for student nurses provided indirect benefit to the College of Nursing; in 1965-66, for example, the Nursing Student Loan Program authorized by the Nurse Training Act of 1964 provided $63,000 to University of Iowa nursing students.[19]

Uncertainties in federal funding raised serious concerns both in the College of Nursing and elsewhere across the health science campus in the 1970s. University of Iowa President Willard Boyd reported to the State Board of Regents in February 1974 on major reductions in federal support for instructional programs, citing total losses of more than $1.5 million in the health science colleges, including $367,000 in the College of Nursing. Boyd predicted even larger reductions through 1976.[20] In fact, the College of Nursing's capitation funds, for example, fell to $90,000 in 1976 and to $78,600 the following year, down from $172,000 in 1973. In addition to legislated funding cuts, repeated executive department impoundments and recissions plagued university and College of Nursing budgeting processes. Nonetheless, Dean Evelyn Barritt reported in a May 1977 interview that the college was perhaps not hurt as badly as were other health science colleges.[21]

In September 1965, the American Nurses Association released its "Position Paper on Education for Nursing" endorsing the bachelor's degree as the appropriate entry level qualification for the registered nurse,[22] a document that caused more than a little controversy. At the University of Iowa College of Nursing, it sparked a ripple of excitement and a good deal of discussion as well. Then dean Laura Dustan was an outspoken proponent of baccalaureate education, maintaining that the well-trained nurse "who can reason, make judgments and has the ability and courage to ask questions" was "the outcome of a university education."[23] Such assertions, however, like the ANA position paper, received a cool response from increasingly embattled advocates of diploma programs.

In 1967, the Iowa State Nurses Association sponsored a debate in Marshalltown, Iowa, setting Dean Dustan against Thomas Hale, executive vice president of the Albany (NY) Medical Center Hospital.[24] Dustan charged that hospital-based diploma programs were products of a bygone era, organized to benefit hospital administrators and physicians and ill-suited to the demands placed on the modern professional nurse. In addition, Dustan argued that nursing should be joined to the higher education system because of rising costs in nursing education, because of nurses' need for a solid grounding in the social and physical sciences, and because of the clear advantages in recruiting capable students to college and university programs. In turn, Hale castigated what he called "nurse educationists," a pejorative term clearly meant to apply to Dustan. Such educationists, Hale said, were remote from the practice of nursing itself and, in their rush to enhance the academic aspects of nursing education, had lost touch with the art of nursing. In Hale's view, diploma schools were essential to meet the rising demand for skilled nurses, and he argued that Dustan's prescription would result in "inadequate numbers of nurses, inadequately prepared" for the practice of nursing.

By 1974-75, diploma schools' share of basic nursing enrollments had fallen to 26.2 percent, from 69.1 percent in 1965-66; and their share fell to just 18.2 percent in 1979-1980. The slump in diploma schools' share of nursing graduates was even more pronounced, slipping from 74.8 percent in 1965-66 to 19.0 percent in 1979-80. Worse still, diploma schools claimed only 15.7 percent of all admissions to basic nursing education programs in 1979-80. In terms of admissions, enrollments, and graduate numbers, diploma schools in Iowa followed the same general trends, although at a slower pace. Diploma programs at Iowa hospitals admitted 740 students in the fall of 1967 and 497 in the fall of 1979. In the same period, total enrollments fell from 2,004 to 1,342, while the number of graduates fell from 594 to 469.

By and large, the data suggest that those who argued that hospital schools were essential in training adequate numbers of bedside nurses failed to appreciate the extraordinary growth potential in associate degree programs. For example, Thomas Hale's 1967 prediction that baccalaureate programs would be unable to meet the rising demand for nurses was no doubt correct, but the combined increase of some 152,000 in baccalaureate and associate degree enrollments from 1966 to 1979 not only balanced the loss of 50,000 diploma school enrollments but also provided a net increase of 100,000 in basic nursing students.

At the University of Iowa College of Nursing, baccalaureate enrollments and graduates increased significantly from 1965-66 to 1979-80 (Table 4.2), reaching a peak of 584 in the fall semester of 1974-75. The decline in undergraduate enrollments in the later 1970s paralleled a nationwide slump attributed commonly to a significant decrease in student interest in nursing careers, but reduced enrollments at the University of Iowa also reflected stricter admissions standards for sophomore students, a greater focus on graduate education in the College of Nursing, and increasing enrollments at other baccalaureate programs around the state. At the same time, the bulge in junior and senior enrollments in the middle and late 1970s reflected in part the effect of the articulation project—

described immediately below—that brought students to the College of Nursing after completion of two years of preparatory courses at other institutions around the state. In 1974-75, for example, the total enrollment of 584 included seventy-two upper division transfer students. Throughout the period, Iowa residents accounted for a sizable majority of the undergraduate student body, rising from sixty-seven percent in 1967-68 to eighty-three percent in 1972-73, suggesting that Iowa residents accounted for nearly all the increase in enrollments in the intervening years.

One of the most striking features of enrollment patterns at the College of Nursing between 1965-66 and 1979-80 was the increase in male enrollments, rising from 1-2 percent to 8-10 percent and reaching as high as 11.5 percent in 1976-77.[25] In contrast, despite the considerable time and attention devoted to affirmative action programs from the late 1960s, enrollments of ethnic minorities remained low. The 1979-80 student body included a single African-American student, two Native American students, and four students listed on enrollment reports as Asian/ Pacific Islander. Of

TABLE 4.2. The University of Iowa College of Nursing Baccalaureate Enrollments and Degrees, 1965-66 to 1979-80[a]

	Pre-Nursing	Sophomores	Juniors	Seniors	Not Classified	Total	Male/Female	Degrees
1965-66	---	145	95	125	34	404	6/398	108
1966-67	---	145	125	104	38	416	4/412	100
1967-68	312	160	142	116	0	418	2/416	116
1968-69	332	143	159	131	1	434	4/430	126
1969-70	311	147	158	141	3	454	5/449	143
1970-71	279	151	179	164	2	496	4/492	145
1971-72	312	119	190	185	0	501	7/494	173
1972-73	333	121	219	218	5	563	24/539	185
1973-74	394	105	201	254	5	565	31/534	221
1974-75	458	59	230	290	5	584	42/542	238
1975-76	437	41	190	276	3	510	38/472	222
1976-77	421	30	167	252	7	456	47/409	159
1977-78	480	31	187	277	2	497	45/452	184
1978-79	507	42	168	299	6	515	35/480	216
1979-80	470	42	195	227	4	488	35/453	202

[a]Enrollment figures are for fall semester.

Source: 1965-66 and 1966-67 data, Dean of Admissions and Records, Comparative Enrollment Reports; thereafter, annual series "A Profile of Students Enrolled at the University of Iowa."

course, those figures corresponded in rough measure to the ethnic makeup of the state of Iowa itself, a state in which whites made up 98.5 percent of the population in the 1970 federal census. Nonetheless, the fact remains that Iowa's 33,000 African-Americans were poorly represented in College of Nursing enrollments, particularly when ANA and NLN counts of African-American enrollments in baccalaureate programs nationwide rose from 197 in 1965-66 to 6,318 in 1978-79.

While an ardent champion of baccalaureate education over the older diploma schools, Dean Laura Dustan conceded the limitations, geographic and socioeconomic, in baccalaureate nursing education. In 1968, just three baccalaureate nursing programs existed in Iowa, leaving large areas of the state without ready access to nursing education at the baccalaureate level. In contrast, one of the virtues of hospital-based nursing education had been its ability to put nursing education—whatever its limitations—within easy reach of most young women and those few young men who sought it. Dustan conceded in a 1970 article that "the nursing education system is failing rather badly at the baccalaureate level,"[26] a realization that led her to champion an "articulation project" designed to blend the benefits of locally accessible education with the baccalaureate nursing program at the University of Iowa.[27]

The subject of articulation, described informally as a "feeder system," appeared sporadically in faculty discussions from the time of Dustan's arrival in the fall of 1964, and the college began preliminary negotiations in 1966 with Upper Iowa College (now Upper Iowa University), negotiations aimed at devising a coordinated program that would allow students to enroll for two years of prenursing study at Upper Iowa before transferring to the university.[28] The College of Nursing's executive council and curriculum committee continued work on the articulation idea in 1967-68, and Dean Dustan notified the faculty in the fall of 1968 that she intended to apply for a Public Health Service special projects grant under the title "A Design for Articulation: A New Approach to Increasing Opportunities for Baccalaureate Nursing Education."[29] College of Nursing faculty gave their approval to the articulation project at an October 1968 meeting, despite concerns about the quality of available basic science courses in many private and community colleges.[30] Dustan's grant proposal described the fundamental "disarticulation" among the various existing nursing education programs, noting that much of the problem arose from the fact that diploma, practical nursing, and associate degree programs were all terminal programs, rather than stepping stones to higher level degree programs. As a consequence, graduates of such programs who later sought baccalaureate degrees "must first backtrack to pick up the required foundational courses before they are ready to undertake the upper division major." Dustan's goal was to develop lower division transfer curriculums in cooperating two- and four-year institutions that would mesh with the upper division offerings at the University of Iowa.

Approved by the National Advisory Council on Nurse Training in May 1969 and funded in June at nearly $462,000 for the five-year period through 1973-74, the articulation project soon enrolled five private colleges, five community colleges, and the two other state institutions of higher education—Iowa State University and the University of Northern Iowa, the latter having previously broached the idea of instituting a baccalaureate nursing program of its own.[31] Much of the grant money was earmarked for support of additional faculty positions and for the hiring of an assistant project director. The first seven articulation students enrolled at the university in the summer of 1970; twenty more followed in 1971; and the College of Nursing prepared to accommodate as many as fifty transfer students by 1973. A second goal of the program was to encourage the development of four-year nursing programs at other institutions across the state; thus, the articulation project was not designed to funnel all, or even most, of the student nurse population to the university but to foster broader support for baccalaureate nursing education. Partly as a result of that effort, the number of baccalaureate programs in Iowa grew from three to five between 1968 and 1971.

Planning for the articulation project coincided with the demise of the practical nursing program operated—to mixed reviews—by the College of Nursing since January 1953. Dean Laura Dustan, in a December 1965 communication to University of Iowa President Howard Bowen, noted that "education at this level belongs in area-technical schools" and that the College of Nursing, therefore, "anticipated that this program will probably be discontinued at an appropriate future date."[32] In an April 1966 note to the dean of academic affairs, Dustan further confided, "Between the two of us, our program in practical nursing is really a service program for the University Hospitals."[33]

In June 1966, with sixteen practical nursing programs in operation in the state and six more slated to open in the fall, Dustan notified the university administration of her intent to close the practical nursing program.[34] Besides the apparent abundance of alternative educational opportunities, Dustan questioned the propriety of housing a vocational program in the university; moreover, in the dean's estimation, the local program, which was more expensive than other such programs, had survived to that point largely because of "internal pressures." Terminating the College of Nursing's responsibility for practical nursing education, the dean argued, would free resources for the college's core missions of baccalaureate, graduate, and continuing education. At its July 1966 meeting, the State Board of Regents concurred, terminating the practical nursing program effective in August 1967.

The growth in graduate education in nursing paralleled the growth in baccalaureate education during the 1960s and 1970s. In 1965-66, the National League for Nursing counted fifty-six master's degree programs and ten doctoral programs in nursing. By 1974-75, the number of master's degree programs had grown to eighty-six, with total enrollments in excess of 9,600 and nearly 2,700 master's degrees awarded during the academic year. In the ten years from 1964-65 to 1974-75, master's level enrollments increased 241 percent nationwide, although the proportion of part-time students rose from twenty-six to forty-four percent. Federal funding was an important factor in the expansion of graduate nursing education, with the Professional Nurse Traineeship Program playing a dominant part. At the University of Iowa College of Nursing, pushed by an expanded menu of graduate offerings, the number of master's candidates rose dramatically as nursing faculty sought to shore up the shaky graduate programs inherited from earlier in the decade. Enrollments rose from twenty-one in the fall of 1965 to seventy in the fall of 1969 to ninety-one in the fall of 1979, and the number of master's degrees awarded jumped from just five in 1964-65 to a peak of fifty-one in 1975-76.

Across the nation, growth in graduate education at the doctoral level was agonizingly slow, owing in part to limited funding, in part to the lack of qualified faculty for such programs, in part to resistance from other university colleges and departments, and in part to the debate within nursing over the proper nature of such doctoral programs.[35] A 1981 study divided the history of doctoral education among nurses into three periods.[36] In the first period, from 1926 to 1959, 132 nurses had received doctorates, including eighty EdDs and forty-seven PhDs. In the second period, from 1960 to 1969, an additional 449 nurses earned doctoral degrees; however, the proportion of PhDs, mostly in the sciences and a handful in nursing, grew significantly, with the mix including 191 EdDs and 215 PhDs. Finally, in the 1970s, the opening of sixteen doctoral programs in nursing, twelve offering research-oriented PhD programs and four offering clinically-oriented Doctor of Nursing Science degrees, marked a new era, bringing the total of nursing doctoral programs to twenty-two in 1980. By the latter year, according to figures compiled by the American Nurses Association, more than 1,960 nurses were enrolled in doctoral programs of all kinds, both nursing and otherwise, with 53.8 percent in PhD programs, 34.3 percent in EdD programs, and 5.3 percent in DNSc programs. In 1980, the University of Iowa College of Nursing was one of the large majority of American nursing colleges that did not yet offer a doctoral program.

The College of Nursing Building Campaign

Dean Laura Dustan took special delight in relating an anecdote about her on-campus interview in the fall of 1963. Her introduction to the College of Nursing quarters in the south end of Westlawn, Dustan later remembered, induced in the soon-to-be-dean "a feeling of depression," a sensation heightened as she sat with search committee members in one particularly dismal room and flicked peeling paint from a wall.[37] At that awkward moment, in Dustan's recollection, one committee member blurted, "The reason we need a dean is to have someone who will get a new building for the College of Nursing." That project was to consume the greater part of Dustan's energies for the next several years, an effort that highlighted both the yet uncertain status of nursing within the larger university and the unwavering dedication of Dustan and her cohorts in pursuit of a dream.

The idea of a nursing building was not new in 1963; it had been a subject of discussion since at least the 1940s. Serious planning began in the late 1950s and early 1960s, fueled largely by prospects for federal funding in support of health professions education. In a September 1960 staff meeting Dean Mary Mullane apprised her College of Nursing colleagues of the promising outlook for federal construction funds, citing legislation then under consideration in Congress.[38] In November 1961, the university's central administration included a nursing building on a list of general university projects, and Mullane directed nursing faculty to prepare lists of departmental needs for teaching, research, and office space.[39] Mullane impressed upon President Hancher the likely need to curtail projected growth in nursing enrollments in the absence of more suitable quarters, and, shortly thereafter, Mullane began preliminary design consultations with the university architect.[40] In the fall of 1963, the National League for Nursing inquired of the college's building plans in the wake of passage of the Health Professions Educational Assistance Act,[41] and, in November, Acting Dean Florence Sherbon submitted to the US Public Health Service a letter of intent to apply for building funds. However, the project was not yet a high priority for the university or for the state legislature, which would have to appropriate matching funds.[42]

Howard Bowen's assumption of the presidency in September 1964 opened an era of ambitious planning and construction across the University of Iowa campus, construction driven by the arrival of thousands of students from the baby-boom generation. President Bowen was, in Laura Dustan's words, "a builder," and, by the time he left office in 1969, he had engineered the funding of construction projects valued at some $125,000,000.[43] In November 1964, Dustan met representatives of the US Public Health Service in Dallas, Texas, to explore the potential of the newly passed Nurse Training Act to fund College of Nursing programs in general and new construction in particular.[44] In discussions with the USPHS Division of Nursing head, Jessie Scott, Dustan emphasized the importance of the University of Iowa College of Nursing, at the time one of the nation's five largest nursing schools. According to Dustan, Scott had argued that a new building would be less expensive in the long run than an extensive remodeling of Westlawn, particularly since the Nurse Training Act provided funding for two-thirds of the cost of new construction but only half the cost of remodeling existing facilities. However, Scott had warned that because of the marginal condition of the physical plant at most schools of nursing she anticipated "a great flurry of requests for construction funds," a warning that, to Dustan, injected an element of urgency to planning at the University of Iowa.

A 1959 study had estimated the need for graduate nurses in Iowa at 8,500 by 1970, projecting total enrollments of as many as 950 undergraduate and 400 graduate students at the University of Iowa College of Nursing.[45] In light of such projections, Dean Laura Dustan early in her tenure convened an *ad hoc* faculty committee charged with assessing the College of Nursing's longterm needs, and, in response to a request from President Bowen, the committee had formulated a ten-year plan for the college. In the committee report and in a followup letter to Dean of Academic Affairs Willard L. Boyd,[46] the nursing dean and faculty pointed out that the College of Nursing was, at that time, one of just two baccalaureate programs in the state. Therefore, development of the college was of the utmost importance for the growth of Iowa nursing. In addition, they pointed out that the College of Nursing was the state's only resource for graduate education in nursing. In light of those considerations, Dustan envisioned a near doubling of undergraduate enrollments to 730 or more by the mid-1970s, compared to current enrollments of 400-450, with the aim of graduating 220-230 nurses per year. She also envisioned a substantial expansion of graduate education, with total enrollments—graduate and undergraduate—rising to 830 in 1975 and with graduate enrollments continuing to grow through the latter half of the decade.

In both undergraduate and graduate areas, new and enlarged facilities, initially estimated at 67,500 square feet, were keys to planned growth. The single largest consideration, in view of the small-group style of teaching in nursing education, was the 13,500 square feet devoted to demonstration-practice and seminar rooms in the committee on long range planning and building's fall 1964 plan. The second largest component, nearly 11,000 square feet, was designated for faculty offices. Quick action by the legislature on a request for matching funds would, Dean Dustan hoped, allow construction to begin in 1968, with completion in 1970. In February 1965, Dustan asked the university administration to approve half-time status for Etta Rasmussen so that Rasmussen—then on a quarter-time basis at the university as state supervisor of practical nursing programs—could develop building plans.[47]

From the outset, however, the College of Nursing building project was embroiled in an all too familiar pattern of university politics, a pattern that involved funding priorities and also extended to the building site itself. Then home to several unsightly World War II era quonset huts, the site next door to Westlawn was nonetheless highly desirable, and Laura Dustan and Etta Rasmussen at one point vowed to "camp out" on the spot if need be in order to preserve it for the College of Nursing.[48] In November 1965, a spokesman for the university's health science campus planning committee assured the nursing faculty that the College of Nursing's needs had been included in its recent capital investment proposal prepared for the university president.[49] Nonetheless, the College of Nursing building ranked just twelfth on a university-wide capital improvements priority list in early 1966, a designation protested by Dean Dustan at a February 16 meeting of the Building Advisory and Campus Planning Committee and in letters to the committee chair and to President Howard Bowen.[50]

The College of Nursing had, Dustan complained in her letters, supported priority funding for a basic science building, a project for which the state legislature had appropriated $3.5 million in 1965.[51] In doing so, the college had accepted assurances, first, that the basic science building was a prerequisite to the planned expansion in nursing enrollments and, second, that the Board of Regents would seek $1 million for the proposed nursing building at the next session of the General Assembly in 1967. Now, however, the building committee had not only insulted the college with its current priorities but had also recommended renovation of Westlawn rather than construction of a new building. Under the circumstances, Dustan observed, the chances of winning state funding for even the latter unacceptable alternative seemed dim. In reply to Dustan's concerns, President Bowen reiterated his administration's support for the college. "You may be sure that the position of the College of Nursing in the priorities is being seriously restudied," he wrote.[52] In turn, Dustan assured the president that she did not want to appear to be unreasonable and that she would uphold the interests of the university as a whole; her intent was to insure that all parties understood the college's position.[53]

Dustan had earlier reminded Bowen's chief lieutenant, Willard Boyd, that funding under the Nurse Training Act would expire in June 1969, with no assurance of an extension. "If grants are awarded on a 'first come, first served' basis," she pointed out, "the University of Iowa may be running late."[54] With the full support of the Bowen administration, the college submitted its application for construction funds to the Division of Nursing in the fall of 1966, in the hope that if all went well both in Washington and in the state legislature construction might still begin as early as 1968.[55] After initial screening of the application, a consultant from the Division of Nursing made a site visit to the university in December 1966 to assess the details of the application and to offer advice. The division subsequently asked for further documentation before approving the application in March 1967.[56]

Ignoring the university's lobbying efforts, the Iowa General Assembly in 1967 failed to appropriate matching funds for the College of Nursing building, a crushing disappointment made even worse for nursing partisans by the legislature's approval of nearly $4 million for a new dentistry building. In a July 1967 letter to Dean Dustan, President Bowen admitted that the chances of including the nursing building in the 1967-69 biennial construction program were almost nil.[57] However, buoyed by a two-year grant extension from the US Public Health Service Division of Nursing,[58] Bowen expressed confidence that construction funds would somehow be forthcoming from the state. The president advised College of Nursing officials in late summer 1967 to proceed with planning, and Bowen notified Dustan of his intent to juggle the university's construction budget to find the needed $1 million, news that Dustan then passed on to the Division of Nursing.[59] The Board of Regents in January 1968 selected Herbert and Associates of Des Moines as architects, and President Bowen appointed a College of Nursing building committee to conduct a detailed study of space needs for the college's various operations.

By early 1968, then, the building project was moving ahead, but without a firm funding commitment from the state. Moreover, further setbacks lay ahead. Inflation in construction costs since the initial design work and adjustments proposed by the building committee led later in 1968 to a significant redesign and a reduction in the overall size of the proposed building, chiefly involving elimination of a 300-seat auditorium and some proposed seminar rooms.[60] Those changes prompted another review by the Division of Nursing and a meeting of Dustan and architect Charles Herbert with representatives of the Division of Nursing and officials of the Kansas City regional office of the US Public Health Service.

Meanwhile, in March 1968, with the funding problem still unresolved, Dean Dustan emphasized to President Bowen that without larger facilities, there was little room for growth in undergraduate nursing enrollments, forcing the college, Dustan said, to hold sophomore admissions to a maximum of 160-170.[61] In an April 1968 letter to the Board of Regents, citing the need to act soon or risk losing federal funding, President Bowen proposed that the board reallocate to the College of Nursing $1.2 million from the state legislature's 1967 capital appropriation, drawing specifically upon funds originally approved for the College of Dentistry. Bowen's proposal was an unusual expedient, to say the least, one justified, in his eyes, by the approaching expiration of the extension granted by the Division of Nursing in 1967, coupled also with the realization that pending applications for federal construction funds under the Nurse Training Act far exceeded program resources.[62] Bowen acknowledged that there was some risk that the state legislature would not replace the $1.2 million in its prospective 1969 capital appropriation for the university; however, he assured the Board of Regents that the risk was minimal. At its April meeting, the board accepted Bowen's proposal. A few days later, the dean of dentistry, who appears to have learned of the board's action only through press reports, protested the reallocation, to no effect.[63]

In June 1968, after the university had provided copies of the architect's working drawings to the Division of Nursing, the division's director notified university officials of the formal award of $1,295,362.[64] The board of regents approved preliminary building plans the following month, holding to the earlier projected cost of $2.5 million.[65] Division of Nursing rules required issuance of the construction contract by June 1969, but several delays in the planning process led the university to seek an extension.[66] In the meantime, as late as June 1969 and in spite of commitments from the Board of Regents, President Bowen was hedging his bets, warning

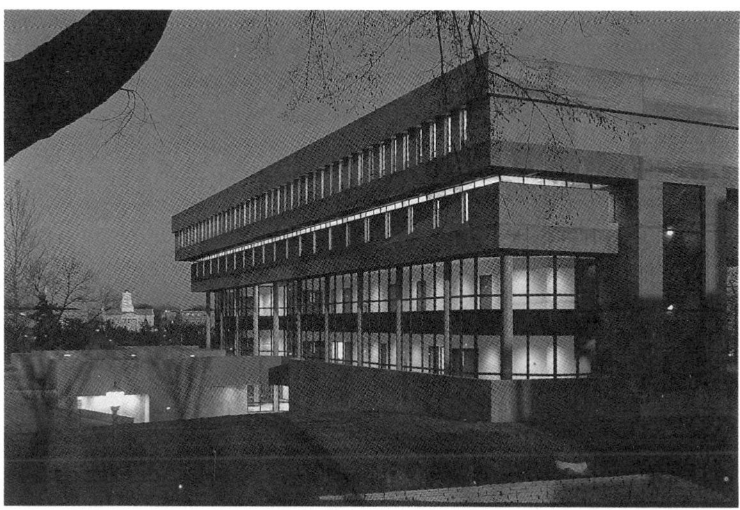

Fig. 4.1. College of Nursing Building (College of Nursing Collection).

Dustan of two "further hurdles" in the way of the building project.[67] The first was a legal challenge to the bonding authority recently granted by the state legislature to the University Hospitals,
upon which hinged hospital-based teaching facilities for the College
of Nursing. Bowen's second concern was that "bids on some of the
other buildings may go wild and require retrenchment somewhere
in our building program"—"somewhere" apparently referring to the
College of Nursing. To the relief of Bowen, Dustan, and others,
however, the Board of Regents awarded the general construction
contract in September 1969, and ground-breaking ceremonies followed on October 14.

Constructed of precast concrete and completed in 1971, the
new College of Nursing Building rose five stories on a limestone
outcropping above the Iowa River, facing the liberal arts campus to
the east and the expanding University of Iowa Hospitals and Clinics
complex to the west. Dean Dustan was effusive in her praise of
President Howard Bowen and Dean Willard Boyd for their stubborn support of the College of Nursing's cause,[68] and both Bowen
and Boyd in turn maintained that Dustan deserved the bulk of the
credit. "I merely stood by and apparently did not get in your way,"
Bowen wrote in one exchange.[69]

The dedication ceremony on Saturday, December 4, 1971, pre-
ceded by a daylong program of clinical sessions on Friday, included

special recognition awards for distinguished service to the University of Iowa given to Lola Lindsey and Lois Corder, both long connected to the School of Nursing, and to Mary Mullane and Myrtle Kitchell Aydelotte, the first two deans of the College of Nursing. Dean Laura Dustan's address at the opening of the Friday clinical sessions served as a valedictory of sorts, since she had submitted her resignation a year earlier, effective in January 1972.[70] Dustan's remarks focused chiefly on the chronology of events that had led to the present celebrations, and she noted that the new Nursing Building embodied the dean's role as an institutional steward, providing management and service to the college. Dustan likened the ten-year plan developed in 1964 to a four-legged stool, with the goal of expanded and improved nursing education programs supported by modern facilities, an upgraded curriculum, faculty development, and enlarged student enrollments. The dean's part in bringing together those four components was, she maintained, the ultimate test of stewardship, accomplished with the help of many others both inside and outside the college. Notwithstanding successes in the building campaign and in other areas, however, Dustan admitted to two "soft spots" in her record at the University of Iowa. The first lay in faculty development, which had, for a variety of reasons, lagged behind her hopes. The second was her relations with the larger community of Iowa nurses, for whom she had been "a continuing problem and disappointment" because of her uncompromising support for baccalaureate education.

Following Dustan in the Friday morning program, Anne Kibrick, president of the National League for Nursing, argued that the fuller utilization of the skills of registered nurses was an essential factor in the efficient functioning of the health care system.[71] Nurses, Kibrick pointed out, were the largest group of health care professionals and, arguably at least, the most enthusiastic and dedicated, and Kibrick predicted that nurses in the 1970s would be asked to shoulder greater responsibility and accountability as concern turned toward health maintenance and disease prevention. In turn, she predicted, nurses would move toward independent practice and reimbursement, prepared by more flexible educational programs featuring individualized courses of study designed with student input. At present, Kibrick noted, just ten percent of practicing nurses held baccalaureate or higher degrees while only a relative handful of nursing educators held doctoral degrees and just thirty-seven percent held master's degrees. In her view, the future of nursing practice and education hinged on a substantial expansion in graduate programs to train a new and enlarged generation of nursing leaders.

Howard Bowen, having left the University of Iowa in 1969 to become chancellor of the Claremont University Center in California, was the featured speaker at the Saturday dedication luncheon. In his remarks, Bowen, like Kibrick, predicted fundamental changes in store for the health care system.[72] A combination of consumer and political pressures, Bowen assured his listeners, would shift the focus of health care in coming years toward "health maintenance and enhancement," a shift that in turn meant "great new opportunities for nurses" accompanied by significant inducements—such as daycare and flexible hours—to "make possible lifelong careers for women" in nursing. At the same time, Bowen emphasized that looming manpower shortages in health care necessitated increased enrollments in the health science colleges, a need that the new Nursing Building would help to address. In closing, Bowen, lauded the outgoing dean for her "monumental accomplishments" at the University of Iowa.

In the long history of nursing education at the University of Iowa, the December 1971 building dedication was indeed a critical moment. In practical terms, the new quarters afforded much needed facilities for nursing education, while, in symbolic terms, the College of Nursing's removal from Westlawn also capped the long separation of nursing education from the University Hospitals. In a congratulatory letter to Dean Dustan, one longtime College of Medicine faculty member noted that the dedication was "an occasion we will all remember for a long time," one that stood as a "tribute to the perseverance of Myrtle [Kitchell] and you in creating the College of Nursing." It was also, he remarked, a triumph over "the hurdles thrown up by my stuffy colleagues" in opposition to nursing's independent development.[73]

The Basic Curriculum and the Student Body

From her arrival in 1964, Dean Laura Dustan made clear that the college's most important concerns were, for the short term, preparation for the upcoming NLN accreditation visit and, for the long term, developing building plans. Accordingly, she notified faculty members in December 1964 that substantive curriculum revision lay three years down the road. Nonetheless, several curriculum issues commanded immediate faculty attention, some of them carryovers from previous years. Three of them were particularly pressing—the phaseout of the general nursing and psychiatric nursing programs to create a single undergraduate curriculum, the suitability of basic science courses designed expressly for nurses, and the quality and evaluation of students' clinical work. In addition, preliminary work on a full-blown curriculum revision, a project that stretched into the next decade, was underway by 1966.

The phaseout of the general program and the integration of registered nurse students, mostly graduates of diploma programs, into the basic curriculum was the first curriculum issue to be resolved. Since the early 1950s, College of Nursing faculty had conceded the importance of affording baccalaureate opportunities to registered nurses; however, the general program proved an unending source of headaches, largely because of controversy over the assignment of transfer credit for diploma-level courses and debate over the clinical competence of registered nurse students. By the early 1960s, the trend in nursing schools across the nation was toward a single, integrated baccalaureate track combining both general and basic programs, a trend strongly encouraged by the National League for Nursing.

At the University of Iowa, the College of Nursing general curriculum committee in 1962-63 began an examination of related NLN materials and also undertook an examination of schools that had already made the conversion to a single program.[74] The following year, the curriculum committee recommended several changes with respect to course requirements for registered nurse students, both diploma and associate degree, including twenty-seven semester hours of specified upper level courses to be taken in residence at the university, a maximum of thirty-five semester hours of transfer credits, creation of a new course for general students titled "Nursing of Adults and Children" to integrate information from the physical and behavioral sciences, the addition of microbiology to the expanded list of resident course requirements, and the inclusion of both basic and general students in the same sections of senior nursing courses.[75] The full faculty adopted those recommendations in May 1964, effective for entering students in the fall of 1965, creating a single baccalaureate curriculum and granting registered nurses admission with advanced standing.

A corollary issue, the evaluation of registered nurse students' preparation for upper division nursing courses, proved especially troublesome. Originally, College of Nursing faculty voted to use performance in the new course Nursing of Adults and Children as a tool to assess students' needs for additional work in the various nursing specialty areas—that is, medical-surgical, pediatric, obstetric, and psychiatric nursing. However, a spring 1965 report by two faculty members argued that it was inappropriate to use one clinical course of limited scope to predict performance in other, more specialized clinical areas. The report recommended instead that advanced standing be left in the hands of individual clinical departments, a proposal modified by a full subcommittee of the curriculum committee to require that students take the regular final examinations in each of the junior level clinical courses in order to qualify for the full thirty-five hours of advanced credit and attain senior status.[76] Based upon that recommendation, the college faculty ultimately instituted a system of "challenge exams" for registered nurse students in each of the specialty areas.

Continued difficulties led to a review of the entire process in the spring semester of 1969. By that time sixty-eight registered nurse students had taken the challenge exams, and sixty-two had earned the full thirty-five semester hours credit.[77] Notwithstanding their success in the challenge exams, registered nurse students complained of what they perceived as unnecessary repetition, particularly in the required practicums, which they viewed as devaluing their previous training and experience. Many preferred to enroll in more liberal arts courses rather than to repeat courses and experiences already mastered. While faculty appreciated the often intense motivation of registered nurse students, undergraduate curriculum committee minutes contained one instructor's observation that they seemed "more defiant this semester than before," the word defiant changed in a later version to "defensive."[78] In response to student complaints, Dean Dustan recommended in May 1969 that the faculty appoint an *ad hoc* committee to study the usefulness to registered nurse students of the Nursing of Adults and Children sequence.[79]

The integration of psychiatric nursing into the basic curriculum at the University of Iowa was a second part of the problem of curriculum integration. From 1952 to 1958, as described in the previous chapter, psychiatric nursing was a baccalaureate track open to registered nurse students who opted for extensive coursework in psychology and psychiatric nursing theory and practice in lieu of the comprehensive junior and senior year nursing courses. As noted previously, the psychiatric nursing option was eliminated as of 1958, leaving the question of psychiatric nursing's place in the basic curriculum in limbo. By the mid-1960s, however, with federal funds then available for the integration of psychiatric nursing into a single basic curriculum, the University of Iowa nursing faculty in December 1965 began work on the problem,[80] aided by a $35,000 federal grant. As a result of that effort, psychiatric nursing became a major part of the senior year basic curriculum (Figure 4.2).[81]

The status of basic science courses designed expressly for nurses was the second curriculum-related issue to come under scrutiny in the mid-1960s. In November 1965, Dean Dustan praised College of Medicine Dean Robert Hardin for his support for common basic science courses offered to undergraduate students across the health sciences rather than applied courses tailored to specific audiences.[82] Dustan and her faculty colleagues expressed special concern with regard to microbiology and anatomy, areas in which the designation "for nurses" had on occasion posed problems for students applying for admission to graduate programs. Assuming the availability of facilities and the cooperation of the offering departments, the mainstreaming of nursing students was, on the surface, a relatively simple matter. However, it also raised hidden problems, the most important of which dealt with departmental prerequisites for the more advanced courses. The chair of the Department of Microbiology, for example, warned Dustan that his department's general course in microbiology included among its prerequisites eight to ten semester hours of organic chemistry.[83] For the time being, then, the college sought a compromise, generally working to drop the designation "for nurses" from course descriptions whenever possible while encouraging cooperating departments to upgrade course offerings for nursing students.

Fig. 4.2. Fall 1967 Basic Nursing Curriculum

Freshman Year [College of Liberal Arts]

First Semester	Semester Hours	Second Semester	Semester Hours
Rhetoric	4	Rhetoric	4
Historical-Cultural Core	4	Historical-Cultural Core	4
Chemistry	4	Chemistry	4
Intermediate Algebra	3	Psychology or Sociology	3
		Elective	2
Total	15	Total	17

Sophomore Year

First Semester	Semester Hours	Second Semester	Semester Hours
Foundations of Nursing	3	Foundations of Nursing	3
Foundations Practicum	2	Foundations Practicum	2
Physiology	4	Microbiology	4
Sociology or Nutrition	3	Human Growth & Development	4
Anatomy	4	Psychology or Nutrition	3
Total	16	Total	16

Junior Year

First Semester	Semester Hours	Second Semester	Semester Hours
Medical-Surgical Nursing	6	Maternity Nursing	3
Medical Practicum	3	Maternity Practicum	3
Surgical Practicum	3	Nursing Care of Children	3
Literature	4	Care of Children Practicum	3
		Community Sociology	3
		Elective	3
Total	16	Total	18

Senior Year

First Semester	Semester Hours	Second Semester	Semester Hours
Psychiatric Nursing	6	Nursing in the Social Order	3
Psychiatric Practicum	3	Senior Nursing	
Public Health Nursing	3	Senior Nursing Practicum	5
Public Health Practicum	3	Literature	4
Fundamentals of Community Health	2		
Total	14	Total	17

The third of the immediate curriculum problems, the nature and evaluation of student clinical experience, was an issue of long standing in the College of Nursing. From the 1950s, nursing faculty had agonized over fundamental issues regarding students' clinical experience, focusing on the concepts and behaviors to be taught and on the assessment of skills learned, but clinical training in nursing suffered the same lack of structure and consistency that generally plagued clinical training in medicine. With the implementation of the four academic year curriculum in 1961, clinical education in the University Hospitals took place in a more controlled environment; however, in need of additional clinical resources, the college also arranged for a variety of clinical experiences at off-campus sites. At different times in the 1960s, the local Veterans Administration Hospital, Mercy Hospital in Iowa City, Des Moines and Sioux City public health nursing facilities, the Iowa Security Medical Facility at nearby Oakdale, the Iowa City Extended Care Center, and the Visiting Nurse Associations of Iowa City, Dubuque, Davenport, and Cedar Rapids all provided students clinical experience. By the late 1970s, nursing students benefited from practical experience at some fifty off-campus sites.

The increasingly diverse menu of clinical experiences only magnified existing problems associated with clinical experience, and a faculty committee agreed in February 1965 to suggest fundamental structural reforms in clinical training. The committee's first goal was to "develop an acceptable evaluation tool,"[84] and, by the opening of the fall 1965 semester, the committee had devised a lengthy statement of philosophy encompassing the purpose of clinical training and the goals of student evaluation. The committee had also constructed a list of desirable characteristics to be incorporated in a system of evaluation: growth in the performance of essential nursing skills, ability to communicate both orally and in writing, and personal growth and development.[85] Finally, the committee asked for the entire faculty's involvement in crafting an evaluation tool, with the committee's preliminary work serving as a basis for discussion at a September 1965 faculty workshop.

A 1965-66 survey of sophomore students' opinions of clinical experiences afforded in the various wards and departments of University Hospitals provided a grassroots perspective on clinical training.[86] However, the results could not have been reassuring, even allowing for expected student hyperbole and unrealistic expectations. While students gave high marks to some departments, notably ophthalmology and ear-nose-and-throat, they offered devastating criticisms of some others, especially during the fall semester, with the women's orthopædic ward faring the worst. In the latter case, ten students rated ward personnel as "unfriendly," and eleven labeled them "not helpful." In the spring semester, in contrast, nineteen students rated women's orthopædic ward staff as "friendly" and eighteen rated them as "helpful." In general, three clear lessons emerged from student responses: first, a good many sophomore students approached their clinical experiences with strong apprehension because of their lack of skills and preparation; second, clinical supervision was, to say the least, spotty; and, third, the quality of the clinical experience varied widely, not only from one ward to another but also on the same ward from one semester to another. The results of that student survey led to the institution of much more structured undergraduate clinical experiences, defined and enforced by standard interagency agreements between the College of Nursing and the various participating agencies, including the University Hospitals.

Even as the nursing faculty dealt in piecemeal fashion with a range of curriculum issues, a fundamental revision of the basic curriculum gathered steam from the middle to the late 1960s. As early as 1963, faculty had engaged in extended discussions focused on the kinds of positions for which the college prepared its students and the kinds of skills needed,[87] discussions that led the undergraduate section of the curriculum committee in 1965-66 to begin a study of the philosophy and objectives underlying the baccalaureate curriculum.[88] In April 1966, the committee embarked on a five-part approach to curriculum revision, beginning with the functions of the professional nurse and moving to consideration of instructional objectives, strategies for achieving the objectives, applications of theoretical knowledge to the stated objectives, and development of tools of evaluation.[89]

A detailed survey of 1965 baccalaureate graduates—the first from the four academic year program—provided a practical basis for much of the initial discussion of curriculum revision.[90] Sixty-four of eighty-six graduates, or seventy-four percent, returned the lengthy questionnaires. Thirty-three were married at the time of the survey, but there were just three children among the married cohort. Sixty-one of the respondents were employed, reporting a mean annual salary of $5,165. Forty-three of the respondents were hospital staff nurses; nine were in public health nursing, five in teaching positions, and two in graduate school. Twenty-one respondents anticipated enrollment in graduate school within two years.

Fifty-five respondents, or 85.9 percent, agreed that the baccalaureate program had afforded adequate preparation for their present positions, and all but one agreed that she had been wise to choose a baccalaureate program over the alternatives, many citing the more comprehensive nature of the baccalaureate educational experience. Also, many compared their own academic preparation favorably to that of their present colleagues. Nonetheless, respondents offered a good many negative observations regarding their student experiences. In particular, they complained of a lack of career guidance, and of "undesirable repetition or duplication" in many nursing courses, suggesting, some said, a lack of coordination in course design and instructional content. "It often seemed different instructors did not know what the other was doing or had done," was a typical comment. In addition to better organized and coordinated courses, respondents hoped to see a better qualified faculty and a more "practical" focus in clinical instruction. The last—an echo of timeworn grievances among medical students—was juxtaposed with requests for more intellectually challenging classroom work and more exposure to the liberal arts.

The curriculum committee also reviewed curriculum development at other schools of nursing, and, at the advice of Dean Willard Boyd, also considered curriculum reform efforts then underway in the University of Iowa Colleges of Medicine and Dentistry.[91] In November 1966, the committee invited Associate Executive Dean of Medicine Daniel Stone and Dean of Dentistry Donald Galagan to describe the aims of curriculum revision in their respective colleges, and both men stressed the importance of defining an essential core of knowledge while allowing students greater flexibility in moving toward chosen areas of specialization.[92] In January 1967, the College of Nursing held a faculty conference focused on future trends in health care and curriculum development, featuring several speakers from outside the college. In the wake of the conference, faculty discussion centered on what students should know, what kind of education they should have, what outcomes were desirable, and how to approach curriculum change. Faculty also agreed to create five subcommittees to assess specific curriculum issues.[93]

Teaching methodology was a central concern in discussions of curriculum revision. A spring 1967 progress report of an *ad hoc* committee on student characteristics put the issue succinctly.[94] "Are we," committee members asked, "recognizing and applying effectively known theories which enhance learning?" Answering their own question in the negative, committee members observed that the lack of rigorous attention to instructional methodology left nursing students "unsure of our expectations" and led faculty to demand behaviors that students were "not emotionally or academically equipped to produce." That report was one subject of discussion during two successive days of curriculum committee meetings dealing with the definition of nursing, the object of the nursing curriculum, the characteristics of a professional leader, the conceptual underpinnings of the nursing curriculum, and the role of the total faculty in curriculum planning.[95]

Ongoing and increasingly intense curriculum study, coupled with related faculty development issues, put added pressures on an already strained College of Nursing budget and led to creation of yet another special committee, this one to seek funding from outside agencies.[96] Subsequently, the college received a grant from the US Public Health Service Division of Nursing in the summer of 1968 to support a formal curriculum project group that assumed primary responsibility for curriculum revision. Mildred Freel—released from teaching responsibilities—became project director, and six clinical faculty served as assistant directors. The project group took much of the burden off the existing makeshift structure of subcommittees and *ad hoc* committees, whose members at times appeared to be overwhelmed by their assigned tasks.[97]

After devoting much of the summer of 1969 to the basics of curriculum reorganization, the project group led a faculty curriculum conference in October 1969, and, by the fall of 1970, the project group had made significant progress in identifying essential curriculum content, in defining desirable behavioral outcomes, and in preparing recommendations regarding the liberal arts components of the curriculum.[98] At faculty meetings in the spring of 1971, special task forces on supporting content, resources, and theoretical framework reported their recommendations to the full nursing faculty. The following autumn, the faculty adopted a series of statements regarding the philosophy of nursing education, the nature of the learning process, the roles of students and instructors, the place of the liberal arts in nursing education, the importance of varied classroom and clinical experiences, and the development of professional responsibility in the student nurse.[99]

In 1972 and 1973, the extended curriculum revision begun in 1966 resulted in the finished "process curriculum," the central concepts of which were the nursing process and the health-illness continuum (Figure 4.3). Nursing students would, in the language of the finished document, "approach nursing as a process directed toward the maintaining as well as regaining of health of individuals and groups."[100] Instituted for sophomore students in the spring of 1974, the new curriculum defined six knowledge areas that provided the base for nursing practice: physiological, psychological, psychosocial, sociological, environmental, and general education. The curriculum included two new liberal arts courses: a five-semester-hour course in animal biology and a four-semester-hour course in anthropology. At the heart of the curriculum were the core nursing courses, numbered I through V, designed to take students in stepwise fashion through the phases of the nursing process—assessment, planning, intervention, and evaluation—and to inculcate leadership skills. Moreover, although it specified basic requirements, the curriculum was designed to maximize flexibility for individual students.

Significant changes in teaching methodology accompanied the process curriculum. The new curriculum aimed to create an integrated learning experience with continual cross references among the basic sciences, humanities, and clinical areas; more important, it recognized learning itself as a process and sought to lead students from basic concepts to more complex applications through a system of programmed instruction, a concept that gained considerable currency throughout the health sciences in the late 1960s and early 1970s. Self-study was an important element of the new curriculum and the new learning model, and a learning resources center, created and directed by Mildred Freel, provided students the opportunity to enhance their learning skills at a self-directed pace. At the same time, the college established an instructional design and production department to assist in the development of instructional materials.

For the nursing profession, the process curriculum was important because it embodied a concerted effort on the part of nursing faculty—an effort obscured to some extent in formal descriptions of the curriculum and even of the revision process—to define fundamental nursing concepts, roles, and behaviors and to incorporate those insights into the student's learning experience. This was, as Dean Evelyn Barritt later noted, a significant step away from a time-honored medical model for nursing education and, by exten-

Fig. 4.3. Process Curriculum, 1974

General Education Requirements	Semester Hours
Rhetoric	8
Historical-Cultural	4
Literature	4
Electives	19
Total	40

Supporting Content Requirements	Semester Hours
Animal Biology	5
Chemistry	5
Anatomy	4
Physiology	4
Microbiology	4
Nutrition	3
Psychology	4
Sociology	4
Anthropology	4
Human Development and Behavior	3
Total	40

Nursing Courses	Semester Hours
Introduction to Health Care Services	3
Nursing I	5
Nursing II	8
Pathology	4
Nursing III	8
Nursing IV	8
Nursing V	8
Nursing in the Social Order	3
Nursing Electives	6
Total	53

sion, for nursing practice as well. In subsequent years, that trend toward nursing education grounded in concepts peculiar to nursing played an increasingly larger role in curriculum design, in nursing research, and in the overall professional development of nursing.

Apart from curriculum renovation, the 1960s and 1970s brought significant changes in the nursing student body and in student life. Perhaps most obviously, the inception of the four academic year curriculum and the end to compulsory hospital service in 1961 at last fulfilled Myrtle Kitchell Aydelotte's goal, by then more than a decade old, of fully integrating nursing students into the university community. Students enjoyed more free time for participation in campus organizations and events, and, liberated from the nurses' dormitory in Westlawn, they also mingled with their peers in university dormitories and in off-campus housing throughout their student years. In academic terms, nursing students compared favorably to the rest of the university student body, perhaps resulting from a growing pool of applicants, more rigorous screening procedures by the college's admissions committee, and an enhanced image of the nursing profession in society at large. In 1965-66, according to the university's "Profile of Students," the College of Nursing carried the highest mean grade point average of all undergraduate colleges and, at 2.65 for the fall semester and 2.77 for the spring semester, stood well above university averages of 2.41 and 2.43 respectively.

Nursing student organizations, too, displayed a new vitality in the late 1960s and 1970s, reflecting at least in part the growing sense of pride and mission in the college and in the nursing profession. The rejuvenation of the Student Nurse Organization (SNO) in the late 1960s and its affiliation with the Iowa Association of Nursing Students (IANS) were symptomatic of that revival, and a University of Iowa student was elected IANS president in 1970. Student organizations, first the SNO and later the Association of Nursing Students (ANS), served important social functions, including staging dances and picnics, while student representatives also engaged in a range of service activities, including high school recruitment campaigns, drug education programs, and charitable fund-raising. In 1974, the ANS inaugurated an annual "student day" featuring an all-day program of featured speakers and informational sessions. Finally, the SNO and ANS published student newspapers, *PRN* and later *The Drawsheet.*

Gamma Chapter, Sigma Theta Tau, enjoyed a similar resurgence. From its founding in 1929, Gamma Chapter had performed a largely social purpose, but the 1960s and 1970s saw mushrooming membership and increasing emphasis on more professional concerns, especially scholarship and research. From seventy in 1965-66, Gamma Chapter's membership roll grew to 181 in 1975-76 and to more than 370 in spring 1978. By spring 1980, the chapter had inducted a total of 1,442 members since its inception in 1929.[101] The chapter began planning a scholarship fund in the early 1960s and announced the first scholarship award in April 1968. Similarly, the chapter established a research fund in the 1970s that provided small grants to defray direct costs of faculty and graduate student research. Gamma members also participated in a three-year Nurse Faculty Research Development in the Midwest program funded by the National Institutes of Health and in a Mid-America Research Conference series. Likewise, the chapter cosponsored with the College of Nursing an annual research forum in which faculty and graduate students shared their work. One of the chapter's most visible projects was funding and equipping a heritage room in the new Nursing Building, a space that served as faculty lounge and seminar room and also provided areas for the display of historical artifacts. In 1979, Gamma Chapter celebrated its golden anniversary, highlighted by the attendance of three members from the chapter's original roll and by the reenactment of the secret initiation ritual conducted annually from 1929 to 1942.

One of the most significant changes in the nursing student body from the mid-1960s was the increased enrollment of males. The influx of males, albeit still in limited numbers, was of symbolic as well as demographic importance, a fact recognized by Dean Laura Dustan at a summer capping ceremony for sophomore students in 1971. Noting that male nurses did not wear the traditional cap, Dustan renamed the event a "recognition ceremony" and presented the two male students with lapel insignias designed in the form of a Maltese cross. Noting also that nursing had long been considered "women's work," the dean observed that men entering the profession "had to be courageous believers" willing "to swim against the current of public opinion."[102] When those two male students became seniors in 1973, the University of Iowa Hospitals and Clinics employed just three male registered nurses and two male practical nurses,[103] but College of Nursing enrollments included twenty-seven males—twelve sophomores, nine juniors, two seniors, and four graduate students. In addition, ten males were then completing their sophomore years at articulation project institutions.[104] Male nursing students were often non-traditional in ways other than gender; many, for example, were older students drawn to nursing by experience in the army and navy hospital corps.

The presence of larger numbers of males in the nursing student body mirrored in an unusual way a university-wide emphasis on affirmative action, a policy applied to recruitment of both students and faculty. Begun in the late 1960s during the administration of President Howard Bowen, affirmative action efforts forced the College of Nursing, along with the rest of the university, to address the issue of attracting minority and disadvantaged students and devising programs to meet their special needs. In fall 1968, the faculty's undergraduate curriculum committee devoted considerable time to an assessment of methods of working with disadvantaged students, but the committee displayed a general reluctance to develop formal policies that would set apart specific students or categories of students from the rest of the student body.[105] In 1971, the college's faculty association voted to create an ad hoc committee to work with the university's office of special support services regarding specific recommendations for the admission of minority students; as noted previously, however, the results, in terms of minority enrollments, were meager.[106]

The Growth of Graduate and Continuing Education

The widening of graduate educational opportunities in nursing was an especially pressing issue during the late 1960s and 1970s, both because of the accelerating trend toward specialization in nursing practice and because of the desperate need of qualified candidates for faculty positions in schools of nursing. In a 1971 survey of Iowa nursing schools, just twenty-nine percent of all faculty at baccalaureate, associate, and diploma programs held master's degrees or higher.[107] In the face of such numbers, the University of Iowa College of Nursing, like many other university-based nursing schools, pursued a "grow-your-own" policy of grooming promising graduate students for faculty positions.[108] However, such a policy depended first and foremost on bolstering the college's own graduate programs that had fallen on hard times in the late 1950s and early 1960s.

In the interregnum between Dean Mary Mullane's 1962 departure and the arrival of Laura Dustan in the fall of 1964, the College of Nursing graduate curriculum committee began preliminary work aimed at upgrading the existing graduate program. In analyzing the content of the three clinical majors—medical-surgical, psychiatric, and maternal and child health—the committee noted significant duplication of content and the lack of a "common philosophy, purpose and objective."[109] In due course, the committee composed statements of philosophy and purpose and a list of objectives to impose a measure of uniformity across the majors. Graduate study, the committee observed in its statement of philosophy, "is designed to develop the scholarship and leadership potentialities of nurses."[110] Graduate instruction, the statement continued, was "a process through which opportunity is provided and used for critical study and analysis of the content of nursing, examination of source materials with ever-increasing intensity, development and testing of hypotheses, and the formulation of intellectual and moral judgments dictated by and consistent with high-level responsibility."

In assessing the graduate curriculum, nursing faculty referred often to findings from a 1961 National League for Nursing survey of graduate programs, a survey that cited serious deficiencies in the educational preparation of both graduate students and graduate faculty and also cited major disparities in graduate programs. In late May 1964, a NLN consultant in graduate education visited the University of Iowa campus for two days of intensive on-site investigation.[111] The consultant noted in her report that the College of Nursing lagged well behind other colleges and departments of the university in terms of faculty academic preparation, research, and publication, but, she noted, she "did not push too hard on this point," explaining that "in view of the frequent changes in the deanship over the past several years...the faculty was doing very well to even hold itself together." The consultant's report included several recommendations, the most important of which were closer integration of research into the graduate program, including improving the research skills of faculty, closer attention to the screening of applicants for graduate study, and greater efforts to instill a sense of responsibility for learning in graduate students.

In April 1965, the College of Nursing graduate faculty approved a statement of purpose for the graduate program,[112] asserting that the aim of graduate education was "to provide students opportunities for the scholarly pursuit of nursing" and "to prepare them to assume appropriate professional leadership roles." In a companion statement of philosophy, the faculty declared their support for "a sound undergraduate base of general and professional education" as a prerequisite to graduate work and endorsed clinical specialization as an essential element of graduate education.

In December 1965, barely a year in office, Dean Laura Dustan reported to President Howard Bowen the anticipated approval of a new graduate program in nursing service administration and the reactivation of the then moribund program in pediatric nursing, a combination that would give the college four graduate majors by 1970.[113] The college had no present plan to develop a doctoral program in nursing, the dean reported, but she hoped that such a program might be feasible by 1980. In a later report, Dustan noted that the College of Nursing had contributed just five of the 1,379 master's degrees awarded nationwide in 1964-65; similarly, only nine of the college's thirty-five master's degree faculty held degrees from the University of Iowa.[114] Thus, in Dustan's interpretation, Iowa was a "debtor state" in the preparation of nursing faculty, evidence, she argued, of the "colossal public apathy and inattention" accorded nursing education, particularly graduate education, in the state.

The college's graduate faculty in the fall of 1965 approved the proposal for a master's program in hospital nursing service administration, a program submitted by Eva Erickson, who had been recruited by Dean Mullane specifically to reinstitute such a program. Erickson's proposal stressed the need to "prepare professional nurses for careers in top-level nursing service management positions in complex hospital settings," noting that each of Iowa's 170 hospitals needed a nursing service administrator.[115] In addition, nearly sixteen percent of such positions already budgeted in six midwestern states were vacant, evidence that "qualified persons are not available for appointment." Erickson's proposal drew some criticism from faculty who, like their colleagues in other nursing schools, favored the clinical specialization embraced in the college's philosophy of graduate education and who feared that the nursing service administration program would provide insufficient grounding in basic nursing. In response, Dean Dustan explained that the program would operate on an experimental basis for five years with highly selective admission requirements, and on that basis the program received interim approval from the Graduate College and from Dean of Academic Affairs Willard Boyd in the fall of 1965, enrolling its first six students in the fall of 1966.[116]

The college's graduate offerings won accreditation from the National League for Nursing's Department of Baccalaureate and Higher Degree Programs in the spring of 1966, an important step, as Dean Dustan pointed out, to obtaining federal funding for graduate education.[117] NLN site visitors did express reservations on several counts, perhaps most importantly the lack of faculty research productivity. In fact, the lack of faculty research was one of two fundamental problems hindering development of graduate programs at the College of Nursing through the 1960s and, to a significant extent, through the 1970s. A second and related problem was that of faculty recruitment, discussed in more detail in the following section. While a majority of faculty, by their own declaration, preferred a graduate program focused on clinical specialization, Myrtle Kitchell Aydelotte and colleague Ann Whidden noted in 1966 that the quality of instruction in clinical specialties was in fact a major weakness of the college.[118] In much the same vein, Laura Dustan predicted in 1965 that "a doctorate will be required of those who head up graduate programs in the future."[119]

In that environment, discussion of the purpose and scope of graduate program offerings consumed increasing amounts of faculty time at the University of Iowa. The research component common to all four graduate majors received special scrutiny because of the central importance of research skills in the training of nursing faculty. In 1967, the graduate faculty adopted a coordinated two-semester sequence of courses in research methodology, statistics, and nursing research to replace two existing courses entitled social research and research in nursing. The rationale behind the change was straightforward: first, that the previous courses were grounded in sociology and "emphasized the techniques of investigation to the neglect of the questions to be asked," and, second, that, assuming the existence of a body of nursing knowledge, research techniques should be taught from a nursing perspective.[120] However, graduate students repeatedly complained of a lack of support in gathering data and compiling study results and of a lack of overall faculty guidance and interest in their work. Likewise, students and faculty alike cited conflicting expectations among faculty members in charge of the research sequence on the one hand and faculty members advising on work in particular areas on the other. Meanwhile, faculty at one point worried about a perceived increase in plagiarism and improper footnoting in graduate student work.[121]

Nursing service administration also attracted renewed attention, reflecting the still unresolved struggle over the proper direction—clinical or functional—of graduate education and indicative, in a larger sense, of a profession still seeking to define itself. Originally conceived as a five-year experiment, the nursing service administration program awarded degrees to fifty-three students from February 1968 to August 1971; in October 1971, Eva Erickson reported that fifteen graduates were employed as directors of nursing services, nine were employed as assistant or associate directors, and thirteen were employed as nursing supervisors or head nurses.[122] Because the college had won a five-year federal grant in 1968 to support the program, faculty agreed to its continuance until the termination of the grant in 1973. The faculty did, however, schedule a full-scale review of the program for 1972-73, promising a spring 1973 decision on its future.[123]

That decision dragged into the 1973-74 academic year, as a graduate council committee in turn reviewed the review. In January 1974, the committee submitted some thirty questions to program director Eva Erickson, expressing concern over the validity and focus of the nursing service administration curriculum and its actual impact on hospital practice. Erickson responded with a spirited defense of her program.[124] Answering a committee inquiry regarding the nearly twenty percent of program graduates in a recent survey who "indicated a concern about the worth of graduate education," Erickson pointed to the thirty-six percent of graduates from the nursing in children major who had raised the same doubts about that program in a similar 1973 survey. In answer to another area of committee concern, she argued that the flexibility of the nursing service administration curriculum did not betray a lack of focus but was one of the program's strengths, permitting students to tailor their education to their needs and interests. Erickson conceded that she had no hard data on the program's actual impact on nursing practice; nonetheless, she maintained that anecdotal information from graduates and from employers suggested a significant effect. Erickson's case was apparently persuasive; in any event, the nursing faculty granted the nursing service administration major new life.

Graduate enrollments in the College of Nursing grew rapidly in the late 1960s and 1970s, rising to seventy-eight in the fall of 1970 and to 116 in the fall of 1975, although in the latter year just fifty-six were full-time students. Throughout the period, the college maintained the four graduate majors in medical-surgical nursing, psychiatric nursing, nursing service administration, and nursing of children, the last revived in 1969 under the guidance of June Triplett. Throughout the period, too, the funding of graduate education was an ongoing worry. Much of the financial support for graduate programs came in the form of program grants from the US Public Health Service Division of Nursing and from federal nurse traineeship grants. In 1969-70, for example, a College of Nursing committee estimated the university's contribution to graduate education at $75,750, most of that in the form of program directors' salaries. In the same year, more than $88,000 in federal grants supported nursing service administration and psychiatric nursing majors, and the college also received over $205,000 in federal traineeship grants.[125] Heavy reliance on federal funds, however, particularly in an era of threatened retrenchment, increasingly complicated planning and budgeting processes through the 1970s.

In summer 1970, representatives from the College of Nursing and the College of Medicine's Department of Pediatrics proposed a pediatric nurse practitioner program (PNP).[126] The proposal was, as Dean Laura Dustan understood it, merely a draft to be reviewed and revised in the event that federal funds became available to support such programs. Nonetheless, sent to the Department of Health, Education and Welfare for preliminary recommendations, the proposal "met with enthusiasm," and appeared to be on the verge of funding by fall 1971 under provisions of the Nurse Training Act authorizing funding for advanced-practitioner projects.

That gratifying response placed the dean in the awkward position of having submitted a curriculum proposal for funding that had not yet been reviewed by the full College of Nursing graduate faculty. Somewhat embarrassed, Dustan advised graduate faculty in October 1971 that the program offered "a unique opportunity for collaboration" between nursing and medicine and would also bolster the college's existing nursing of children graduate curriculum. Planned around sixty semester hours of formal course work supplemented by clinical practice, the proposed program required the college to add to its faculty a pediatric nurse practitioner as program co-director and required the College of Medicine to provide instructional resources available both to the nurse practitioner program and to the nursing of children major. Funded by a grant issued by the Maternal and Child Health Service of HEW, the three-semester pediatric nurse-practitioner program began operation in 1972.

At the behest of the dean of the Graduate College, a university review committee in January 1975 presented "An Academic Review of the Master of Arts Program in Nursing,"[127] a report that highlighted both the strengths and weaknesses of graduate training in the College of Nursing. The review committee began with the observation that "graduate education in nursing remains in an early stage of development," a situation made worse by the shortage of doctorally prepared faculty. In contrast to patterns in older disciplines, the review committee noted that nurse educators had invested much more energy and attention in the undergraduate curriculum than they had in graduate education and that, partly as a result, undergraduate and graduate programs were poorly integrated, as were the four current graduate offerings. The review committee commended in particular the research component in each of the programs, although suggesting better integration of research issues and skills into the overall curriculum. On the whole, the committee also commended the flexibility of individual programs, which permitted students to choose "highly eclectic plans of study." At the same time, the committee cited faculty teaching loads and faculty development as major concerns, particularly in light of the gulf between university-wide standards for academic credentials, research, and publication and prevailing standards in the College of Nursing. In conclusion, the review committee strongly recommended the continued development of existing graduate majors rather than extension into new areas of study, fearing that the latter course would weaken the quality of offerings and worsen faculty workloads. The committee also recommended the integration of the four existing majors into a single program combining a common core curriculum with specialized options.

By the mid-1970s, out-reach programs to make graduate education more accessible to practicing nurses were major topics of discussion at a national level, and, in 1974, a special committee of the University of Iowa College of Nursing graduate council began a study of "new routes to graduate education," meant to identify alternatives to the conventional residential graduate programs. While the extension concept enjoyed significant faculty support, it also raised serious questions regarding quality, logistics, and resources,[128] even as surveys of prospective target audiences gave evidence of widespread interest among practicing nurses. A January 1975 survey of 350 nurses in the Quad-Cities area (Davenport and Bettendorf, Iowa, and Rock Island and Moline, Illinois) attracted 140 favorable responses, with the greatest interest in a master's degree program in medical-surgical nursing.[129]

A larger statewide survey of 1,779 Iowa nurses elicited interest from more than 500 respondents, most of whom were graduates of baccalaureate programs.[130] On the basis of such surveys, the graduate council committee recommended implementation of off-campus, part-time programs in Des Moines and in the Cedar Rapids/Waterloo areas, and the full graduate council accepted the committee's report in March 1975.[131] With support from a federal grant, the college began offering a medical-surgical graduate program in Des Moines in January 1976, with all nursing courses taught by College of Nursing faculty and courses in related fields offered at Drake University and Iowa State University.

Fresh on the heels of the major revision of the undergraduate curriculum, nursing faculty began in the mid-1970s a thorough revision of the graduate curriculum, a revision that generated some tension within faculty ranks over issues ranging from definitions of the fundamental concepts of graduate education and the essential elements of the graduate curriculum to the allocation of teaching assignments in the revamped program. From the outset, the relative isolation of the four program majors, each with its own faculty and staff, goals, and requirements, was a cause of special concern, a concern noted by the university review committee report of January 1975. In 1974, the College of Nursing's graduate program administrative council began work on a theoretical framework to apply to all nursing graduate programs, centered on the premise that graduate education assisted students "to increase their ability to analyze, synthesize, create and use specialized knowledge and to develop scholarship and leadership for the purpose of improving nursing practice."[132] In 1974-75, an *ad hoc* graduate council committee began a comprehensive study of the graduate curriculum in the context of current national trends in graduate education.[133] In the fall of 1975, pursuant to that committee's report, the graduate council as a whole established a series of task forces to deal with admission criteria, admission procedures, core courses, a common research component, and thesis advising.

The ensuing commitment of faculty time to graduate curriculum revision became an issue in itself; a fall 1976 survey of faculty opinion reflected concern over "heavy, but uneven" workloads, "ad hoc committees which seem to self generate," and work schedules "not at all conducive to scholarly endeavors."[134] That survey also offered abundant testimony that the present organizational format of the graduate program contributed "to isolationism and separatism" and to "overlapping of course content" within the different graduate majors. In short, as one faculty respondent put it, the result was four distinct graduate programs, "not the graduate program." Faculty also criticized the task force approach as too fragmented, affording no overarching plan or goal. Moreover, the chair of the graduate council admitted that progress toward curriculum revision had been slow, hindered by uncertainties regarding task force assignments, poorly defined problems, and various unnamed "diversions from productivity."[135]

As the curriculum revision moved haltingly forward, the graduate council requested an evaluation of each of the current majors, defining elements that were necessary, those deemed negotiable, perhaps to be included in core courses shared by all majors, and those that might be dispensable.[136] Once again, the nursing service administration major held much of the spotlight, and Eva Erickson, who had headed the program since its inception a decade earlier, once more defended a program that she saw as essential "to prepare professional nurses for top level administration of the delivery of nursing care in a complex health care facility."[137] Erickson contended that a separate administration program was imperative in order that the teaching of basic nursing administration concepts be undertaken by "one with expertise" in the field, but she conceded that some portions of the present curriculum, including the clinical component, could be part of a graduate core curriculum, while others could be taught by other university departments and colleges. The graduate faculty, reiterating its longstanding majority preference for clinical over functional specialization, recorded a preliminary vote to require clinical training in medical-surgical nursing for nursing service administration students, although leaving open the possibility of student petitions for alternative assignments.[138]

With reports from the various task forces taking shape, the graduate council agreed in November 1976 to have a single committee attempt to synthesize task force findings and to make recommendations.[139] Two months later, a curriculum consultant admonished the faculty that the time had come to make some hard decisions.[140] "The graduate program has been reviewed long enough," she said; "it is time to stop [talking about the problems] and tackle them." The consultant counseled setting short time-lines—no more than two months—for completion of specific tasks so that faculty could adopt at least the broad outline of a revised curriculum in spring 1977. She then recommended formation of three new task forces, the first to develop a new conceptual framework for graduate education that would be more acceptable to all majors; the second to collect data on local and regional needs for graduate education and the nature of the health care system; and the third to consider both the nature of the graduate student clientele and their needs and the learning theories underlying teaching strategies. Finally, she recommended a restructured graduate program consisting of a core, made up chiefly of research and nursing and leadership theory, along with "clusters of options" to allow students "to design individualized pathways through the program."

In fall 1977, with questions surrounding broad concepts and goals at last resolved, the graduate council adopted a series of specific measures regarding admission standards, curriculum organization and content, and graduation requirements.[141] The council envisioned a program of forty-five semester hours, including fifteen semester hours in core courses, fifteen semester hours in specialized courses, nine semester hours in supporting courses, and six semester hours allotted for thesis credit. Faculty continued to work on the new curriculum through the spring and summer of 1978, chiefly on the design of specific course offerings, the distribution of teaching assignments, and the specific duties of three proposed admissions committees. Although six task force committees continued to work through the 1978-79 academic year,[142] the college implemented the new graduate curriculum in fall 1978, offering just three areas of specialization, all of them clinical in focus—child health nursing, adult health nursing, and community/family health nursing—but with considerable flexibility in tailoring students' programs to individual interests, including functional concentrations in education, administration, and advanced practice.

Prospects for a doctoral program in the College of Nursing also attracted the first serious discussion in the 1970s. In the early and mid-1970s, nursing representatives from eleven participating universities in the Committee on Institutional Cooperation (CIC)—the Big Ten universities plus the University of Chicago—held a series of meetings regarding common problems, the prospects of sharing information and resources, and, in particular, the issue of establishing doctoral programs. University of Iowa College of Nursing Dean Evelyn Barritt and Professor Ada Jacox participated in the group and reported on CIC discussions to the College of Nursing faculty.[143] By early 1974, the University of Wisconsin, the University of Illinois, and Ohio State University had all announced plans for nursing doctoral programs; by autumn 1974, Indiana University and the University of Michigan, too, had announced such plans. In November 1974, CIC members met specifically to discuss "possible collaboration between schools of the CIC network around doctoral programs." Early in 1975, the group prepared a formal proposal for a study of resources for doctoral education in nursing in the midwest for submission to the US Office of Education.[144]

By 1976, the University of Iowa College of Nursing had created a committee to study the feasibility of a doctoral program, with Assistant Dean for the Graduate Program Marilyn Molen as chair. Molen's committee developed a series of position papers assessing questions such as the demand for doctoral education in Iowa and the surrounding area, the resources needed to conduct a viable doctoral program, and the comparative virtues of PhD and DSc programs.[145] The committee concluded that some form of doctoral program was not only feasible but "imperative" at some point in the near future,[146] arguing that "doctoral preparation for nurses is rapidly becoming the direction of the future" and that "this College has the responsibility and potential resources to provide quality doctoral education for an emerging profession." While admitting that demand for doctoral education in Iowa was "not intense," the committee warned that terminal master's programs, like that at the University of Iowa, would likely become less attractive both to students and potential faculty.

The committee's final feasibility report presented in April 1977 took the form of a strategic planning guide, aiming to achieve the needed ingredients for a doctoral program within the next decade.[147] The committee focused especially on the educational preparation and research productivity of faculty, both essential elements in the maintenance of a credible doctoral program and both, as committee members recognized, areas of obvious deficiency in the college. The report noted that the 11.4 percent of current nursing faculty with the doctorate compared favorably with the national average of 9.5 percent in nursing baccalaureate programs; however, the latter figure included a wide range of institutions, most without graduate programs of any kind. To redress the problem of faculty preparation, the committee recommended intensified programs of faculty development and faculty recruitment, both of which would require substantial support from the university administration. On the companion problem of research productivity, the committee noted that just three nursing faculty were then engaged in funded research and that prospects for a doctoral program rested on a sizable increase in such activity "in the next few years." In 1977, then, College of Nursing faculty were aware that a doctoral program was yet some years away; nonetheless, Marilyn Molen saw the revamped master's program and efforts to recruit better prepared faculty as encouraging steps toward that goal.[148]

Like the college's other educational endeavors, the scope of continuing education programs widened in the 1960s and 1970s as did program enrollments. By the early 1960s, the college offered an extensive program of non-credit conferences and workshops; the 1961-62 schedule, for example, included eleven dates and seven separate topics, including "Evaluation of Hospital Nursing Service

Personnel," "Administration of Diploma Programs in Nursing," and "Supervision of Nursing Care of Geriatric Patients." Those offerings were generally two to ten days in length; many featured special lecturers from other colleges and departments of the university, especially the College of Medicine, and also from other institutions. Likewise, the college scheduled some of its continuing education offerings at off-campus sites and in many cases co-sponsored events with other agencies, such as the Iowa Hospital Association and the Iowa Heart Association. Finally, the college also participated in regional efforts to coordinate continuing education programs.

By the late 1960s, under Pearl Zemlicka's direction, continuing education had expanded to ten or more topics each year and blended general issues, such as "Management Principles Applied to Nursing Services" and "Science Principles and Curriculum Building," with more specialized issues, such as "Nursing Care of the Patient with Myocardial Infarction" and "Growth and Development of Children." To a significant extent, continuing education was self-financing; in 1966-67, for example, continuing education programs attracted more than 400 registrants who paid some $12,000 in registration fees, compared to direct expenses of $8,900. However, as was the case throughout the college, federal funding was an important factor in the growth in continuing education. The university's dean of the Division of Extension apprised the college in October 1965 that Title I of the Higher Education Act of 1965 authorized matching funds, disbursed by the US Office of Education, "for general university extension programs" conducted as part of a statewide plan and "geared to aid in the solution of a community problem."[149] The college subsequently secured Title I funds for several projects, especially those related to the improvement of nursing service organization and administration, and 136 Iowa nurses enrolled in Title I programs in 1969-70.

Through much of the 1960s, the College of Nursing faculty curriculum committee assumed responsibility for continuing education, attempting to provide more formal philosophical and methodological foundations for those programs and also seeking input from potential audiences regarding needs and interests. Late in the decade, a service affairs committee inherited responsibility for continuing education along with broader issues surrounding the college's public service role. The service affairs committee developed a comprehensive position paper on continuing education and also devised goals, both short and long term, for the program. With a reorganization of the faculty in the early 1970s, a continuing education council superseded the service affairs committee, and, in the later 1970s, the college added an assistant dean for continuing education. Beginning in 1976-77, the college sent annual continuing education announcements to all nurses holding Iowa licenses, some 19,000 in Iowa and 6,000 outside the state, and those programs—thirty-five on campus and eighteen off campus—attracted 2,750 nurses.[150]

Governance and Faculty Development

Diminutive, yet feisty, witty, and occasionally irreverent, Laura Dustan had an uncommon capacity to charm supporters and critics alike. Certainly, University of Iowa President Howard Bowen and his successor Willard Boyd appear to have been much taken with Dustan, using the simple salutation "Dear Laura" in much of their correspondence with the dean. In her December 1970 letter of resignation, Dustan noted that she had been offered "a unique professional opportunity" to become assistant commissioner for nursing services for the New York State Department of Health. However, she observed also that the college deserved "the opportunity for periodic reassessment of its leadership, of its objectives, and of its future directions."[151] Thanking President Boyd for his "firm support" in his years first as dean, then vice president, and now president, she testified that her tenure at the University of Iowa had "been the most challenging and stimulating of my entire professional career" and that "a part of my heart" would remain always in Iowa. In response, the president commended the dean for her exemplary service to the college and the university, especially for the new building then under construction and for the "spirit" pervading nursing faculty and students.[152]

Planning to step down in January 1972, Dustan recommended Etta Rasmussen's appointment as acting dean, a recommendation based on Rasmussen's long experience in the college, her previous stints as acting dean, her reputation among the nursing faculty, and her recent service as assistant dean.[153] After Dustan's departure, the university provost confirmed Rasmussen's appointment and named a seven-member deanship search committee, with professor Ada Jacox as chair. The search committee considered several candidates, including Mary M. Lohr, since 1966 dean of the University of Illinois College of Nursing and a former member of the University of Iowa nursing faculty; Eileen M. Jacobi, then executive director of the American Nurses Association; Rosemary Ellis, a professor at Case Western Reserve University; Evelyn R. Barritt, dean of the Capital University School of Nursing in Columbus, Ohio, and previously assistant executive director of the Ohio State Nurses' Association; and Virginia Jarratt, dean of the Harris College of Nursing of Texas Christian University.[154] The search committee solicited comments and recommendations from several quarters on those and other candidates. Former Dean Myrtle Kitchell Aydelotte declined to name specific individuals but noted in general that the circumstances of nursing were "fraught with change, dilemma, and turmoil," and the former dean counseled that the new dean should "be inquiring, analytical, open-minded, courageous, and innovative." In light of the important decisions facing nursing education, Aydelotte warned, "The boat may have to be rocked."[155]

Lohr, Jacobi, and Jarratt visited the campus in late spring 1971, and Jarratt in particular garnered strong support from the selection committee, from nursing faculty, and from nursing students. In late July, however, the selection committee reported that all three initial candidates were either unavailable or unacceptable.[156] Evelyn Barritt made a campus visit in the fall, and the selection committee, with support from faculty and students, recommended her appointment in December 1971, an appointment confirmed by the Board of Regents in March 1972.[157] A native of Royal Oak, Michigan, Barritt had an Iowa connection, receiving an associate of arts degree from Graceland Junior College in Lamoni, Iowa, in 1949. She then earned a diploma in nursing from the Independence, Missouri, Sanitarium and Hospital School in 1952 before earning a bachelor of science degree in nursing in 1956, master of arts in 1962, and doctor of philosophy in higher education administration in 1971 from Ohio State University. Asked by the search committee for her opinion of Barritt, Rozella Schlotfeldt described her as a "magnificent person" who was "bright, sensible, and a diplomat."

For her part, Barritt pointed to a series of educational innovations she had overseen at Capital University.

Evelyn Barritt came to the deanship at the College of Nursing with the professed goal of enhancing the image of nursing education as a scholarly enterprise. Likewise, she shared with her predecessor Laura Dustan a desire to improve women's position within the university community. Despite Howard Bowen's and Willard Boyd's emphasis on affirmative action and despite changes in policies and procedures meant to give women a greater voice in university affairs, the dean of nursing remained through the 1960s and 1970s the only female collegiate dean on campus. Laura Dustan recounted with particular relish a commencement procession in which the deans, as was customary, marched in chronological order based on the year of their colleges' establishment, a scheme that left "little Laura Dustan bringing up the rear." In her remarks to the commencement audience, Dustan took as her theme the enjoinder from the book of Matthew: "Many that are first shall be last; and the last shall be first." And, as predicted, the closing recession—with the deans marching in reverse order—placed the dean of nursing first, striding directly behind President Bowen to the accompaniment of a ripple of laughter from an appreciative audience.

Humor aside, both Dustan and Barritt, like many other women before and since, chafed at the male-dominated university culture. That culture made adjustment difficult for nursing faculty, who were often young, single women, and Dustan at one point suggested that shortterm university housing might ease their integration into university circles.[158] Dustan also sought to increase the level of sensitivity regarding gender issues on the university campus. On one occasion, she complained of a particularly tasteless display of sexism in the medical students' publication *Autopsy*. "Are we supposed to look to these men (?) as <u>leaders</u> of the health team?" she asked in a letter to Willard Boyd.[159] On another occasion, when a local newspaper consigned to the "women's section" a story on a College of Nursing research project on the alleviation of pain, the dean objected to the editor that pain had "no sex linkage," and therefore the story hardly belonged "on the page reserved for the announcements of engagements, marriages, recipes, and the like."[160] At the same time, as noted earlier, women's second-class status was an undercurrent in the campaign for the new Nursing Building, putting Dustan and her colleagues ever on the alert to fend off challenges for priority in funding and in site selection.

Having grown to maturity in the late 1930s, Dustan did not count herself an ardent feminist, at least not as that term was understood in the late 1960s and early 1970s. In contrast, however, the campus newspaper touted her successor Evelyn Barritt as a model of the "new woman," combining marriage and family responsibilities with professional aspirations.[161] Like Dustan, Barritt was a determined champion of women's place in the larger university community, for example, serving on a university-wide affirmative action task force charged with the review of each of the university's colleges and academic areas and, closer to home, objecting to the lack of female representation in planning for what was to be the first of several major expansion projects at the University of Iowa Hospitals and Clinics. In the latter case, Barritt denounced the existing planning structure "as a combination physician-male chauvinistic program"[162] For the same reason, Barritt sought to include female representation on the University of Iowa Hospitals and Clinics advisory committee.

"Modern woman" or not, Laura Dustan, much like Myrtle Kitchell, claimed allegiance to the principles of inclusion and responsiveness in her design of an administrative structure for the College of Nursing. In a tongue-in-cheek reminiscence at the December 1971 dedication of the Nursing Building, Dustan professed to remember just two instances of "authoritarian" rule during her tenure as dean, one of which had turned out badly and one of which, in contrast, had been a striking success. The first involved a change in student uniforms from traditional pinstripe to blue, a change accomplished at the expense of considerable faculty time and energy but one that students most emphatically deplored. After seeing "Dustan's dusters" lampooned in a student skit, the dean resolved in future to leave the question of uniforms to student committees. Her second anecdote involved a change in the nursing faculty's informal dress code, a change accomplished by example in the fall of 1970 when "the Dean of the College of Nursing appeared at her office in a pantsuit." The following morning, Dustan reported, "the College of Nursing blossomed with pantsuits."

Early on, Dustan effected a reform of the college's administration (Figure 4.4). In September 1965, she notified faculty of the elimination of the existing director of programs for graduate nurses, a move reflecting the adoption of a single baccalaureate curriculum, and the naming of an assistant dean to assume responsibility for graduate and practical nursing programs. The undergraduate program, with five clinical departments, came under the purview of the dean and an administrative assistant. By that time, the college's administrative staff had also grown considerably, including a dozen secretaries assigned to the dean, the assistant dean, the administrative assistants, and to each of the college's educational programs.

Several factors led Dustan to propose significant organizational changes in the late 1960s, changes accepted in principle by the university's central administration. Dustan argued that increased enrollments in undergraduate and graduate programs, coupled with an enlarged faculty roster and the enhanced stature of the college had "overtaxed" the existing administrative structure, making it impossible to provide the kind and degree of support necessary for a

Fig. 4.4. College of Nursing Administration, September 1965

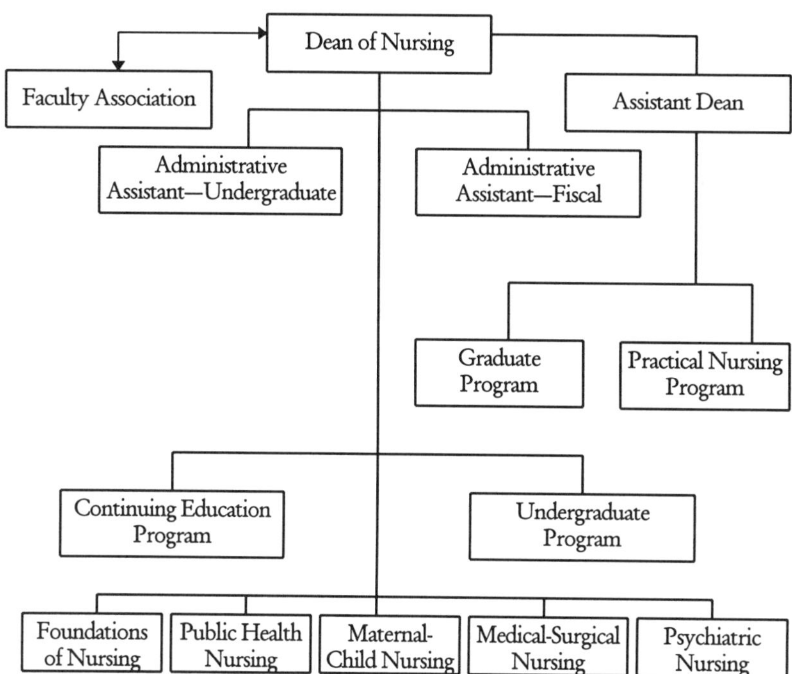

"rigorous, satisfying, and creative" educational enterprise.[163] Moreover, the dean noted that the longstanding departmental structure of the college, roughly paralleling that in the College of Medicine, was "not well suited to the way in which the College actually operates." Originally meant to bring together as a unit all faculty involved in specified content areas, the structure tended also to compartmentalize faculty, Dustan argued, and it ignored the fact that not all undergraduate concentrations were connected to corresponding graduate programs and vice versa. Dustan then proposed to complement the existing assistant dean of graduate programs with an assistant dean of undergraduate programs to oversee undergraduate education programs that would be divided into functional course groups rather than the current specialty departments. A part of Dustan's plan came unhinged, however, when the university failed to fund the undergraduate assistant dean position, forcing Dustan to shuffle personnel in a fall-back plan.

Early on in her tenure, Dustan reorganized the faculty body, creating a Faculty Association governed by formal by-laws and charged with defining "philosophy, purpose, and objectives" for the college, recommending "policies relating to student and faculty affairs," formulating "curriculum patterns and policies," and promoting "the welfare of the students and faculty." As chair of the Faculty Association, the dean served also as chair of an executive council, consisting of the faculty secretary, the chairs of three standing committees (curriculum, student affairs, and faculty affairs), and one elected representative for every ten faculty members. According to the by-laws, the executive council's role was to advise the dean "on such matters as she presents" in addition to receiving reports and recommendations from association committees, appointing members of standing committees, and creating and charging *ad hoc* committees.[164] In 1967, an amendment to the by-laws extended the definition of faculty to include all full- and part-time personnel with the rank of instructor and above as well as assistants in instruction with more than one year's experience. In 1969, the association included two classes of members, regular and associate, the latter—who had the privilege of attendance and voice but not the vote—were lecturers and assistants in instruction in the first year of their appointments. By 1971, the by-laws included two further changes, first, adding the phrase "to promote nursing research activities" to the faculty association's purposes and including the same language among the functions of the faculty affairs committee and, second, allowing for the appointment of undergraduate student members to standing committees.[165]

Early in Evelyn Barritt's tenure, the Faculty Association became the College of Nursing Association.[166] Under by-laws adopted in May 1973, membership encompassed four classifications: active members, including all persons participating "in the major functions of teaching, research, and service"; adjunct members with primary appointments outside the college; associate members, comprising ten undergraduate and two graduate students elected representatives as well as student appointees to the various association councils; and affiliate members from outside the college elected to membership by the association. The association assigned chief responsibility in designated areas to five councils—undergraduate affairs, graduate affairs, continuing education, faculty affairs, and research. Council chairs, elected by the association for two-year terms, were full professors in the college. Meanwhile, changes in the administrative structure of the college under Evelyn Barritt included appointment of an assistant dean of undergraduate academic affairs, an assistant dean of undergraduate curriculum affairs, and an assistant dean for the graduate program, plus, at a later date, an assistant dean for continuing education.

Throughout the period from 1965 to 1980, faculty development was the most troubling issue in the college. In a 1966 letter to University of Iowa President Howard Bowen, Myrtle Kitchell Aydelotte noted bluntly that, in the aggregate, the present nursing faculty was weak in "academic preparation, clinical competence, and scholarly productivity."[167] Moreover, Dean Laura Dustan was well aware of the problem and called faculty development her greatest frustration as dean; in a 1967 report to the North Central Association, Dustan listed among her college's problems the educational backgrounds of faculty and their lack of commitment to research.[168] In a June 1967 note, Dustan also observed that turnover among nursing faculty averaged as much as one-third each year and that "without question, faculty recruitment is the most difficult, frustrating, and time-consuming aspect of my position as Dean"[169]—a sentiment likely shared by her predecessors and successors in more or less equal measure.

A 1969 faculty affairs committee study assessing factors that had led current faculty to seek appointments to the college shed some light on the basic problem in faculty development, particularly the issue of low research productivity.[170]   Thirty-seven of sixty-one faculty members gave "opportunity to utilize own knowledge and skills in area of choice" as the most important factor in their decision to join the faculty, outdistancing all other factors by a considerable margin. The second most important reason, "nature of teaching load and assignment," was closely related. Beyond that, serendipity appears to have been a major factor in faculty decision-making, with twenty-two respondents already living in the area prior to joining the faculty and eighteen more coming to the university because of a spouse employed or in school in the area. Meanwhile, just one respondent listed "opportunity to engage in research" as most important in her decision-making, and twenty-seven listed research as having had "no influence." Overall, respondents gave research opportunities the same ranking as "availability of leisure time activities."

In 1970, according to a College of Nursing accreditation report to the National League for Nursing, the college boasted only one full professor, Myrtle Kitchell Aydelotte, in addition to Dean Dustan, and Aydelotte was full-time nursing service director at University Hospitals. The faculty also included ten associate professors, just four of whom held doctoral degrees, three of them in education and one in sociology. A fifth associate professor was then a doctoral candidate in education at Columbia University Teacher's College. Of the other five, all had received their first nursing degrees in the 1930s, four of those from diploma programs, and all currently held master's degrees in nursing education, nursing service administration, or public health. The college listed twenty-five faculty at the rank of assistant professor, all holding master's degrees in nursing, education, or public health. A total of thirty-seven faculty, then, held the rank of assistant professor or above in 1970. The college also employed seventeen faculty at the level of instructor, sixteen holding master's degrees and one—an administrative assistant for the undergraduate program—holding a bachelor's degree. Finally, the faculty list included thirteen assistants in instruction, all of whom, possessed bachelor's degrees.[171]

In terms of the proportion of faculty holding advanced degrees, the college had made significant strides in the 1960s. However, the situation was still far from ideal; in particular, the college had made little progress on the research front by 1970. In part, the latter reflected the relatively low levels of available funding for nursing research, primarily from federal agencies. In 1969-70, for example, the University of Iowa College of Medicine attracted more than $6 million in research grants; by that standard, funding for nursing research, amounting to scarcely more than a few thousand dollars, was minuscule. Nursing faculty in 1971 contacted university authorities seeking additional local support for nursing research, including seed money to develop research ideas.[172]

The availability of funding was not the only issue; research productivity was also a function of educational preparation and professional acculturation, with the doctoral degree serving, however imperfectly, as a barometer of research interest and potential. In contrast, master's degree programs—whether in one of the clinical specialties or in nursing education—rarely provided a rigorous grounding in research problems and methods. A 1972 review committee report noted that in the previous five years College of Nursing faculty had participated in just four federally funded research projects.[173]

The college's 1974 accreditation report listed seventy-nine faculty, including assistants in instruction, a 22.4 percent increase in four years. Forty-seven of the seventy-nine held the rank of assistant professor or above, an increase of 27.0 percent over 1970. The faculty count included five full professors, all of them possessing doctoral degrees; ten associate professors, five of them possessing doctoral degrees; thirty-two assistant professors, all possessing master's degrees; twenty-two instructors, all likewise possessing master's degrees; and ten assistants in instruction possessing bachelor's degrees. Of the ten doctoral degrees, seven were in education, one in anatomy, one in psychology, and one in sociology. Overall, eighty percent of the growth in faculty numbers since 1970 had come in the ranks of instructor and assistant professor.

As faculty numbers grew and as nursing education achieved a greater measure of maturity, questions surrounding promotion and tenure claimed a prominent and sometimes divisive place in faculty affairs, especially the relationship between tenure and promotion standards in the college and prevailing standards elsewhere in the university. In January 1967, the College of Nursing Faculty Association considered instituting a peer review policy for assessing and recommending promotions. In response, Dean Laura Dustan reviewed the history of promotion decisions, noting that such decisions had previously been handled by department chairs and the dean. Dustan also emphasized that the college must, in its promotion decisions, keep in mind university standards for research and publication.[174] A year later, the faculty adopted new policies for promotion, serving both as formal criteria for promotion and as guidelines for faculty self-development.[175]

The new policies emphasized that teaching and research were "the central functions of the faculty" and that other "professional contributions"—to the college, the university, or the profession—were "subsidiary to these fundamental tasks." However, in a significant departure from the university faculty manual, the criteria accepted the master's degree, rather than the doctorate, as the minimum credential for promotion to the level of assistant professor, along with "promise of scholarly productivity, supported by publication or equivalent"—an exemption granted for a period of five years by then Vice President for Academic Affairs Willard Boyd. Special projects and "activities which contribute to the improvement of competency in teaching nursing" could substitute for the stated research requirement. The new promotion criteria vested responsibility for promotion recommendations in three faculty committees: one committee made up of full professors to recommend candidates for that rank; a second committee made up of associate and full professors to recommend candidates for associate professor; and a third committee made up of assistant, associate, and full professors to recommend candidates for assistant professor. Each committee was to "select the names of persons to be considered for promotion and/or tenure" and to seek written information on candidates from the dean and other faculty as necessary. Committee recommendations, along "with supporting information," were due in the dean's office by the end of February each year.

Under normal university procedure, faculty recommendations regarding promotions went first to the dean of the college, who then passed on those recommendations, with comments, to the university provost, with ultimate authority over promotion and tenure residing in the university's governing Board of Regents. However, nursing faculty raised questions regarding candidates' rights to be informed of the outcome of peer-group deliberations before final decisions by the provost and Regents. At a November 1969 meeting of the faculty association, Provost Ray Heffner advised against such an "interruption" of the promotion process, emphasizing the tentative nature of all promotion and tenure decisions at the level of peer-group review.[176]

Thanks to the new guidelines and the college's five-year exemption from more stringent university requirements, the promotion and tenure conundrum receded into the background for a time. However, in April 1973, the College of Nursing's faculty affairs committee notified faculty colleagues of the impending expiration of the exemption and asked for input regarding various aspects of the promotion procedure.[177] Reviewing the situation in August 1973, Dean Barritt urged the importance of "continued education for all faculty."[178] In January 1974, the renamed faculty affairs council submitted modified promotion criteria to the full faculty for consideration and adoption,[179] recommendations that still did not impose the doctoral requirement for appointment at the rank of assistant professor but did specify the doctorate as a requirement for the granting of tenure and promotion to associate professor.

The council's recommendations also failed to specify a limit on time spent at the rank of assistant professor, disregarding a university policy requiring that assistant professors achieve tenure—that is, an earned doctorate and promotion to associate professor—within a seven-year period or face mandatory termination. For the College of Nursing, that was as important as the issue of promotion itself, since many faculty at the rank of assistant professor lacked the normal credentials and experience for tenure and were near or, in some cases, beyond the time limit specified for promotion or termination. The university administration resolved that issue by granting the college yet another exemption, this one, in effect, setting the "tenure calendar" to zero in all such cases, effective July 1, 1974.[180] The aim, as Special Assistant to the President David Vernon explained in what became known as the "Vernon memo," was "to be completely fair to the Nursing faculty" yet ultimately "to treat College of Nursing faculty members as we do faculty members in other academic units of the University." Aiming to bring promotion and tenure decisions in the college into line with general university guidelines by 1980, Vernon was optimistic that "with a fresh start and with full understanding of the expectations,...the faculty members in the College can and will meet the standards."

Given the frank expectations expressed in the "Vernon memo," issues surrounding promotion and tenure consumed an increasing proportion of nursing faculty time and energy in the years that followed. The 1974 appointment of May Brodbeck as the university's vice president for academic affairs and dean of the faculty was a significant event in the unfolding promotion and tenure drama, marking—in the view of historian Stow Persons—a commitment by the central administration to closer scrutiny of faculty recruitment and promotion decisions throughout the university and to the more uniform enforcement of university regulations in that regard.[181] Brodbeck circulated a no-nonsense communication regarding promotion policy to all university faculty in November 1975, a communication based on the latest edition, not yet released, of the university faculty handbook.[182] Under the revised guidelines, appointments at the assistant professor rank were not "ordinarily" to exceed seven years, with faculty given a one-year terminal appointment at the end of six years. Moreover, faculty promoted from instructor to assistant professor, a common pattern in the College of Nursing, were not to exceed a combined seven years prior to tenure or termination. Also, Brodbeck noted that for faculty currently exceeding the seven-year limit "a review leading to a tenure or termination decision should be initiated immediately." Brodbeck cited provisions in the handbook enjoining deans to make promotion recommendations "in consultation with the collegiate faculty," although without specifying the nature or degree of consultation. Finally, Brodbeck provided a detailed list of supporting materials to accompany all promotion recommendations forwarded to her office, including reports of collegiate promotion review committees.

Brodbeck's communication was evidence that the university's central administration intended to implement more uniform promotion policies across the board, an issue of special concern to the College of Nursing where, in Stow Persons' count, more than thirty assistant professors and instructors had reached at least the sixth year of their appointments with little prospect of gaining tenure. In December 1975, the college's faculty affairs council held an emergency meeting to discuss responses to the new guidelines and attempted to schedule a meeting with both Vice President Brodbeck and President Willard Boyd to explore several issues, including the impact of the latest guidelines on the "Vernon memo" of 1974 and the degree of latitude open to the college in making promotion decisions.[183] One alternative, proposed by Dean Barritt to Brodbeck and to the nursing faculty, was creation of a clinical associate category, a non-tenured teaching faculty of "persons with records of excellent clinical teaching and service to this institution."[184] Clinical associates would not, Barritt assured the faculty, be "second-class citizens" in terms of salary or participation in college affairs. At one point at least, Brodbeck was apparently receptive to creation of such a clinical track, but nursing faculty, by and large, were not.[185]

At a December 16, 1975, meeting, Vice President Brodbeck assured nursing faculty of her understanding of the special problems facing the college, not least the importance of retaining faculty of demonstrated quality whose credentials fell short of accepted norms, the small recruiting pool of potential nurse faculty—scarcely 700 nationwide—holding the doctorate, and her willingness to work with the college's faculty affairs council to arrive at a satisfactory compromise.[186] The nursing faculty created an ad hoc committee on promotion and tenure, made up of the faculty council and six additional members, to pursue further discussions with Brodbeck. Among the many issues raised by committee members in anticipation of talks with the vice president, perhaps the most important were whether or not the university was prepared to commit the resources necessary to hire greater numbers of nursing faculty with doctoral degrees, assuming that such candidates could be found, and whether or not the college could devise equivalent standards, short of the doctoral degree, to meet the intent of university requirements for faculty promotion. Again and again, committee members voiced concern over the difficulties in the way of faculty self-development and research in the face of existing teaching commitments and administrative tasks. At one point, however, Dean Barritt objected to that line of argument, asking if the intended message was "that our faculty were incapable of any scholarly work by 1980."

Committee members agreed to prepare a "white paper" for Vice President Brodbeck, the finished draft of which provided essential background information "concerning nursing in general and the College of Nursing in particular."[187] Reviewing the peculiar history of nursing education, the committee pointed out that more than eighty percent of registered nurses nationwide currently lacked baccalaureate credentials and only 0.2 percent held doctoral degrees. Also, just forty-six nurses had received doctoral degrees in 1974. Under the circumstances, the committee argued, "no university nursing program...could realistically expect doctoral preparation as a prerequisite for all faculty appointments at the assistant professor level." Nor, they argued, could the college "possibly adhere to a rigid time limit for pre-tenured probationary status and expect to maintain a stable faculty."

The committee counted twenty-two assistant professors currently exceeding six years in rank but considered "vital to the continued implementation of the newly adopted integrated curriculum." An additional twenty-eight faculty at the rank of assistant professor and instructor could well exceed the six-year limit by 1980. The committee then cited the extraordinary changes underway in the health care system, changes that placed ever greater responsibilities on professional nurses and, by extension, on university educational programs. Against Dean Barritt's earlier advice, the committee argued that the time and effort invested by nursing faculty in basic teaching functions, in curriculum revision, and in general self-improvement made it difficult, if not impossible, for them to pursue research and formal coursework toward advanced degrees.

After several meetings with the college's faculty affairs council, Vice President Brodbeck addressed a special meeting of the full nursing faculty in February 1976. The vice president congratulated her audience for "very excellent work" on the difficult issues at hand; however, she expressed concern that all faculty fully understand the promotion process and the expectations surrounding it. Nursing faculty were assured that the much-discussed "Vernon memo" had not been superseded and that all faculty appointed prior to 1974 were still under its protection. Nonetheless, Brodbeck emphasized, no faculty member was therefore assured of a six-year contract; all non-tenured faculty were subject to reappointment at the expiration of current contracts. In a real sense, then, particularly with regard to peer review and evaluation, the promotion-tenure issue grew to encompass annual reappointments of non-tenured faculty.

Through the remainder of the spring and into the autumn of 1976, College of Nursing faculty wrestled with the details of the promotion-tenure-reappointment policy, especially with the issue of candidates' rights of access to materials compiled in their personal files. On the latter point, the faculty agreed in February that files would be open until submitted to the appropriate peer review committee.[188] However, barely a month later, faculty reconsidered the just-adopted procedures when one candidate for promotion objected that letters had been placed in her file literally on the eve of her peer review committee meeting.[189] That was not, she maintained, in keeping with either the spirit or the letter of the declared open-files procedure. Lengthy faculty discussion, recorded and transcribed verbatim, led to objections from others that specified deadlines had been ignored and that peer review committees had, contrary to stated policy, solicited oral information regarding specific candidates. At the same time, however, one faculty member interjected that she had sat "through these things [peer review committee proceedings] for now seven years" and that the new procedures represented "a decided improvement" over the past.

In the end, a majority of faculty agreed that there existed significant procedural shortcomings in the just approved guidelines. The faculty then charged the faculty affairs council to clarify the time sequence and the data collection and evaluation procedures and to present its proposals at the first fall meeting of the College of Nursing Association. In a separate motion, faculty also agreed that, for that year only, candidates could have belated access "to the data gathered from persons designated by them and from persons designated by the peer [review] group." In addition, the association agreed to support candidates' attempts "to correct inaccurate data," although the procedure for doing so was not at all clear, since the promotion recommendations had already gone to the office of the vice president for academic affairs.

In October 1976, the faculty affairs council, as instructed, submitted its procedural revisions to the full faculty for consideration, procedures based in large part on the university handbook.[190] At an October 22 meeting attended by Vice President Brodbeck and devoted entirely to the promotion and tenure issue, the nursing faculty, after lengthy discussion and minor amendments, adopted the new promotion guidelines.[191] The most important provisions were, first, to designate the faculty affairs council as faculty advocate during the promotion and tenure procedure; second, to ensure that "all evaluative data to be utilized by the peer group are open to the candidate" and that candidates might add pertinent material to their files; third, to set a detailed schedule for the promotion procedure, beginning with selection of candidates for promotion by the second Monday in October each year; fourth, to allow peer review committees to seek outside evaluations; and, finally, to provide detailed rules of operation for peer review committees. After reviewing the promotion process during the 1976-77 academic year, the faculty affairs council suggested and the College of Nursing Association adopted a range of minor amendments in May 1977.[192]

For all the effort that went into it, the new promotion procedures did not address the fundamental problem of the looming 1980 expiration of the grace period granted nursing instructors and assistant professors under the 1974 "Vernon memo." And while the 1970s did bring some improvement in the level of research and scholarly publication within the college, the degree of faculty participation in those endeavors varied widely. Likewise, few faculty took steps toward attaining doctoral credentials. In the meantime, a high faculty turnover rate, especially among junior faculty, continued to plague the college and further complicated the issue of faculty development. In 1975-76, for example, the college recorded thirty faculty resignations, constituting roughly a third of instructional staff, including ten assistant professors, twelve instructors, and seven assistants in instruction.[193]

In 1973, the faculty had organized a research committee—later named the research council—to develop funding sources for faculty and graduate student research projects and to compile guidelines for the evaluation of research proposals. The college also administered a grant from the Graduate Fund for Nursing Education and a College of Nursing Faculty Development Fund, which together helped to nurture scholarly work through small research grants and support for visiting professors of national stature. There were also a handful of instances in which faculty successfully pursued external grants. One of the earliest—an effort headed by Ada Jacox and funded in 1971 by a two-year grant of $82,000 from the US Public Health Service Division of Nursing—studied patient responses to pain and the efficacy of nursing intervention in the alleviation of pain. The Division of Nursing in 1973 renewed funding for that project for an additional three years. In addition to her research, Ada Jacox served as mentor to several young faculty and graduate students, and her departure in 1977 was, by all accounts, a significant blow to the research aspirations of the college.

Two 1976 College of Nursing studies, the first surveying faculty appointment factors and the second surveying faculty retention factors, showed some similarities and some differences in faculty attitudes toward research compared to the 1969 study described earlier.[194] As in 1969, "opportunity to utilize own knowledge and skills in area of choice" and "courses included in teaching assignment" were strong positive factors in faculty appointment and retention in 1976, while research opportunities again were relatively insignificant in faculty career decisions. Importantly, especially in light of the ongoing concern over promotion and tenure, more than half of all faculty respondents in 1976 pointed to "opportunity for promotion in rank and tenure" as "moderately or strongly influencing me to want to leave," even though a large majority of faculty also cited "opportunities for continued education through formal courses" at the university as positive influences in their career choices. From the point of view of faculty, the heavy teaching loads, both undergraduate and graduate, and limited resources to provide release time for individual development were major obstacles to scholarly productivity. Also, faculty commonly cited the lack of research space, an issue not considered in the design of the new Nursing Building, as a hindrance to the development of a research orientation in the college, even though the University of Iowa Hospitals and Clinics, with Myrtle Kitchell Aydelotte as director of nursing services, answered some of the research space need.

Overall, the faculty appointment and retention study only highlighted the lack of an established research culture in the College of Nursing. That situation, which reflected the situation in the nursing profession at large, was surely the largest single obstacle to enhanced scholarly productivity. Importantly, too, Evelyn Barritt's background in research and publication was limited at the time of her appointment to the deanship, a fact that had concerned Aydelotte and perhaps other senior faculty at the time. In the absence of a well established research culture, research expectations were minimal and would-be researchers found few peer models and discouragingly little real encouragement within the college.

Those and other issues were central to a blowup in the college in the spring and summer of 1979. Many of the details of events are hidden by documents either missing from the archives or closed to inspection; nonetheless, most of the essential facts are a matter of public record.[195] In April 1979, displeased with Dean Evelyn Barritt's leadership, a group of senior nursing faculty petitioned university President Willard Boyd for an administrative review of the college, citing "decreasing academic vitality and the accelerated decline in the stature of the College of Nursing." In later court depositions, dissenting faculty stressed that they had not sought the dean's dismissal. A few days later, the group met with Boyd, and, in early May, Vice President Brodbeck named a university committee headed by law professor William G. Buss to review the college.

Dissenting faculty met with President Boyd a second time in June, a meeting apparently scheduled to discuss general grievances but one which, instead, centered on charges that the dean or her agents had eavesdropped on faculty conversations. Those charges stemmed from a recent incident in which the dean's secretary had interrupted a telephone conversation between one member of the dissident group and her lawyer. So-called "wiretapping," then, became a part of the controversy, although at least one of the principals later dismissed the incident in question as a trivial matter. Whatever the case, the university review committee concluded in August that "the mutual enmity" between the dean and some faculty "is very bitter and runs very deep." On August 24, 1979, President Boyd and Vice President Brodbeck asked for Dean Evelyn Barritt's resignation—submitted on August 29 and accepted by Boyd the following day.[196]

That bare-bones recitation surely obscures much about the matters at hand. Certainly, for a group of faculty to approach the university president in such a fashion was an extraordinary occurrence. That alone suggests serious problems in the college but offers little insight into the nature of those problems. Certainly, too,

Evelyn Barritt struck many observers as enthusiastic, energetic, and capable; moreover, she attained a degree of national recognition during her tenure, serving as president of the American Association of Colleges of Nursing in 1976-78. Yet available evidence, both documentary and anecdotal, suggests long-festering tensions between the dean and some faculty members, tensions perhaps stretching back to Barritt's initial appointment to the deanship. Those tensions were readily apparent by the mid-1970s, but the dean, for whatever reason, ignored the deepening rift within the college, or so some observers attest.

Events of the spring and summer of 1979 brought to light disputes over salaries, teaching and administrative assignments, and the dean's administrative style. In addition, faculty raised charges of secret personnel files and intimidation of individual faculty members and complained of the dean's general inability to manage faculty and college affairs. In turn, Barritt charged that an "old girls network" had undermined her authority and poisoned faculty meetings and day-to-day operations in the college. Barritt also traced dissident faculty members' complaints to two principal causes: first, stressful changes in the college—most of which the faculty itself had endorsed and over which the dean had little personal control—and, second, her determination to function as a strong administrator rather than a "matriarchal" figure.

For its part, the university review committee pointed to two precipitating factors in the controversy. The first was conflict over the new graduate program, specifically over last minute changes reportedly instituted during the summer of 1978 without the approval of some senior faculty. The second element related to the long troubling issue of promotion and tenure, an issue that had first arisen in the mid-1970s when some senior faculty had objected to the dean's decision to promote one faculty member to full professor. The issue of promotion and tenure came to a head in the spring of 1979 when the dean departed from peer review committee recommendations with regard to five faculty members—two reportedly recommended for promotion by the dean but not by peer review committees and three recommended by peer review committees but not by the dean.[197] Student concerns, too, became an issue and led to a late summer meeting between student leaders and President Boyd, who conceded that "faculty and administrative politics had led to an atmosphere of mistrust and little open communication within the College of Nursing."[198]

With Evelyn Barritt's resignation in hand and without consultation with the nursing faculty, President Boyd named Sue Rosner, an associate professor of psychology, as acting College of Nursing dean in September 1979. In January 1980, Evelyn Barritt became dean of the University of Miami School of Nursing and filed suit against eight University of Iowa faculty members, charging that they had "intentionally and maliciously" harmed her reputation. One defendant filed a countersuit in February complaining of salary problems and "irregularities in the promotion-tenure process." Fed by rounds of motions, depositions, and other maneuvers, the legal contest dragged on until an out-of-court settlement of Barritt's suit in September 1981, a settlement neither initiated nor welcomed by the defendants but negotiated by the state attorney general's office which was, by law, charged with the legal defense of university employees in work-related cases.

In the meantime, the College of Nursing faced the imminent expiration of the six-year grace period framed in 1974, and it was clear by fall 1979 that few of the affected faculty could meet university requirements for promotion and tenure. Facing a hard choice and obviously sympathetic to the college's plight, Vice President Brodbeck chose "the humane alternative," in historian Stow Persons' words, and proposed to grant tenure at present rank to the remaining twenty-two assistant professors and one instructor still on faculty and covered by the 1974 memo.[199] An extraordinary departure from university norms, Brodbeck's decision, as she must have known would be the case, triggered vigorous objections from the university's faculty senate and some dissent within the College of Nursing as well.[200] In response, the university faculty senate established a select committee on academic standards to investigate the situation and to make recommendations.

The eighteen members of the faculty senate committee maintained in their report that "longstanding University standards of performance in teaching, research, and service pertaining to faculty appointments, promotions, and tenure are the cornerstone on which the University as a major educational institution rests."[201] To depart from the standards "in any significant degree" would, the committee held, "compromise the mission of the University and jeopardize its standing among major universities." The committee admitted that those standards had arisen in "more established disciplines" with "the great advantage" of longstanding research programs and practices and that accommodation to those practices by "newer disciplines" such as nursing was a difficult matter. Nonetheless, the committee argued that the College of Nursing's integrity as an academic institution depended on its "standing on an equal footing with the other collegiate faculties of the University."

The committee then recommended that the college "continue its efforts to attract well qualified appointees" and "encourage and assist the scholarly development of its present faculty." As for the probationary faculty at the heart of the controversy, the committee said that the college "should review the qualifications" of each and take appropriate action on a case-by-case basis. In the committee's view, those deemed to have satisfied university requirements should be recommended for promotion and tenure; those who "have made significant scholarly progress" and showed promise of satisfying promotion requirements within three years should be given contract extensions; those who "have made valuable contributions as teachers" but showed little propensity for scholarship should be given clinical (that is, non-tenure track) status; and those who showed little promise as teachers and even less as scholars should be terminated. Vice President Brodbeck apprised tenured nursing faculty of the university faculty senate's ruling in a January 1980 memo,[202] terms later reiterated by both Brodbeck and Acting Dean Rosner.

While a thorough assessment of the problems that beset the College of Nursing in the late 1970s awaits the release of further documentation, much of what transpired was undoubtedly the product of tensions growing out of an important transition in nursing education. In the 1950s and early 1960s, instruction was necessarily the chief focus at newly established colleges of nursing, pushing research and publication into the background. Under the circumstances, demonstrated teaching skills were the prime considerations in faculty recruitment, and a good many early nursing faculty—many of whom had obtained master's degrees only after obtaining faculty appointments—appear to have thought that caregiving was in itself sufficient justification for nursing's collegiate status and that research was of secondary importance. However, as baccalaureate nursing programs achieved a degree of maturity in the late 1960s and 1970s, as graduate programs expanded, and as nursing educators sought academic respectability within the university setting, questions surrounding faculty credentials, scholarly productivity, and promotion and tenure became acute. Yet resources devoted to nursing research remained slim, and the pool of nurses holding doctoral degrees was insufficient to cover the faculty needs of the more than 300 baccalaureate programs in operation by the mid-1970s. As late as 1980, a survey of a random sample of NLN-accredited schools concluded that just twenty percent of institutions maintained the doctoral degree—and, presumably, research and publication—as a formal requirement for tenure.[203]

For whatever reason, University of Iowa nursing faculty as a group made little headway toward meeting university requirements for promotion and tenure during more than a decade of grace from 1968 to 1979. In the blowup that resulted, dean and faculty blamed one another for the failure, the former charging insufficient faculty interest in self-improvement and the latter claiming insufficient attention by the dean to faculty development and recruitment. There were also other factors involved in this complex story, including limited university support for faculty development programs and the remarkable investment of faculty time and creative energies in undergraduate and graduate curriculum revisions. On the latter score, the College of Nursing was surely unique among the health science colleges—all of which carried through major curriculum revisions in the same period—in the proportion of faculty time devoted to curriculum matters.

Nurse-educators' peculiar fondness for curriculum issues surely reflected the fact that so many held advanced degrees in education, which, as one critic put it, fed an insatiable appetite "to adopt, to revise, to alter, and to innovate" in curriculum matters.[204] A remarkably comprehensive bibliography of published nursing research from 1950 to 1974 counted just sixty-five having to do with clinical research, while 166 publications—more than sixteen percent of the total—were education-related.[205] At the same time, the stark contrast between nursing and other health science colleges in terms of investment in curriculum issues reflected the comparatively underdeveloped research imperative in nursing, which, for better or worse, left more time for activities such as curriculum innovation.

In any event, the pressures of the moment surely made the crisis that rocked the University of Iowa College of Nursing in the late 1970s in some degree inevitable, while the specific outcome—notably the public dispute between the dean and senior faculty—likely owed much to local circumstances and personalities.

Conclusion

The decade and a half from 1965 to 1980 constituted yet another major transitional period for nursing education in America and at the University of Iowa College of Nursing, a transition marked by ambitious growth in the numbers of baccalaureate programs and their graduates and by concerted efforts to redefine the basis of nursing education. The period likewise saw the blossoming of graduate education in nursing, measured by the proliferation of graduate programs, including the addition of several new doctoral programs in nursing, and the refinement of graduate curriculum content. Just as important, the late 1960s and 1970s saw the emergence—sometimes halting and painful—of a new emphasis on the production by nurses of a distinct body of nursing knowledge, a trend that promised both an end to nursing's long reliance on a knowledge base derived chiefly from medicine and a new era of professional autonomy for nurses and nursing. One result, not always a happy one, was to assign greater importance to academic preparation and scholarly productivity in academic nursing's reward system.

Behind the developments in nursing education lay an unprecedented expansion of the American health care economy, expansion fueled by rapid technological innovation and by the investment of an ever greater share of national resources in health care goods and services. Indeed, health care was among the fastest growing economic sectors during the years from 1965 to 1980, as total health care expenditures in the United States increased nearly 500 percent in the period, rising from $41.7 billion to $249.0 billion and from 6.0 percent to 9.5 percent of gross national product.[206] Federal Medicare expenditures alone rose from $4.5 billion in 1967 to $35.7 billion in 1980. In Iowa, personal health care expenditures rose from $196 million in 1966 to $724 million in 1978, while per capita expenditures on hospital care rose from $68 to $307, and per capita expenditures on nursing home care rose from $22 to $112.

Both nationally and in Iowa, such statistics translated into extraordinary growth in the nursing profession and presented nurses with important new opportunities. Nonetheless, nursing in general and nursing education in particular faced stubborn problems as the 1970s drew to a close. On the whole, the health care system, increasingly focused on concerns over cost containment rather than issues of accessibility, still denied nurses adequate recognition and compensation for their professional services. Meanwhile, nursing education faced a lack of adequately trained faculty, a still weak research culture, and inadequate funding for nursing research. Such problems were all too evident at the University of Iowa College of Nursing, an institution which, far from unusual in that regard, remained one of America's best.

At the dawn of the 1980s, then, forecasts of nursing's future were mixed. Some leaders saw recent events as portents of a new era of professional growth and recognition for nurses; at the same time, others pointed to obstacles that still limited nursing's potential and that seemed, despite progress in many other areas, to defy resolution. Rozella M. Schlotfeldt, a 1935 graduate of the University of Iowa School of Nursing and a leader of long standing in the nursing field, argued in 1981 that by the year 2000 nurses could well be the chief primary care providers in the American health care system, a role buttressed by improved nursing education, both undergraduate and graduate, and enhanced nursing scholarship.[207] Schlotfeldt admitted that her prediction hinged on nursing's escape from the medical model of nursing care, a model based in illness, disability, and therapeutic interventions in times of crisis, and also on nurses' willingness to embrace professional accountability. In contrast, Gloria R. Smith, dean of the University of Oklahoma College of Nursing, answered Schlotfeldt's optimism with the warning that such rosy scenarios ignored "the lessons of the last quarter century,"[208] particularly the daunting structural and economic obstacles to nurses' professional claims within the existing health care system.

In fact, as today's health care consumers are only too well aware, events overwhelmed the predictions of optimists and pessimists alike. At the end of the 1970s, for example, national health insurance, which would grant federal agencies a central role in determining the price and distribution of health care benefits in a bigger and better—but otherwise little changed—health care economy, was still a much-discussed topic and still, whatever its weaknesses and however strong its enemies, carried an air of inevitability. Yet, as the spiral of health care costs continued unabated through the 1980s and into the 1990s and as the American political climate turned firmly against expanded government mandates, an uneasy coalition of third parties—from the federal government itself to health insurance companies and major corporate purchasers of health care coverage—turned the health care debate, the health care economy, and, by extension, the future of nursing in new and unexpected directions. By the mid-1990s, despite an aborted attempt at revival by the Clinton administration in 1993-94, the idea of national health insurance was scarcely more than a fading memory, displaced by a variety of private, market-oriented experiments in the organization and philosophy of health care delivery, experiments that, in turn, brought a host of new challenges for the nursing profession and for nurse educators.

Notes

1. "Summary Report and Recommendations: National Commission for the Study of Nursing and Nursing Education," *Nursing Outlook* 18 (February 1970), pp. 46-47.
2. American Nurses Association, *Facts About Nursing, 1966*, p. 204, and *Facts About Nursing, 1980-81*, p. 308.
3. US Public Health Service, *Health: United States, 1984* (Washington, DC: US Government Printing Office, 1984), p. 147.
4. *Health: United States, 1984*, p. 149.
5. Unless otherwise noted, all statistics dealing with nursing education, employment, and economics in this chapter are taken from annual compilations by the National League for Nursing and American Nurses Association published in *Nursing Outlook*, *Facts About Nursing*, and *Nursing Data Book*. Perhaps inevitably, there are small variations from one source to another; likewise, there are differences in the numbers reported in a single source at different times.
6. Joanne Comi McCloskey, "What Rewards Will Keep Nurses on the Job," *American Journal of Nursing* 75 (January 1975), pp. 600-602.
7. *Nursing Outlook* 28 (September 1980), p. 530.
8. For a larger discussion of nurses and collective bargaining, see Kalisch and Kalisch, *The Advance of American Nursing*, pp. 459-466.

9.   See "The Professional Model," *American Journal of Nursing* 75 (February 1975), pp. 288-292.

10. For a fuller treatment of the development of the nursing service, see Tali Neumann, *The Administrations of Marie E. Tener, Helen F. Watters, Myrtle Kitchell Aydelotte, and Mary E. Fuller: Four Directors of Nursing Service, the University of Iowa Hospitals and Clinics, 1949-1979*, Master's Thesis, The University of Iowa, 1987.

11. "Nursing Is Coming of Age...Through the Practitioner Movement," *American Journal of Nursing* 75 (October 1975), pp. 1834-1843.

12. Cathryne A. Welch, "Health Care Distribution and Third-Party Payment for Nurses' Services," *American Journal of Nursing* 75 (October 1975), pp. 1,844-1,847.

13. See Rosemary T. McCarthy, *History of the American Academy of Nursing, 1973-1982* (The Academy, 1985).

14. National League for Nursing, *Study on Cost of Nursing Education: Part I. Cost of Basic Diploma Programs* (New York: NLN, 1964).

15. For contemporary observations on the student body, see Marilyn D. Willman, "Changes in Nursing Students," in Janet A. Williamson, ed., *Current Perspectives in Nursing Education: The Changing Scene* (St. Louis, MO: C. V. Mosby Company, 1976), pp. 74-79.

16. "Ford Pocket-Vetoes Nurse Training Act," *American Journal of Nursing* 75 (February 1975), pp. 195, 222.

17. Mary Anderson Hardy, "The American Nurses' Association Influence on Federal Funding for Nursing Education, 1941-1984," *Nursing Research* 36 (January/February 1984), p. 32.

18. RC Hardin to David Bolender, December 3, 1971, Box 9, Folder "Medical—Dr. Hardin 1970-," College of Nursing Papers, The University of Iowa Archives.

19. Staff Report, October 29, 1965, Box 3, Folder "Administrative Staff 1965-66," College of Nursing Papers, The University of Iowa Archives.

20. WL Boyd to RW Richey, February 28, 1974, Box 10, Folder "President Boyd—General 1973," College of Nursing Papers, The University of Iowa Archives.

21. *Daily Iowan*, May 11, 1977.

22. American Nurses Association, "American Nurses' Association's First Position on Education for Nursing," *American Journal of Nursing* 66 (March 1966), pp. 515-517.

23. "UI College of Nursing Plans Construction of New Building," *The Daily Iowan*, September 20, 1967. See also LC Dustan to College of Nursing Faculty, July 11, 1966, Box 4, Folder "Faculty Association 1966-67," College of Nursing Papers, The University of Iowa Archives.

24. For participants' position statements, see Laura Dustan, "Education for Nursing: Apprenticeship or Academic?" and Thomas Hale, "Wanted:

Nurses to Nurse Patients," *Nursing Outlook* 15 (September 1967), pp. 26-32.

25. All numbers on University of Iowa College of Nursing enrollments are from Dean of Admissions and Records, Comparative Enrollment Reports, The University of Iowa Archives.

26. Laura C. Dustan, "Needed: Articulation Between Nursing Education Programs and Institutions of Higher Education," *Nursing Outlook* 18 (December 1970), pp. 34-37.

27. See a description of the program compiled by assistant project director Adrian Schoenmaker in Box 15, Folder "Building Dedication," College of Nursing, The University of Iowa Archives.

28. See Executive Council Minutes, November 14, 1966, and March 21, 1967, Box 3, Folder "Executive Council, 1966-67," College of Nursing Papers, The University of Iowa Archives.

29. A copy of the proposal—twenty-eight pages in length—is in Box 71, 1968-69, HR Bowen Papers, The University of Iowa Archives.

30. Minutes of the Faculty Association, October 11, 1968, Box 71, 1968-69, HR Bowen Papers, The University of Iowa Archives.

31. Executive Council Minutes, March 20, 1967, Box 3, Folder "Executive Council, 1966-67," College of Nursing Papers, The University of Iowa Archives.

32. LC Dustan to HR Bowen, December 20, 1965, Box 3, Folder "Executive Council 1965-66," College of Nursing Papers, The University of Iowa Archives.

33. LC Dustan to WL Boyd, April 13, 1966, Box 9, Folder "President Bowen—General, 1966-67," College of Nursing Papers, The University of Iowa Archives.

34. LC Dustan to WL Boyd, June 15, 1966, Box 9, Folder "Correspondence with Dean Dustan (Concerning PN School Closing-1966)," College of Nursing Papers, The University of Iowa Archives.

35. See, for example, Margaret A. Newman, "The Professional Doctorate in Nursing: A Position Paper," *Nursing Outlook* 23 (November 1975), pp. 704-706; Rozella M. Schlotfeldt, "Professional Doctorate: Rationale and Characteristics," *Nursing Outlook* 26 (May 1978), pp. 302-311.

36. Juanita F. Murphy, "Doctoral Education In, Of, and For Nursing: An Historical Analysis," *Nursing Outlook* 29 (November 1981), pp. 645-649.

37. Dustan included the story in her remarks as part of the dedication preparation on December 4, 1971; see Box 15, Folder "Dean Dustan's—Dedication, December 4, 1971," College of Nursing Papers, The University of Iowa Archives.

38. Administrative Staff Meeting Minutes, September 15, 1960, Box 2, Folder "Administrative Group Minutes, September 1, 1960-August 31, 1961," College of Nursing Papers, The University of Iowa Archives.

39. "List for Determination of Priorities in SUI Building Program," attached to VM Hancher to Administrative Council members, January 4, 1962, Box 15, Folder "General Statement of Building Needs"; Faculty Minutes, November 3, 1961, Box 5, Folder "Faculty Minutes, 1953-62," College of Nursing Papers, The University of Iowa Archives.

40. Administrative Staff Meeting Minutes, January 16, 1962, Box 2, Folder "Administrative Staff Meetings, July 1, 1962-June 30, 1963 [sic]," College of Nursing Papers, The University of Iowa Archives.

41. Administrative Staff Minutes, October 10, 1963, Box 3, Folder "Administrative Staff Minutes, 1963-64," College of Nursing Papers, The University of Iowa Archives.

42. Administrative Staff Minutes, May 14, 1964, Box 3, Folder "Administrative Staff Minutes, 1963-64," College of Nursing Papers, The University of Iowa Archives.

43. Stow Persons, *The University of Iowa in the Twentieth Century*, p. 184.

44. LC Dustan to WL Boyd, November 27, 1964, Box 71, 1964-65, HR Bowen Papers, The University of Iowa Archives.

45. Untitled Paper, November 6, 1959, Box 5, Folder "College of Nursing Faculty Minutes 1953-62," College of Nursing Papers, The University of Iowa Archives.

46. For a summary, see LC Dustan to WL Boyd, December 1, 1965, Box 15, Folder "General Statement of Building Needs," College of Nursing Papers, The University of Iowa Archives.

47. LC Dustan to WL Boyd, February 19, 1965, Box 9, Folder "Dean Boyd—General, 1964-66," College of Nursing Papers, The University of Iowa Archives.

48. Laura Dustan, Telephone Interview, September 5, 1995.

49. Faculty Minutes, November 8, 1965, Box 5, Folder "Faculty Meeting Minutes, 1964-65," College of Nursing Papers, The University of Iowa Archives.

50. LC Dustan to ET Jolliffe, February 21, 1966, and LC Dustan to HR Bowen, February 21, 1966, Box 71, 1965-66, HR Bowen Papers; Faculty Association Minutes, March 18, 1966, Box 5, Folder "Faculty Minutes, 1965 [sic]," College of Nursing Papers, The University of Iowa Archives.

51. "U of Iowa Health Sciences Campus Plans Outlined," *The Cedar Rapids Gazette*, November 13, 1965.

52. HR Bowen to LC Dustan, February 25, 1966, Box 71, 1965-66, HR Bowen Papers, The University of Iowa Archives.

53. LC Dustan to HR Bowen, March 1, 1966, Box 71, 1965-66, HR Bowen Papers, The University of Iowa Archives.

54. LC Dustan to WL Boyd, February 8, 1966, Folder "Executive Council, 1965-66," College of Nursing Papers, The University of Iowa Archives.
55. Faculty Minutes, October 21, 1966, Box 5, Folder "Faculty Meeting Minutes, 1964-65," College of Nursing Papers, The University of Iowa Archives.
56. Faculty Association Minutes, December 16, 1968, Box Folder "Faculty Association September 1966-June 1969," College of Nursing Papers, The University of Iowa Archives.
57. HR Bowen to LC Dustan, July 5, 1967, Box 71, 1967-68, HR Bowen Papers, The University of Iowa Archives.
58. LC Dustan to HR Bowen, July 14, 1967, Box 71, 1967-68, HR Bowen Papers, The University of Iowa Archives.
59. LC Dustan to DE Reese [chief of Construction Grants Section, Division of Nursing], September 19, 1967, Box 71, 1967-68, HR Bowen Papers, The University of Iowa Archives.
60. LC Dustan to DE Reese, November 19, 1968, Box 71, 1968-69, HR Bowen Papers, The University of Iowa Archives.
61. LC Dustan to HR Bowen, March 25, 1968, Box 9, Folder "President Bowen General, 1967-68," College of Nursing Papers, The University of Iowa Archives.
62. "Regents Reallocate Dentistry Funds For New Nursing College Building," *The Daily Iowan*, April 12, 1968.
63. Donald Galagan to HR Bowen, April 15, 1968, Box 9, "President Bowen General, 1967-68," College of Nursing Papers, The University of Iowa Archives.
64. See HR Bowen to JM Scott, July 1, 1968, Box 71, 1968-69, HR Bowen Papers, The University of Iowa Archives.
65. "Nursing Building Tops List of Okd UI Projects," *The Daily Iowan*, July 13, 1968.
66. LC Dustan to DE Reese, March 18, 1969, Box 71, 1968-69, HR Bowen Papers, The University of Iowa Archives.
67. HR Bowen to LC Dustan, June 6, 1969, Box 71, 1968-69, HR Bowen Papers, The University of Iowa Archives.
68. See, for example, LC Dustan to HR Bowen, July 3, 1968, Box 71, 1968-69, HR Bowen Papers, The University of Iowa Archives.
69. HR Bowen to LC Dustan, July 9, 1968, Box 9, Folder "President Bowen General, 1968-69," College of Nursing Papers, The University of Iowa Archives.
70. Laura C. Dustan, "A Consideration of the Present," Box 15, Folder "Friday Speech," College of Nursing Papers, The University of Iowa Archives.
71. "Utilizing Potential of Nurses Vital to Health Care," *Iowa City Press-Citizen*, December 4, 1971.

72. "Bowen Predicts Major Changes in Health Services," *Iowa City Press-Citizen*, December 6, 1971; "'Pressure for Health Service Reform Well-Nigh Irresistible,'" *The Cedar Rapids Gazette*, December 5, 1971.

73. P Seebohm to LC Dustan, December 7, 1971, Box 15, Folder "Dedication Committee," College of Nursing Papers, The University of Iowa Archives.

74. Curriculum Committee Minutes, November 16, 1962, Box 3, Folder "General Nursing Curriculum Committee 1962-63," College of Nursing Papers, The University of Iowa Archives.

75. E Hutchins to College of Nursing Faculty, April 24, 1964, Box 71, 1963-64, VM Hancher Papers, The University of Iowa Archives.

76. See "Report: Subcommittee to Consider Criteria for Establishing Advanced Standing for R.N. Students" and General Nursing Curriculum Subcommittee to Basic Curriculum Committee, "Credit for previous nursing study of R.N. students," May 20, 1965, Box 3, Folder "Curriculum Committee Undergraduate 1965," College of Nursing Papers, The University of Iowa Archives.

77. M Freel to Curriculum Committee, February 27, 1969, Box 3, Folder "Curriculum Committee 9/66-2/69," College of Nursing Papers, The University of Iowa Archives.

78. See Undergraduate Curriculum Committee Minutes, February 28, 1969, March 14, 1969, and March 28, 1969, Box 3, Folder "Curriculum Committee Undergraduate 9/1966-2/1969" [sic], , College of Nursing Papers, The University of Iowa Archives.

79. See Report of the Curriculum Committee to Faculty Association, 1968-69, Box 4, Folder "Faculty Association 9/1966-6/1969," College of Nursing Papers, The University of Iowa Archives.

80. Executive Council Minutes, January 21, 1966, Box 3, Folder "Executive Council Minutes 1965," College of Nursing Papers, The University of Iowa Archives.

81. Executive Council Minutes, February 25, 1966, Box 3, Folder "Executive Council Minutes 1965," College of Nursing Papers, The University of Iowa Archives.

82. LC Dustan to RC Hardin, November 22, 1965, Box 3, Folder "Undergraduate Curriculum Committee 1965-66," College of Nursing Papers, The University of Iowa Archives.

83. JR Porter to LC Dustan, June 15, 1966, Box 3, Folder "Curriculum Committee 1966-67," College of Nursing Papers, The University of Iowa Archives.

84. Ad Hoc Curriculum Evaluation Committee, February 22, 1965, Box 3, College of Nursing Papers, The University of Iowa Archives.

85. "Preparation for Development of Methods for Evaluation of the Nursing Student in the Practicum Courses of the Basic Curriculum," Box 3,

Folder "Curriculum Evaluation Committee, Ad Hoc II, 1964-65," College of Nursing Papers, The University of Iowa Archives.

86. "The Evaluation of Clinical Facilities: Report of Sophomore Students' Responses on 5-9-66 to Opinionnaire," Box 3, Folder "Undergraduate Curriculum Committee 1965," College of Nursing Papers, The University of Iowa Archives.

87. General Nursing Curriculum Committee Minutes, February 11, 1963, Box 3, Folder "General Nursing Curriculum Committee 1962-63," College of Nursing Papers, The University of Iowa Archives.

88. MK Aydelotte to Undergraduate Section of Curriculum Committee, October 1, 1965, Box 3, Folder "Undergraduate Curriculum Committee," College of Nursing Papers, The University of Iowa Archives.

89. Approach to Major Study of Curriculum, April 11, 1966, Box 3, Folder "Curriculum Committee 1965-66," College of Nursing Papers, The University of Iowa Archives.

90. "Final Report of the Questionnaire Survey of the June and August, 1965, Graduates of the Four Academic Year Baccalaureate Program, February 1966," Box 5, Folder "Faculty Minutes 1965," College of Nursing Papers, The University of Iowa Archives.

91. LC Dustan to M Freel, October 24, 1966, Box 3, Folder "Curriculum Committee-Undergraduate, 9/1966-2/1969," College of Nursing Papers, The University of Iowa Archives.

92. Box 3, Folder "Curriculum Committee-Undergraduate, 9/66-2/69," College of Nursing Papers, The University of Iowa Archives.

93. "Summary of Discussion Faculty Conference, January 30-31, 1967," Box 3, Folder "Curriculum Committee 1966-67," College of Nursing Papers, The University of Iowa Archives.

94. "Progress Report—Ad Hoc Committee on Student Characteristics," April 12, 1967, Box 3, Folder "Curriculum Committee 1966-67," College of Nursing Papers, The University of Iowa Archives.

95. "Summary of Discussion April 12, 1967, and April 13, 1967," Box 3, Folder "Curriculum Committee Undergraduate 9/66-2/69," College of Nursing Papers, The University of Iowa Archives.

96. Minutes of the Undergraduate Program Section of the Curriculum Committee, May 10, 1966, Box 3, Folder "Undergraduate Curriculum Committee 1965," and December 19, 1967, Box 3, Folder "Curriculum Committee—Ad Hoc Committee Folder," College of Nursing Papers, The University of Iowa Archives.

97. For example, in February 1968 the Curriculum Evaluation Committee discontinued an attempt to identify the "common threads" joining all the course offerings in the present curriculum, proposing to turn over to the curriculum committee all its materials on the subject, including a 66-page summary of specific skills taught in the clinical courses. See Curricu-

lum Evaluation Committee Minutes, February 2, 1968, Box 3, Folder "Curriculum Evaluation Committee, Ad Hoc II 1965-68," College of Nursing Papers, The University of Iowa Archives.

98. Mildred Freel, "Curriculum Project Report to Executive Council," September 3, 1970, Box 4 Folder "Executive Council 1970-71," College of Nursing Papers, The University of Iowa Archives.

99. Faculty Association Minutes, January 21, 1972, Addendum 1, Box 5, Folder "Faculty Association 1971-72," College of Nursing Papers, The University of Iowa Archives.

100. "Undergraduate Process Curriculum," Box 5, Folder "Grad. Council Minutes Sept. 1974-May 1975," College of Nursing Papers, The University of Iowa Archives.

101. Gamma Chapter Annual Reports, Gamma Chapter Collection, The University of Iowa College of Nursing.

102. "Male Nurses 'Liberated' At Recognition Ceremony," *Iowa City Press Citizen*, July 21, 1971.

103. "Male Student Notes Role in Nursing Profession," *Daily Iowan*, January 23, 1973. It should be noted that the University Hospitals routinely hired male nursing staff in limited numbers as early as the 1930s.

104. "Record Number of Men Studying Nursing at UI," *Iowa City Press Citizen*, February 3, 1973.

105. See Curriculum Committee Undergraduate Section Minutes, October 18, 1968, and November 22, 1968, Box 3, Folder "Curriculum Committee—Undergraduate 9/1966-2/1969," College of Nursing Papers, The University of Iowa Archives.

106. Faculty Association Minutes, May 24, 1971, Box 4, Folder "Faculty Association Minutes," College of Nursing Papers, The University of Iowa Archives.

107. Minutes of Special Open Meeting of the Ad Hoc Committee for Review of the Graduate Program, October 28, 1971, Box 6, Folder "Minutes and Correspondence 1970-71," College of Nursing Papers, The University of Iowa Archives.

108. The reference appears in LC Dustan to HR Bowen, July 3, 1968, Box 9, Folder "President Bowen—General 1968-69," College of Nursing Papers, The University of Iowa Archives.

109. Graduate Faculty Curriculum Meeting, February 17, 1964, Box 6, Folder "Graduate Program Curriculum Committee 1963-64," College of Nursing Papers, The University of Iowa Archives.

110. Graduate Program in Nursing Spring 1964, Box 6, Folder "Graduate Program Curriculum Committee 1963-64," College of Nursing Papers, The University of Iowa Archives.

111. See Consultation on Graduate Education, May 28-29, 1964, and J Campbell to RE Boyle and Staff, June 17, 1964, Box 6, Folder "Graduate

Program Curriculum Committee 1963-64," College of Nursing Papers, The University of Iowa Archives.

112. Graduate Faculty Minutes, April 6, 1965, Box 5, Folder "Faculty Meeting Minutes Spring 1965," College of Nursing Papers, The University of Iowa Archives.

113. LC Dustan to HR Bowen, December 20, 1965, Box 3, Folder "Executive Council 1965-66," College of Nursing Papers, The University of Iowa Archives.

114. LC Dustan, "Statement on Graduate and Professional Instruction," Box 9, Folder "Dean Boyd—General 1964-66," College of Nursing Papers, The University of Iowa Archives.

115. Proposed Program in Nursing Service Administration, November 12, 1965, Box 6, Folder "Graduate Nursing Faculty Minutes 1965," College of Nursing Papers, The University of Iowa Archives.

116. LC Dustan to HR Bowen, July 18, 1966, Box 4, Folder "Faculty Association 1966-67," College of Nursing Papers, The University of Iowa Archives.

117. *Ibid.*

118. A Whidden and MK Aydelotte to LC Dustan, January 26, 1966, Box 9, Folder "Correspondence: Ann Whidden, Dean Dustan," College of Nursing Papers, The University of Iowa Archives.

119. Graduate Faculty Minutes, March 12, 1965, Box 6, Folder "Graduate Nursing Faculty Minutes 1965," College of Nursing Papers, The University of Iowa Archives.

120. Two Semester Course in Nursing Research, Box 6, Folder "Graduate Curriculum Committee 1961-70," College of Nursing Papers, The University of Iowa Archives.

121. Graduate Council Minutes, November 15, 1974, and December 20, 1974, Box 5, Folder "Graduate Council Minutes September 1974 through May 1975," College of Nursing Papers, The University of Iowa Archives.

122. EH Erickson to E Rasmussen, October 20, 1971, Box 7, Folder "Interim Committee State Legislature," College of Nursing Papers, The University of Iowa Archives.

123. Graduate Faculty Minutes, May 25, 1972, Box 7, Folder "Graduate Faculty Association," College of Nursing Papers, The University of Iowa Archives.

124. Ad Hoc Committee of the Graduate Council to EH Erickson, January 23, 1974; Erickson to A Scheffel, January 25, 1974, Box 6, Folder "Graduate Council 1973-74," College of Nursing Papers, The University of Iowa Archives.

125. "Sources of Support for the Graduate Majors, 1969-1970," Box 7, Folder "Program Review Committee," College of Nursing Papers, The

University of Iowa Archives. See also, "Report of the Committee for Collegiate Program Review of College of Nursing," July 10, 1972.

126.   For a review of the history and substance of the proposal, see Laura Dustan, "A Proposal for the Establishment for Training Program for Pediatric Nurse Practitioners and the Enrichment of a Child Health Demonstration Unit," Box 6, Folder "Minutes and Correspondence 1970-71," College of Nursing Papers, The University of Iowa Archives.

127. Box 6, Folder "Graduate Council Minutes 1973-76," College of Nursing Papers, The University of Iowa Archives.

128.   Graduate Council Minutes, September 20, 1974, and October 7, 1974, Box 5, Folder "Graduate Council Minutes September 1974 through May 1975," College of Nursing Papers, The University of Iowa Archives.

129.   Quad-Cities Graduate Study Center, Nursing Survey, Box 6, Folder "Graduate Council Minutes 1973-76," College of Nursing Papers, The University of Iowa Archives.

130.   The University of Iowa College of Nursing Constituent Society, *Nursing News*, Spring 1975, p. 2.

131. Graduate Council Minutes, March 21, 1975, Box 5, Folder "Graduate Council Minutes September 1974 through May 1975," College of Nursing Papers, The University of Iowa Archives.

132.   Graduate Council Minutes, September 20, 1974, and "Conceptual Framework for Master's Program," November 15, 1974, Box 5, Folder "Graduate Council Minutes September 1974 through May 1975," College of Nursing Papers, The University of Iowa Archives.

133. Graduate Council Minutes, February 21, 1975, Box 5, Folder "Graduate Council Minutes September 1974 through May 1975," College of Nursing Papers, The University of Iowa Archives.

134.   Responses of Graduate Faculty to Questions Regarding Concerns About Graduate Program and Task Force Assignments," Box 6, Folder "Graduate Council Minutes 1976-77-78-79," College of Nursing Papers, The University of Iowa Archives.

135.   Graduate Council Minutes, September 10, 1976, Box 6, Folder "Graduate Council Minutes 1976-77-78-79," College of Nursing Papers, The University of Iowa Archives.

136.   Graduate Council Minutes, October 8, 1976, Box 6, Folder "Graduate Council Minutes 1976-77-78-79," College of Nursing Papers, The University of Iowa Archives.

137. EH Erickson to Graduate Council, November 3, 1976, "Response to Request for Information Incorporated in October 8, 1976, Graduate Council Minutes," Box 6, Folder "Graduate Council Minutes 1976-77-78-79," College of Nursing Papers, The University of Iowa Archives.

138. Graduate Council Minutes, April 29, 1977, Box 6, Folder "Graduate Council Minutes 76-77-78-79," College of Nursing Papers, The University of Iowa Archives.

139. Graduate Council Minutes, November 12, 1976, Box 6, , Folder "Graduate Council Minutes 1976-77-78-79," College of Nursing Papers, The University of Iowa Archives.

140. Summary of Report and Recommendations by Holly Wilson, PhD, Curriculum Consultant, January 18, 1977, Box 6, , Folder "Graduate Council Minutes 1976-77-78-79," College of Nursing Papers, The University of Iowa Archives.

141. See Graduate Council Minutes, October 28, November 14, and November 18, 1977, Box 6, , Folder "Graduate Council Minutes 1976-77-78-79," College of Nursing Papers, The University of Iowa Archives.

142. A Whidden to College of Nursing Faculty, October 2, 1978, Box 6, Folder "Graduate Council Minutes 76-77-78-79," College of Nursing Papers, The University of Iowa Archives.

143. See, for example, College of Nursing Association Minutes, May 5, 1975, Box 4, Folder "Faculty Association and College of Nursing Association Minutes," College of Nursing Papers, The University of Iowa Archives.

144. CIC Panel on Nursing Education Minutes, April 19, 1974, and November 26, 1974; "Study of CIC Resources for Doctoral Education in Nursing," January 8, 1975, Box 7, Folder "Committee on Institutional Cooperation 1973-75," College of Nursing Papers, The University of Iowa Archives.

145. See College of Nursing Association Minutes, December 10, 1976, and March 4, 1977, and Ad Hoc Committee to Study the Feasibility of a Doctoral Program in Nursing, Annual Report, April 23, 1977, Box 4, Folder "Faculty Association and College of Nursing Association Minutes," College of Nursing Papers, The University of Iowa Archives.

146. "Position Paper: The University of Iowa Should Offer a Doctoral Program in Nursing," Box 7, Folder "Doctoral Program 1977," College of Nursing Papers, The University of Iowa Archives.

147. "Studying the Feasibility of a Doctoral Program in Nursing at The University of Iowa," Box 7, Folder "Doctoral Program 1977," College of Nursing Papers, The University of Iowa Archives.

148. Draft News Release, August 5, 1977, Box 6, Folder "Graduate Council Minutes 1976-77-78-79," College of Nursing Papers, The University of Iowa Archives.

149. RF Ray to Deans, Directors, and Department Heads, October 12, 1965, and Community Service and Continuing Education Memorandum No. 2, May 9, 1966, Box 3, Folder "Curriculum Committee 1965," College of Nursing Papers, The University of Iowa Archives.

150. College of Nursing Association Minutes, May 4, 1977, Box 4, Folder "Faculty Association and College of Nursing Association Minutes," College of Nursing Papers, The University of Iowa Archives.

151. LC Dustan to WL Boyd, December 7, 1970, Folder 70, 1970-71, WL Boyd Papers, The University of Iowa Archives.

152. WL Boyd to LC Dustan, December 8, 1970, Folder 70, 1970-71, WL Boyd Papers, The University of Iowa Archives.

153. "Proposal for the Administrative Functioning of the College of Nursing, 9/1/71-9/1/72," Box 9, Folder "Provost Heffner—General 1970-71," College of Nursing Papers, The University of Iowa Archives.

154. Box 10, Folder "Committee for Selection of a Dean 1971-72," College of Nursing Papers, The University of Iowa Archives.

155. MK Aydelotte to A Jacox, March 15, 1971, Box 10, Folder "Committee for Selection of a Dean 1971-72," College of Nursing Papers, The University of Iowa Archives.

156. See Selection Committee Minutes, April 11 and May 27, 1971; A Jacox to WL Boyd, June 28, 1971; Selection Committee to College of Nursing Faculty, July 28, 1971, Box 10, Folder "Committee for Selection of a Dean 1971-72," College of Nursing Papers, The University of Iowa Archives.

157. News Release, University of Iowa News Service, March 11, 1972, Box 15, Folder "University News Releases Re College of Nursing," College of Nursing Papers, The University of Iowa Archives.

158. LC Dustan to HR Bowen, November 24, 1967, Box 9, Folder "President Bowen-General 1967-68," College of Nursing Papers, The University of Iowa Archives.

159. LC Dustan to WL Boyd, May 22, 1967, Box 9, Folder "Dean Boyd-General 1966-67," College of Nursing Papers, The University of Iowa Archives.

160. LC Dustan to W Eginton, March 5, 1971, Box 9, Folder "Dean Boyd-General 1970-71," Box 9, College of Nursing Papers, The University of Iowa Archives.

161. "Dean Brings New Image to Nursing," *Daily Iowan*, September 13, 1972.

162. ER Barritt to RC Hardin, February 8, 1973, Box 9, Folder "Medical—Dr. Hardin 1970-," College of Nursing Papers, The University of Iowa Archives.

163. "Proposal for Reorganization of the College of Nursing Administrative Structure," Folder 71, 1969-70, WL Boyd Papers, The University of Iowa Archives.

164. By-Laws of the College of Nursing Faculty Association, Adopted June 1, 1965, Folder 71, 1965-66, HR Bowen Papers, The University of Iowa Archives.

165. *Ibid.*, Revised 1967, 1969, 1969, 1971, Box 4, Folders "Faculty Association Minutes" and "Executive Council," College of Nursing Papers, The University of Iowa Archives.

166. Report for Accreditation of Undergraduate and Graduate Programs in Nursing Offered by the University of Iowa College of Nursing, January 1974, pp. 164-173, Box 1, College of Nursing Papers, The University of Iowa Archives.

167. MK Aydelotte to HR Bowen, April 14, 1966, Box 9, Folder "Miscellaneous Correspondence," College of Nursing Papers, The University of Iowa Archives.

168. Laura Dustan, Institutional Profile Report for North Central Association, December 10, 1967, Box 1, Folder "Accreditation Visits 1967-71," College of Nursing Papers, The University of Iowa Archives.

169. LC Dustan to WL Boyd, June 2, 1967, Box 9, Folder "Dean Boyd General, 1966-67," College of Nursing Papers, The University of Iowa Archives.

170. Resume of Faculty Appointment Factors Study, October 22, 1969, Box 11, Folder "Resume of Faculty Appointment Factors Study," College of Nursing Papers, The University of Iowa Archives.

171. See Executive Council Minutes, September 16, 1966 and LC Dustan to WL Boyd, July 12, 1966, Box 3, Folder "Executive Council 1966-67," College of Nursing Papers, The University of Iowa Archives.

172. LC Dustan to D Spriestersbach, February 19, 1971, Box 4, Folder "Faculty Association Minutes," College of Nursing Papers, The University of Iowa Archives.

173. "Collegiate Program Review of the College of Nursing," January 21, 1972, p. VIb, Box 7, Folder "Program Review Committee," College of Nursing Papers, The University of Iowa Archives.

174. Executive Council Minutes, January 16, 1967, Box 4, Folder "Executive Council, 1966-67," College of Nursing Papers, The University of Iowa Archives. For university guidelines, see "Tentative Guide for Administrative Officers, January 23, 1967," Box 4, Faculty Association 1966-67," College of Nursing Papers, The University of Iowa Archives.

175. LC Dustan to Nursing Faculty, January 23, 1968, "Criteria to Govern Appointment and Promotion to the Rank of Assistant Professor," Box 4, Folder "Faculty Materials 1967-68," College of Nursing Papers, The University of Iowa Archives.

176. Faculty Association Minutes, November 17, 1969, Box 4, Folder "Faculty Association Minutes 1969-70," College of Nursing Papers, The University of Iowa Archives.

177. Faculty Affairs Committee to Nursing Faculty, April 2, 1973, Box 4, Folder "Faculty Affairs," College of Nursing Papers, The University of Iowa Archives.

178. College of Nursing Association Minutes, August 24, 1973, Box 12, Folder "Folder College of Nursing Association," College of Nursing Papers, The University of Iowa Archives.

179. Faculty Affairs Council to College of Nursing Association, January 3, 1974, Box 4, Folder "Faculty Affairs Council 1973-74," College of Nursing Papers, The University of Iowa Archives.

180. DH Vernon to ER Barritt, May 2, 1974, Box 4, Folder "Faculty Association and College of Nursing Association Minutes," College of Nursing Papers, The University of Iowa Archives.

181. See Persons, *The University of Iowa in the Twentieth Century*, pp. 282-284.

182. M Brodbeck to Members of the Faculty, November 10, 1975, Box 4, Folder "Faculty Affairs Council Fall '75 through Summer '76," College of Nursing Papers, The University of Iowa Archives.

183. Faculty Affairs Council to College of Nursing Faculty, December 8, 1975, Box 4, Folder "Faculty Association and College of Nursing Association Minutes," College of Nursing Papers, The University of Iowa Archives.

184. Faculty Affairs Council Minutes, December 10, 1975, Box 4, Folder "Faculty Affairs Council Fall '75 through Summer '76," College of Nursing Papers, The University of Iowa Archives.

185. Promotion/Tenure Ad Hoc Committee Meeting Minutes, December 19, 1975, Box 4, Folder "Faculty Affairs Council Fall '75 through Summer '76," College of Nursing Papers, The University of Iowa Archives.

186. College of Nursing Association Minutes, December 16, 1975, Box 4, Folder "Faculty Affairs Council Fall '75 through Summer '76," College of Nursing Papers, The University of Iowa Archives.

187. Ad Hoc Committee for Development of Promotion and Tenure Procedures, "Preliminary Statement," January 5, 1976, Box 4, "Faculty Affairs Council Fall '76 through Summer '76," College of Nursing Papers, The University of Iowa Archives.

188. College of Nursing Association Minutes, February 13, 1976, Box 4, Folder "Faculty Association and College of Nursing Association Minutes," College of Nursing Papers, The University of Iowa Archives.

189. College of Nursing Association Minutes, March 26, 1976, Verbatim Transcript, Box 4, Folder "College of Nursing Association Minutes," College of Nursing Papers, The University of Iowa Archives.

190. Faculty Affairs Council to Faculty Association, October 19, 1976, Box 4, Folder "Faculty Association and College of Nursing Association Minutes," College of Nursing Papers, The University of Iowa Archives.

191. College of Nursing Association Minutes, October 22, 1976, Box 4, Folder "Faculty Association and College of Nursing Association Minutes," College of Nursing Papers, The University of Iowa Archives.

192. Faculty Affairs Council to College of Nursing Association, April 29, 1977, Box 4, Folder "Faculty Association and College of Nursing Association Minutes"; College of Nursing Association Minutes, May 4, 1977, Box 4, Folder "Faculty Association and College of Nursing Association Minutes," College of Nursing Papers, The University of Iowa Archives.
193. Box 7, Folder "Dean's Meetings 1975-76," College of Nursing Papers, The University of Iowa Archives.
194. 1976 Faculty Appointment Factors Study, May 1976, Box 12, and 1976 Faculty Retention Factors Study, December 1976, Box 11, College of Nursing Papers, The University of Iowa Archives.
195. Details in this account are taken chiefly from newspaper accounts, a university review committee report, and court documents filed under case number 45471, Evelyn Barritt v. Teresa Christy, June Triplett, Mildred Freel, Barbara Thomas, Laura Hart, Hope Solomons, Etta Rasmussen, and Nancy Jordison, filed January 21, 1980, and case number 45471A, Barbara Thomas v. Evelyn Barritt, filed February 13, 1980, Johnson County, Iowa, District Court.
196. "Enmity 'Bitter' and 'Deep' at Nursing School: Report," *The Des Moines Register*, September 11, 1979.
197. In addition to the review committee report, see "Nursing Dean Agrees to Quit in U of I Fuss," *The Des Moines Register*, September 1, 1979. It should perhaps be noted that college of nursing procedures devised by the faculty did not—indeed, the faculty could not—prescribe beyond the peer review process, thus forcing the dean to accept peer review committee recommendations. University rules regarding promotion and tenure specified that the dean consult with faculty regarding promotion decisions but did not preclude her making separate recommendations.
198. *The Drawsheet*, October 3, 1979, Box 15, Folder "The Drawsheet," College of Nursing Papers, The University of Iowa Archives.
199. Stow Persons, *The University of Iowa in the Twentieth Century*, p. 284. See also "23 Nursing Faculty to Get Tenure at UI," *Daily Iowan*, November 6, 1979.
200. See, for example, "Senators Criticize Tenure of Nurses," *Daily Iowan*, November 12, 1979.
201. From Faculty Senate Minutes reprinted verbatim in University of Iowa *FYI*, January 18, 1980.
202. M Brodbeck to Tenured Faculty of the College of Nursing, January 24, 1980, College of Nursing Folders, The University of Iowa.
203. Joanne Kirk Henry, "Nursing and Tenure," *Nursing Outlook* 29 (April 1981), pp. 240-244.
204. Dorothy J. Novello, "Proliferating Curriculums," in Williamson, *Current Perspectives in Nursing Education: The Changing Scene*, pp. 66-73.

205. Susan D. Taylor, "Bibliography on Nursing Research, 1950-1974," *Nursing Research* 24 (May-June 1975), pp. 207-225.
206. Statistics from *Health: United States, 1982* Washington, DC: US Department of Health and Human Services, 1982).
207. Rozella M. Schlotfeldt, "Nursing in the Future," *Nursing Outlook* 29 (May 1981), pp. 295-301.
208. Gloria R. Smith, "Nursing Beyond the Crossroads," *Nursing Outlook* 28 (September 1980), pp. 540-545.

Chapter Five

Nursing Education in an Evolving Health Care System, 1981-1998

For the University of Iowa College of Nursing, the hard-won gains of the 1960s and 1970s, including the Nursing Building campaign, the comprehensive undergraduate and graduate curriculum revisions, and the thorny issues surrounding faculty development and research, were important groundwork for later accomplishments. In the 1980s and 1990s, energized by a new dean, a strengthened academic culture, and important additions to the faculty, the College of Nursing attained newfound prominence in the university and in regional, national, and international nursing affairs. From 1993, *US News and World Report*, in each of its annual rankings of graduate and professional schools, awarded the College of Nursing a place among the top fifteen nursing schools in the United States.

The 1980s and 1990s presented major new challenges to the college and to the nursing profession. Perhaps most important was a fundamental restructuring of the American health care system, a restructuring whose ends are not yet clearly in view. On the one hand, Arnold Relman's "medical-industrial complex"[1]—embracing a panoply of for-profit ventures, from private hospital chains and management companies to commercial dialysis centers, cancer treatment centers, and surgery centers—claimed an increasing share of the health care market. On the other hand, the double-digit rate of inflation in health care costs, an object of increasing attention and concern from the early 1970s, spurred a further shift in the ideology and organization of health care delivery, leading to the adoption of a variety of cost-cutting measures and sparking the growth of an alphabet-soup of alternative delivery systems, such as HMOs (health maintenance organizations) and PPOs (preferred provider organizations) designed to inject cost saving incentives into the provision of health care.

The reorganization of the health care delivery system entailed a major shift in emphasis away from traditional acute care, inpatient hospital services toward clinic and outpatient care and also toward home health care, disease prevention, and health maintenance. The evolving health care market, then, driven by new and more stringent cost controls negotiated by both public and private payers, forced a significant shift in the service patterns of America's hospitals, leading to a dramatic fall in patient admissions between 1980 and the mid-1990s and an even more dramatic increase in outpatient visits. Eventually, shifting hospital service patterns led to major changes in staffing practices, changes with important implications for a nursing profession that had, since the 1930s, become increasingly associated with hospital-centered health care. As more and more hospitals replaced professional nursing staff with "unlicensed assistive personnel" (UAP), a euphemism for marginally trained and poorly paid caregivers,[2] the American Nurses Association held a media briefing in May 1997 to spotlight both "the increased use of unlicensed personnel for patient care" and reports of the dismissal of RNs who protested "harmful staffing decisions."[3] Meanwhile, some observers at least suggested that nursing, in common with the other health care professions, might well face an oversupply of trained personnel in a health care market attuned to supply and demand.

All the while, the changing health care environment accelerated the postwar trend toward specialization and subspecialization in nursing practice, with an associated growth in the ranks of advanced practice nurses of all kinds. Likewise, the explosive rate of innovation in knowledge and technologies changed the role of the professional nurse and, among other innovations, opened a new field of "nursing informatics" involving the application of computerized information systems to health care organization and patient management. At the same time, the expansion of alternative delivery systems—from home health care agencies to community nursing centers—opened new roles to nurses in areas quite different from the now traditional hospital settings. However, nurses' efforts to turn those new professional opportunities to full advantage put a premium on the acquisition of hard data to corroborate the value of nursing services. In part because of that and in part because of arguments that the isolation of nursing faculty from practice was detrimental to teaching and to students,[4] academic nursing centers grew in numbers. A 1990 study counted forty-five academic nursing centers across the nation, blending community service, education, and research.[5]

Through the 1980s and 1990s, events at the University of Iowa College of Nursing reflected both longstanding postwar trends and more recent shifts in the American health care market. By the mid-1990s, undergraduate education had become increasingly less focused on acute care experience and more on community settings, with a significant emphasis on gerontological rural health issues and concerns. Meanwhile, the college's commitment to graduate education, enunciated repeatedly since its inclusion in the college's long term plan in 1964, grew stronger, and graduate enrollments rose sharply along with the range and quality of program offerings. Like undergraduate education, graduate education also became more attuned to primary health care and health promotion.

Also, scholarly research commanded a firm place in the College of Nursing agenda in the 1980s and 1990s, and research and publication, as in other colleges and departments of the university, became important elements in faculty evaluation. A solid base of scholarly productivity in turn supported the establishment of a long-awaited doctoral program in 1988. In the meantime, however, the wave of downsizing and fiscal stringency that affected both public and private spheres in the late 1980s and 1990s carried significant implications for the college, inaugurating an era of leaner budgets, reduced faculty and staff numbers, and increased teaching loads. Likewise, as College of Nursing Dean Geraldene Felton noted in a 1996 forum, the prospects for increased resources in the immediate future appeared dim,[6] even as rapid and far-reaching change in the health care system placed unprecedented adaptive pressures on nursing education.

Nursing, Nursing Education, and the Health Care System

The decade of the 1970s will long be remembered as one of economic stagnation coupled with persistent price inflation. Although health care was a major growth industry and remained so through the 1980s, inflation in health care costs drew ever greater attention to cost containment throughout the health care system.

Initially, much of the impetus behind cost control efforts resulted from spiraling federal expenditures for Medicare and combined federal and state Medicaid costs, but private third parties also took increasingly aggressive cost containment steps by the late 1980s.

The first cost control efforts, dating to the early 1970s, were regulatory in nature. For example, the 1972 amendments to the Social Security Act (PL92-603), which extended Medicare benefits to the disabled and to end-stage renal disease cases, sought also to beef up the utilization review requirements in the original 1965 Medicare legislation by creating Professional Standards Review Organizations (PSROs) at regional and local levels. PSROs, like the Iowa Foundation for Medical Care and the professional practice/utilization review structure set up at the University of Iowa Hospitals and Clinics, had a threefold purpose: to review utilization procedures for Medicare patients, to instill cost consciousness in attending physicians, and to build a database for more accurate assessment of utilization policies. However, critics charged that the PSRO structure, dominated as it was by physicians, held little hope as a cost containment strategy and was, indeed, akin to "the fox guarding the henhouse."[7] The 1972 social security amendments also limited reimbursement rates for many routine hospital services, the rates calculated on the basis of hospital size and location. In addition, the 1972 legislation mandated statewide health care planning. In the same vein, Congress enacted the National Health Planning and Resource Development Act (PL 93-641) in 1974, creating a national structure of Health Systems Agencies and requiring state certificate-of-need programs to scrutinize local hospitals' investments in new services, facilities, and technologies. In Iowa, the state legislature approved certificate-of-need legislation in 1977, establishing the Iowa Health Facilities Council and recognizing the statewide tertiary care function of the University of Iowa Hospitals and Clinics.

In the face of stubborn double-digit inflation in health care, most observers argued by the early 1980s that existing cost control efforts had been, at best, only marginally effective. From 1972 to 1982, Medicare Part A (hospital insurance) expenditures had risen from $6.3 billion to $33.3 billion, an increase of 428 percent. From 1979 to 1983 alone, the overall consumer price index of medical care rose from 239.7 to 357.3 (1967 = 100), and the index of hospital room charges rose from 370.3 to 619.7. Though less dramatic, the same pattern of cost increases continued through the 1980s and into the 1990s. By 1994, Medicare Part A expenditures reached $104.5 billion, and Part B (supplemental medical insurance) added a further $60.3 billion to total federal outlays.

Responding to Medicare cost pressures, Congress in 1983 adopted amendments to the Social Security Act (PL 98-21) that jettisoned the old cost-plus reimbursement formula and created a prospective payment system setting standard charges, with rural-urban differentials, in twenty-three major diagnostic areas encompassing nearly 500 diagnosis-related groups (DRGs). The adoption of prospective payment was a critically important issue to Iowa hospitals, for which Medicare and Medicaid reimbursements in the mid-1980s accounted for some forty percent or more of revenues and most of which, designated as rural facilities, received the lower rural reimbursement rates.[8] For the long term, prospective payment was just as important as a precedent for other third-party payers, especially state agencies and private health insurers, which likewise became increasingly aggressive in unilaterally setting hospital reimbursement rates and negotiating discounts from standard charges. With increasing pressure on hospital reimbursements, the number of hospital beds in the United States fell 11.1 percent from 1980 to 1990 according to American Hospital Association figures; patient admissions declined 13.2 percent; hospital occupancy rates dropped 10.6 percent; and outpatient visits rose 40.0 percent.[9]

The appearance of a variety of alternative delivery systems constituted a second major institutional response to escalating health care costs. The health maintenance organization (HMO), for example, was initially a part of the Nixon administration's "national health strategy" announced in 1971.[10] Touted as a vehicle for the injection of market discipline into health care, the HMO concept in fact floundered in the 1970s, hindered in part by strict federal standards specified in the Health Maintenance Organization Act of 1973. The easing of operating restrictions in the late 1970s and, just as important, the endorsement of the HMO concept in the 1980s by major corporate payers anxious to pare the costs of employee health benefits breathed new life into the heretofore moribund HMOs, which blossomed aggressively in the latter part of the decade and into the 1990s. By 1987, some 700 HMOs provided benefits to thirty-one million enrollees drawn from nearly a quarter million employer groups, up from just 385 HMOs with fewer than seventeen million enrollees in 1984.[11]

A third major institutional response to escalating health care expenditures during the 1980s and 1990s was the expansion of for-profit health care enterprise. In the field of managed care, for example, Blue Cross/Blue Shield organizations took the early lead in establishment and operation of HMOs, but for-profit operators seized increasingly large market shares. As health care became a market commodity, hospital chains, hospital management companies, ambulatory care centers and the like expanded aggressively, setting in motion a wave of mergers and buyouts that led to significant vertical and horizontal integration of the health care marketplace. In Iowa, too, "the discipline of market forces" became a guiding principle behind the organization and delivery of healthcare services. In 1982, a Governor's Commission on Health Care Costs issued a lengthy list of recommendations, with primary emphasis on enhanced competition.[12] Noting that the present health care system lacked "controls to discipline performance," the commission endorsed "movement toward a competitive health care market" in which payers and providers negotiated coverage and reimbursement and in which alternative health care delivery systems played larger roles. In general, however, the restructuring of Iowa's health care economy lagged well behind the pace set in many other states, particularly on the east and west coasts. Still, the number of HMOs and their subscribers in Iowa grew substantially in the 1980s, with total enrollments jumping from virtually none in 1980 to some 141,500 in 1985, and to more than 300,000, or some ten percent of the state's population, in 1990.

At the same time, Iowa hospitals, like hospitals nationwide, saw patient admissions decline sharply, from 550,000 in 1981 to 385,000 in 1990, while the average hospital occupancy rate fell to 64.2 percent in 1991. At the University of Iowa Hospitals and Clinics, for example, patient admissions peaked at 40,669 in 1979 and fell to a low of 33,090 in 1988 before recovering to 37,073 in 1995. In the same period, total inpatient days trended steadily downward, falling from nearly 300,000 in 1983 to 234,592 in 1995. From 1985 to 1995, patients' average length of stay likewise declined, dropping from 7.04 to 5.85 days. As patient admissions to

Iowa hospitals dwindled, total outpatient visits rose dramatically, from just under 2.5 million statewide in 1981 to more than 4 million in 1990. At the University of Iowa Hospitals and Clinics, the number of outpatient visits surged from just over 318,000 in 1980 to more than 451,000 in 1990 and to nearly 530,000 in 1995. Together, the precipitous decline in patient admissions and the strong growth in outpatient numbers were symptomatic of the broader shift then underway in health care delivery patterns.

In 1987, the Iowa Board of Nursing established a 34-member Task Force on Statewide Planning for Nursing to survey the "future health care needs of the people of Iowa" and particularly to assess the role of the nurse in the provision of health care, the numbers of nurses needed, and the type, location, and number of nursing education programs. Released in 1988, the task force report addressed four broad areas of concern, from population health needs and nursing needs and resources to education and public relations.[13] The task force counted 26,245 licensed registered nurses in Iowa as of December 31, 1986. Of those, 4,458 held baccalaureate degrees, 14,754 held nursing diplomas, and 6,940 held associate degrees in nursing (the report listed 93 as "other"). The report also counted 12,672 registered nurses employed full-time and 8,338 employed part-time in nursing; another 483 were employed full-time and 388 employed part-time outside nursing. More than 14,000 Iowa registered nurses were employed in hospitals, more than 2,000 in nursing homes, and more than 1,400 in offices of health care providers. Nearly 4,000 Iowa registered nurses were not employed, either in or out of nursing, and an additional 117 were enrolled in baccalaureate or graduate programs.

The Iowa task force foresaw little change in the state's aggregate population in the years from 1980 to 2000; however, it forecast a 30.9 percent increase in the population seventy-five years of age and older and a 23.0 percent reduction in the 15-24 age group. Based on that demographic shift and on projected trends in health care, the task force anticipated a major shift in employment patterns for registered nurses by the year 2000, with the percentage of registered nurses employed in hospitals dropping from 66.0 percent to as low as 40.8 percent, while the percentage employed in nursing homes could rise from 8.0 percent to as high as 35.6 percent. Overall, the task force predicted that an existing shortage of registered nurses would become "more acute." With regard to education, the report recommended a nursing curriculum centered on critical thinking, problem solving, and organizational and leadership skills; a more flexible curriculum to allow adaptation to external changes and accommodate students' diverse schedules; and closer ties between education and nursing service and health care agencies.

In part because of the increasing utilization of outpatient services and the continued expansion of medical centers in some of Iowa's larger urban areas, overall staff numbers and budgets at Iowa hospitals continued to increase through the 1980s and into the 1990s. At the University of Iowa Hospitals and Clinics, full-time equivalent staff rose from just under 4,700 in 1982-83 to more than 5,700 in 1994-95, and the number of registered nurses rose from 1,151 to 1,560. Hospitals and Clinics total expenditures rose from $132 million to over $400 million during the same period, even as the number of patient beds dwindled from 1,029 to 845. Nonetheless, in late winter and spring 1996, Hospitals and Clinics officials announced the first significant retrenchment since the Depression years of the 1930s, aiming to trim costs by some $65 million over the course of five years largely through the consolidation of some clinical services, reductions in the number of patient beds, especially acute care beds, and the elimination of 200 or more staff positions, many of them in nursing.[14]

Across America, similar hospital staff attrition sparked significant dissent within the nursing profession, with some nurses demanding wholesale resistance to planned staff cutbacks. To make matters worse, a 1995 report of the Pew Health Professions Commission forecast a substantial decline in demand for health professionals in general and nurses in particular, leading the commission to recommend a ten to twenty percent reduction in the number of nursing education programs, these reductions to apply chiefly to associate degree and diploma programs.[15] Moreover, a National Research Council report released in January 1996 noted that hospitals' increased emphasis on cost-efficient care had led often to significant redesign of patient care services, especially nursing services, and to an even greater reliance on nursing assistants, in turn pushing higher-cost registered nurses from direct patient care to supervisory roles.[16] The Research Council report, however, observed that the proliferation of alternative home-based and community-based care systems had significantly changed the patient mix in the nation's nursing homes, increasing the proportion of patients with severe illnesses and creating a need, as yet unmet, for greater participation by nurse specialists and nurse practitioners in nursing home care.

In March 1996, the Division of Nursing of the Health Resources and Services Administration's Bureau of Health Professions counted more than 2.5 million registered nurses in the United States, with 82.7 percent, or just over 2.1 million employed in nursing.[17] Just 31.8 percent of employed registered nurses held baccalaureate degrees in March 1996, while 23.8 percent held hospital school diplomas and 34.6 percent held associate degrees. Hospitals employed nearly 1.3 million registered nurses, or 60.1 percent of the total of employed registered nurses. Various ambulatory care settings accounted for 8.5 percent of employed registered nurses, while 17.1 percent were engaged in some type of community or public health nursing, and another 8.1 percent were employed in nursing homes and other extended care facilities. Among advanced practice nurses, the Division of Nursing estimated some 54,000 clinical nurse specialists, 63,000 nurse practitioners, 30,000 nurse anesthetists, and 6,500 nurse-midwives. Those aggregate numbers reflected a substantial investment of Public Health Service funds in advanced nurse education programs since the mid-1970s,[18] an investment spurred, first, by the general emphasis on primary care that emerged in the 1970s and 1980s, especially concerns over the geographic distribution of primary care services and, second, concerted efforts at cost containment and the associated movement toward managed care.[19]

Not only did advanced practice nurses increase in numbers in Iowa and nationwide; they also sought wider practice authority. For example, nurse practitioners in Iowa were first understood as "physician extenders," scarcely different, that is, from physician assistants—dependent professionals who, under the direct or indirect supervision of physicians, could deliver primary care services at lower cost and could also deliver primary care to underserved populations, often in rural clinics. However, by the late 1980s and early 1990s, pressures from hospitals, HMOs, and other providers for more cost-efficient primary care boosted the professional agenda of Iowa's nurse practitioners and led in 1991 to passage of legislation

(S.F. 363) vesting duly certified nurse practitioners with authority to prescribe drugs in the areas of their specialty.[20] In testimony presented to the state Health Care Expansion Task Force that recommended passage of the enabling legislation, the Iowa Nurse Practitioners Association argued that current state law hindered nurse practitioners' potential and cited more than thirty states in which nurse practitioners already held such prescribing authority. By the mid-1990s, the Iowa Code also contained provisions mandating that third-party carriers include coverage for "necessary medical or surgical care and treatment provided by...an advanced registered nurse practitioner" when such care would be reimbursed if provided by a licensed physician.[21]

From 1980 to the mid-1990s, the demographics of nursing education nationwide continued some long established trends (Table 5.1). First, diploma programs continued their historic slide, dropping in numbers, admissions, total enrollments, and graduates. In the thirteen years from 1980 to 1993, national diploma enrollments fell by 45.8 percent and graduates by 46.2 percent. In the same period, the number of diploma programs in Iowa fell from nine to five, and enrollments diminished to just 888 in 1993. Second, associate degree programs, despite a slump in the middle and late 1980s, maintained an overall strong rate of growth, with enrollments rising 46.0 percent and graduates 54.6 percent from 1980 to 1993. By the latter year, Iowa counted twenty-three associate degree programs, with total enrollments of some 2,300. Third, total enrollments and graduations at America's baccalaureate programs suffered a serious decline in the middle and late 1980s and had, by 1993, barely recovered to levels of the early 1980s. In Iowa, the twelve baccalaureate programs in operation in fall 1993 enrolled 1,308 students and had awarded 304 degrees in the previous year. Finally, practical nursing programs across America, like associate and baccalaureate programs, saw a decline in enrollments and graduates in the middle and late 1980s, with a slow recovery in the early 1990s. In Iowa, however, numbers for practical nursing enrollments and graduates fell less dramatically and recovered more rapidly than the national average, nearly doubling in the ten years from 1984 through 1993.

In contrast to the boom-and-bust cycle in undergraduate education, the 1980s and 1990s saw an explosion in graduate education in nursing. In 1973, according to National League for Nursing tabulations, eighty-six master's degree programs had enrolled some 6,800 students; by 1983, 154 programs enrolled over 18,000 students; and, by 1993, 252 programs counted a total of more than 30,000 students. In those two decades, the number of master's graduates rose from 2,430 to nearly 8,000. Behind the remarkable increase in aggregate numbers of students and graduates lay an equally important trend toward part-time study. As more and more nurses combined full- or part-time employment with the pursuit of graduate education, the proportion of full-time master's students fell from 61.3 percent in 1973 to just 24.8 percent twenty years later. As a result, total enrollments grew more than four times over that twenty-year period, but the number of full-time students increased by just

TABLE 5.1. US Basic and Practical Nursing Enrollments and Graduates, 1980-81 to 1996-97[a]

	Associate Degree		Diploma Nursing		Baccalaureate Degree[b]		Practical Nursing	
	Enroll-ments	Graduates	Enroll-ments	Graduates	Enroll-ments	Graduates	Enroll-ments	Graduates
1980-81	94,060	36,712	41,048	12,903	95,858	24,370	52,565	41,002
1981-82	100,019	38,289	41,009	11,682	93,967	24,081	55,024	43,299
1982-83	105,324	41,849	42,348	11,704	94,363	23,855	57,367	45,174
1983-84	109,605	44,394	42,007	12,200	98,941	23,718	55,446	44,054
1984-85	104,968	45,208	37,256	11,892	95,008	24,975	48,840	36,955
1985-86	96,756	41,333	30,179	10,524	91,020	25,170	39,345	29,599
1986-87	89,469	38,528	22,641	8,272	81,602	23,761	38,510	27,285
1987-88	90,399	37,397	18,927	5,938	73,621	21,504	40,035	26,912
1988-89	95,986	37,837	18,860	4,826	70,078	18,997	42,808	30,368
1989-90	106,175	42,318	20,418	5,199	74,865	18,571	46,720	35,417
1990-91	117,413	46,794	21,969	6,172	81,788	19,264	52,749	38,100
1991-92	123,816	52,896	22,905	6,528	90,877	21,415	56,762	41,951
1992-93	132,603	56,770	23,252	6,937	102,128	24,442	59,095	44,822
1993-94	137,300	58,839	22,235	7,119	110,693	28,912	61,007	45,083
1994-95	135,895	58,749	19,796	7,049	112,659	31,254	59,428	44,234
1995-96	135,235	56,641	16,479	5,703	109,505	32,413	56,028	—

[a] Fall enrollment figures.
[b] Basic students only
Source: National League for Nursing

eighty percent, and graduations lagged well behind growth in total enrollments. The growth in doctoral education in nursing was even more striking. From 1973 to 1993, again according to NLN figures, the number of nursing doctoral programs increased from eight to fifty-four, and total enrollments rose from 375 to 2,751. Unlike the case in master's programs, the proportion of full-time doctoral students held nearly steady, standing at 42.9 percent in 1973 and 39.7 percent in 1993.

Several factors drove the expansion in nursing graduate education. First, graduate education became more accessible not only because of the rapid growth in the number of sponsoring institutions but also because of the opening of new educational venues, including satellite programs that catered directly to practicing nurses. Second, the trend toward increasingly specialized care in hospital settings on the one hand and the increasing reliance on alternative modes of health care delivery on the other fostered demand for advanced practice nurses. Third, the demand for nursing faculty in institutions of higher education continued its longterm growth pattern. A 1983 study counted just over 9,500 faculty in accredited baccalaureate and graduate programs, 80.5 percent holding master's degrees and only 16.1 percent holding doctoral degrees, and the study's authors reported the need for nearly 3,500 additional doctorally prepared faculty over the next five years.[22]

In February 1996, the Iowa Board of Nursing Examiners counted 10,315 diploma nurses, 11,059 associate degree nurses, and 7,950 nurses with baccalaureate degrees (6,106 of those BSNs) licensed and resident in the state. At last count, then, baccalaureate nurses still made up just 27.1 percent of all licensed registered nurses in Iowa, while diploma and associate degree graduates accounted for 35.2 percent and 37.7 percent respectively. The census of Iowa nurses holding graduate degrees in 1996 was quite small: 705 with master's degrees in nursing and an additional 611 with master's degrees in other fields; just sixteen with doctoral degrees in nursing and 124 with doctorates in other fields. All told, nurses with graduate degrees made up only 5.5 percent of all registered nurses in Iowa. The count of advanced practice nurses was similarly small, totaling 464 in November 1995, the largest number of those, 157, certified nurse anesthetists.

Baccalaureate Education at the University of Iowa

The early 1980s brought strong growth in undergraduate enrollments at the University of Iowa College of Nursing (Table 5.2), the figure peaking at 646 in 1984-85. The last half of the decade, as was true across the nation, saw a sharp enrollment decline, the total bottoming at 320 in 1988-89 prior to a significant recovery in the early 1990s. In fall 1980, the college's enrollment report classified 76.7 percent of students as Iowa residents; the undergraduate student body included just four ethnic minorities: one African-American, one Native American, one Asian-Pacific Islander, and one Hispanic-American. In addition, the college enrolled three foreign students, all of them female. In comparison, Iowa residents made up 82.1 percent of fall 1990 nursing enrollments. Minority enrollments, 3.2 percent of the total, included three African-American students, five Asian-American students, and three His-

TABLE 5.2. University of Iowa College of Nursing Baccalaureate Enrollments and Degrees, 1980-81 to 1996-97[a]

	Sopho-mores	Juniors	Seniors	Not Classified	Total	Male/Female	Degrees
1980-81	34	206	274	5	519	37/482	198
1981-82	38	187	289	3	517	31/486	205
1982-83	62	181	267	4	514	25/489	193
1983-84	21	182	272	2	477	23/454	145
1984-85	84	229	331	2	646	38/608	193
1985-86	30	198	315	1	544	31/513	205
1986-87	13	168	321	3	505	27/478	217
1987-88	12	143	244	1	400	18/382	178
1988-89	9	99	210	2	320	21/299	137
1989-90	6	123	204	3	336	23/313	130
1990-91	13	117	213	0	343	18/325	129
1991-92	21	109	239	1	370	17/353	132
1992-93	10	117	276	0	403	31/372	175
1993-94	16	110	281	0	407	40/367	158
1994-95	16	116	297	1	430	39/391	197
1995-96	13	140	303	0	456	42/414	192
1996-97	14	111	292	0	417	32/385	190
1997-98	21	127	274	0	422	39/384	—

[a]Enrollment figures are for fall semester.
Source: "Comparative Enrollment Reports," The University of Iowa Office of the Registrar.

panic-American students. Enrollments in 1990 also included six foreign students, one male and five females. Fall 1994 minority enrollments—one African-American, one Native American, five Asian-Pacific Island, and four Hispanic-American—remained at eleven, representing 2.6 percent of the overall student body. The numbers of BSN degrees conferred by the college followed fluctuations in enrollments, falling from a high of 205 in 1981-82 to a low of 129 in 1990-91 before recovering to 197 in 1994-95. By the end of the 1995-96 academic year, the college had awarded 6,516 BSN degrees since the first graduating class of 1952.

During the 1980s, male enrollments declined at a faster rate than did total enrollments; males made up 7.1 percent of the undergraduate student body in 1980-81 and just 4.5 percent in 1987-88. However, male enrollments, too, recovered in the early 1990s, reaching 9.1 percent of the total in 1994-95, in part the result of an active recruitment campaign. Overall, at least based on scanty student testimony, public reaction to male nurses and male nursing students had changed little since the early 1970s, with friends, family, and patients expressing surprise that males would make such a career choice. Nonetheless, Marilyn Molen, then assistant dean for the graduate program, noted in 1982 that nursing had apparently become "more palatable for men," and she also noted increased interest in clinical nursing on the part of male nursing students, a change from previous years when most male students sought administrative positions after graduation.[23] By the 1990s, male enrollments nationwide reached ten percent, driven, according to testimony in a 1992 *New York Times* report, mostly by rising salaries.[24]

In spring 1982, the College of Nursing published returns from a questionnaire mailed to 1,037 bachelor's degree students graduated since 1975.[25] All in all, those returns suggested a decided turnaround in graduate nurses' career patterns. Of the 574 respondents, more than ninety-two percent were then employed in nursing, three-fourths of those in full-time positions. Seventy percent of responding graduates were engaged in hospital nursing, sixty-eight percent of those as staff nurses. Twenty-seven nurses, or 4.8 percent, had attained master's degrees in nursing; and twenty-eight percent were members of the American Nurses Association. Former students, by and large, strongly endorsed the undergraduate program. Respondents expressed overwhelming satisfaction with their preparation in nursing theory, nearly ninety-six answering "yes" to that survey item; nearly the same proportion, 86.4 percent, responded positively to questions regarding problem solving and critical thinking skills acquired during their undergraduate years. In contrast, 32.4 percent expressed dissatisfaction with their preparation for initial nursing practice, and 41.6 percent faulted their preparation for a specific career area. In addition, a discouraging one-third of all respondents said that they would not choose nursing as a career again.

From the 1950s, the college had considered the education of registered nurse students an important part of its mission, and such students had made up a significant, if varying, part of the student body over the years. In the 1980s and 1990s, the college continued to offer graduates of diploma and associate degree programs the opportunity to obtain the baccalaureate degree both in residence and via satellite programs. Under the auspices of the Iowa Board of Nursing, the original College of Nursing articulation program became the Iowa Articulation Plan for Nursing Education in 1990, aimed at graduates of the state's associate degree programs and five remaining diploma schools. For students satisfying basic science and general education requirements, the college offered a one-year plan of full-time study for completion of the BSN. Although the proportion of registered nurse students on campus dropped to historic lows in the early 1980s, just 0.6 percent of all undergraduates in the fall of 1983, focused recruitment efforts pushed enrollments steadily upward in the early 1990s, the total rising from eleven in fall 1990 to twenty-eight in fall 1995. In addition, the college's satellite education programs became a major part of the articulation effort; by the 1990s, the BSN Degree Completion Satellite Program afforded registered nurses the opportunity to complete the baccalaureate program at three satellite locations using the facilities of the Iowa Communications Network, the state's publicly-financed fiber optic network. Initially, the College of Nursing's outreach efforts roused some objections from the state's other baccalaureate nursing programs, where administrators feared an adverse impact on their own residential and satellite programs.[26] Nonetheless, extension enrollments rose steadily, from five in fall 1986 to twenty-five in fall 1995.

In its basic nursing program, the college offered both four-year (Figure 5.1) and four-and-one-half-year plans of study, the latter assigning students slightly lighter academic loads in most semesters. Overall, in the words of a 1990 college self-study report, the undergraduate nursing curriculum embodied the concept of nursing "as a process directed toward maintaining, attaining, and regaining the health of individuals and groups," with particular attention to the health-illness continuum, growth and development, basic human needs, coping-adaptation, and the nursing process.[27] While that language held echoes of the original 1974 process curriculum, there were significant curriculum changes in the 1980s and the 1990s, changes reflecting shifts both in the health care environment and in the knowledge base of nursing. For example, the addition of a gerontology focus in the late 1980s was driven in part by faculty research interests and in part by the health care needs of Iowa's still significantly rural and increasingly elderly population. Similarly, a shift toward community-based instruction and a lengthening of the clinical component of undergraduate education was another product of the evolving health care market, specifically the diminished reliance on hospital care. In much the same way, the demands of the marketplace in league with advances in health care technologies and nursing research led to heightened emphasis on the utilization of communications and information technologies throughout the curriculum and led also to establishment of an Office of Information and Communication Technologies under the direction of Joann Eland.[28]

A 1994 report assessing progress toward goals in the College of Nursing's most recent five-year strategic plan reiterated much of the above.[29] The report cited growth in the nursing honors program, with an emphasis on research and writing and a variety of enhancements to clinical instruction, including development of "computer simulations to enhance the quality of undergraduate clinical instruction," extension of the senior clinical experience from four to nine weeks, and organization of a technology learning laboratory. In addition, the report cited an ongoing summer cooperative education clinical internship available to high-achieving students and the incorporation of a semester-long intensive clinical internship into the student's final clinical nursing course.

Fig. 5.1. Fall 1995 Basic Nursing Curriculum: 4-Year Model

Freshman Year (College of Liberal Arts)

First Semester	Semester Hours	Second Semester	Semester Hours
Rhetoric	4	Rhetoric	4
Animal Biology	4	Microbiology	4
General Chemistry I	3	General Chemistry II	3
Psychology	3	Sociology	3
Electives	2	Electives	3
Total	16	Total	17

Sophomore Year

Third Semester		Fourth Semester (College of Nursing)	
Anthropology	3	Foundations of Nursing Practice	7
Human Development & Behavior	3	Foundations of Nursing Practice: Clinical and Technical Skills I	2
Physiology	3	Professional Nursing: An Overview	
Nutrition	3	Pathology	4
Anatomy	4		
Total	16	Total	16

Junior Year

Fifth Semester		Sixth Semester	
Nursing Practice in Acute Illness	7	Nursing Practice in Chronic Illness	7
Nursing Practice in Acute Illness: Clinical and Technical Skills II	2	General Education Requirement (Humanities)	3
General Education Requirement: (Historical Perspectives)	3	Intermediate Pharmacology	3
Electives	3	Electives	3
Total	15	Total	16

Senior Year

Seventh Semester		Eighth Semester	
Nursing Practice in Health Promotion	7	Leadership, Management, and Research in Nursing Practice	8
General Education Requirement (Statistics)	3	Historical/Philosophical/Social Foundations	3
Electives	6	General Education Requirement (Foreign Civilization & Culture)	3
		Electives	3
Total	16	Total	17

The increased emphasis on outpatient, clinic, and home health care on the one hand coupled with the *de facto* conversion of hospitals into complex critical care units on the other hand created special problems for nursing educators. The fact that nursing education had originated in the hospital and had, for much of its history, retained a hospital orientation meant that it had evolved as a relatively centralized, highly structured, and closely supervised educational program. However, the shifting locus of health care in the 1980s and 1990s made it more and more difficult to maintain consensus on the core elements of a basic nursing curriculum. That was particularly the case in the area of clinical instruction, where trends in health care led back into the community-based settings characteristic of much of actual nursing practice into the 1930s. While such trends heightened the importance of nurses' care-giving skills and carried the potential of more professional autonomy, they also raised important issues for nurse educators regarding appropriate types of student experience and appropriate means of student supervision. By the mid-1990s, the University of Iowa College of Nursing offered a menu of clinical experiences spanning a range of career possibilities. In 1995-96, some ninety-eight agencies in nearly three dozen Iowa counties provided resources for undergraduate clinical instruction; in addition, the college listed 130 adjunct faculty and 289 staff nurses serving as clinical teaching assistants for nursing students (Figure 5. 2). It should be noted, however, that seventy-nine percent of recent graduates in a 1996 survey were employed in acute care nursing, with just six percent in home health care and five percent in ambulatory care.[30]

The college's 1996 operating plan pinpointed several areas of concern with regard to the undergraduate curriculum, concerns related to the dynamic nature of the health care environment. The plan highlighted the need to provide nurses "a solid foundation in the basic sciences," "a comprehensive series of courses to develop psychosocial, analytical, and communication skills," "a thorough introduction to human values and ethics, as well as health regulation and health law," and "a pragmatic, hands-on extended practice experience to develop the problem-solving logic and dynamics of all of the above." More specifically, the plan focused on the importance of information systems, communications technologies, and

Fig. 5.2. Clinical and Instructional Locations, 1995-96

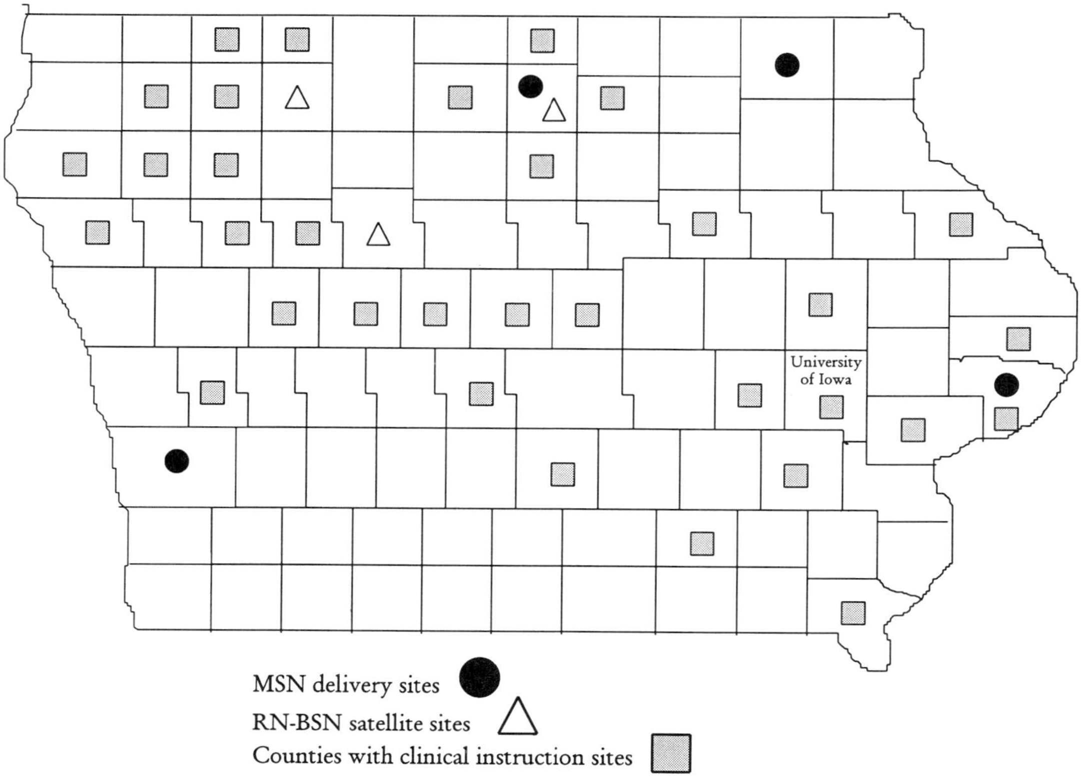

medical devices in contemporary nursing practice and, therefore, the need to keep the curriculum abreast of developments in those areas. However, not just at the University of Iowa but elsewhere as well, creeping specialization—and subspecialization—within nursing practice led many to wonder if the BSN would not soon become, much as the MD, merely a preparatory step for advanced training prior to practice.[31] In 1979, the Frances Payne Bolton School of Nursing of Case Western Reserve University, under the leadership of University of Iowa School of Nursing graduate Rozella Schlotfeldt, instituted a three-year nursing doctorate, a program that had the additional advantage of accommodating students with varied undergraduate backgrounds.[32]

By most measures, the 1980s and 1990s saw improved quality in the undergraduate student body at the University of Iowa College of Nursing. From the mid-1980s to the mid-1990s, applications ran well ahead of admissions, and the ratio of fall admissions to applicants ranged from a low of forty-nine percent in 1994 to a high of seventy-three percent in 1988, with an average near sixty percent. To recognize and encourage academic performance, the college instituted an honors program in fall 1986, requiring a cumulative grade point average of at least 3.25 in all courses and 3.50 in nursing courses. Overall, the college's graduates routinely outpaced statewide and national performance on the NCLEX-RN licensing examination.

The level of professional interest among nursing students—a subject of some concern in the 1960s—showed a noteworthy increase from the 1970s to the 1990s. Membership in the Association of Nursing Students grew, as did the number and scope of chapter activities. Likewise, membership in Gamma chapter, Sigma Theta Tau International, mushroomed at the rate of sixty to eighty per year, with inductees selected from among students and leaders in the local nursing community. In 1993-94, Gamma chapter's total active membership reached 772. Chapter members continued a scholarship program begun in the early 1970s and in the early 1980s also revived a research award program that had briefly fallen dormant, providing small seed grants to nurture the research efforts of students and faculty. From the early 1980s, Gamma chapter and the Association of Nursing Students were joint sponsors of an annual Progressive Nursing Day addressing a broad range of issues in nursing.

Graduate Education

The 1980s and 1990s brought a striking expansion in applications and enrollments in the College of Nursing's master's program. Total enrollments rose from 113 in fall 1980 to 167 in 1985, to 203 in 1990, and to 256 in 1994. In fall 1994, graduate students accounted for 37.3 percent of the total nursing student body. As was the case nationally, much of the enrollment increase came in the ranks of part-time students, many of those served through satellite and outreach efforts. The college's graduate programs attracted proportionately fewer males than did the undergraduate programs, and that proportion dropped significantly with the growth in total graduate enrollments, falling from 6.2 percent in 1980 to 3.5 percent in 1994. Spring 1995 minority graduate enrollments included three Asian/Pacific Islanders, one black, one native American, and four foreign students—a total of 3.5 percent in all categories. Reflecting the increasing proportion of part-time students and also paralleling national trends, the numbers of master's degrees conferred rose more slowly than did aggregate enrollments, rising from twenty-eight in 1980-81 to forty-two in 1994-95. At the end of the 1995-96 academic year, the college had awarded a total of 976 master's degrees since the inception of graduate education in the 1950s.

In the 1980s, the college augmented the three areas of specialization implemented in 1978—child health nursing, adult health nursing, and community health nursing—with two new offerings, gerontological nursing and anesthesia nursing. The college also added a joint MBA/MA degree to its graduate offerings in 1990, a program conducted jointly with the College of Business Administration and requiring sixty-seven semester hours of credit in business and nursing. By the mid-1990s, then, the College of Nursing master's program offered preparation for advanced practice nursing, nursing education, and nursing administration in the five clinical nurse specialties. In addition, the college offered graduate education at the Quad-Cities Graduate Center in collaboration with the University of Illinois and Bradley University and, beginning in 1994, offered master's degree core courses via the Iowa Communications Network to centers in Bettendorf, Mason City, and Council Bluffs.

Implementation of the long-discussed doctoral program was the most important single innovation in graduate education at the University of Iowa College of Nursing during the 1980s and 1990s. Although local skeptics questioned the quality and value of nursing research in general and the college's readiness to support doctoral education in particular, the doctoral program in nursing was, in the eyes of its promoters, necessary to attract resources, students, and faculty to the College of Nursing and to make the college a major center for nursing education and research. A 1985 feasibility study prepared by associate professors Laura Hart and M. Patricia Donahue along with William L. Holzemer, associate professor at the College of Nursing, University of California-San Francisco, assessed both the need for a doctoral program in Iowa and the College of Nursing's resources for such a program.[33]

At the time of the feasibility study, there were just thirty-one nursing doctoral programs in operation across the nation. Likewise, there were just fifty-three nurses in the state of Iowa known to hold doctoral degrees, twenty-seven of those on the University of Iowa College of Nursing faculty, while the study's authors projected a need for 300 or more doctorally prepared nurses in Iowa by 1990. In short, according to the report, "projected need for doctorally prepared nurses continues to exceed the current capacity of nursing programs." Moreover, the report argued that the College of Nursing commanded the resources necessary to sustain a viable doctoral program, most importantly, a cadre of doctorally-prepared faculty with ongoing research programs, solid publication records, and a history of success in attracting external research funding. Finally, a survey of college alumnæ suggested the existence of a large pool of potential doctoral students.

Instituted in 1988 after a three-year struggle to win university approval, the University of Iowa's program, leading to the doctor of philosophy in nursing, paralleled the ambitious nationwide expansion in doctoral education in nursing. From the outset, the University of Iowa program offered concentrations in nursing administration and gerontological nursing (Figure 5.3), areas reflecting the well-established research programs and influence of key senior faculty in the college as well as the dean's conviction that the college must focus its resources in limited areas in order to achieve a desired level of excellence. Aiming at students seeking "careers as researchers, college and university faculty members, consultants, and as leaders in the nursing profession, in health policy-making agencies, and in health care delivery systems," the program's formal requirements included common core courses comprising thirty-six semester hours, coursework totaling twelve semester hours in either the aging or administration area, written comprehensive examinations, and twelve semester hours of dissertation credit, culminating in the finished dissertation and oral defense. In the 1990s, reflecting the increasingly important function of computerized information in nursing, coursework in the doctoral program also included inten-

Fig. 5.3. Doctoral Degree Requirements, 1994-95

Core Requirements		Semester Hours
96:300	Classics in the Social Evolution of Modern American Nursing	3
96:340	Nursing Theory Construction: I-II	6
96:310	Nursing and Health Information Systems	3
96:320	Economics of Health Care Policy	3
96:330	Nursing's Role in Health Care Policy	3
	Cognate Minor Courses	9
	Cognate Research Sequence: research methods and statistics	9
96:490-491	Research Practicums	0
Total		36

Aging Focus		
96:410	Nursing Research of Biological Phenomena and Interventions for the Elderly	3
96:420	Geriatric Mental Health Research	3
96:430	Nursing Research in Sociocultural Phenomena and Interventions for the Elderly	3
96:440	Research Utilization Residency in Care of the Elderly	3
Total		12

Nursing Administration Focus		
96:450	Research Seminar in Nursing Administration I: Organizational Systems Concepts	3
96:451	Research Seminar in Nursing Administration II: Health Care System Concepts	3
96:460	Innovations in Nursing Management	3
96:480	Residency in Nursing Service Administration	3
Total		12

sive coverage of information systems and data management. Enrollments in the doctoral program grew rapidly, rising from seven in fall 1988 to twenty-eight in fall 1993. The university awarded the first four doctoral degrees at the spring 1992 commencement. By 1996, the program—then one of fifty-four in the United States—had graduated fourteen doctoral students.

The nursing service administration focus, culminating in the PhD, of course represented the third reincarnation of nursing service administration at the College of Nursing. Its revival in the 1980s was part of a national trend that owed much to the increasing administrative and managerial complexities in health care, increasing cost pressures throughout the health care system, and the availability of federal funding for graduate programs in nursing administration. At the same time, it also owed much to local circumstances. When Joanne Comi McCloskey, currently one of two University of Iowa Foundation Distinguished Professors in Nursing, came to the College of Nursing faculty in 1981 from the University of Illinois-Chicago, just one graduate level course remained from the nursing service administration graduate major initiated and sustained by Eva Erickson from the mid-1960s to the late 1970s. Possessing, by her own admission, only limited background in the area, McCloskey consented to take over that course. By the fall of 1983, she was teaching two administration-related courses, Nursing Administration: Process and Strategies and Leadership in Nursing Theory and Application.

Spurred by graduate student interest in administration and leadership topics, McCloskey pushed over the years for additional courses and faculty, and nursing service administration, under the rubric of organizations and systems, emerged as one of four initial areas of concentration in a 1984 faculty reorganization discussed below. In her subsequent role as area chair, McCloskey held significant administrative authority over teaching assignments and hiring, first bringing Myrtle Kitchell Aydelotte back to the college and then adding Meridean Maas to the group. In subsequent years, McCloskey and her colleagues pursued federal program grants, which financed, among other things, the Nursing Administration Laboratory housing an expanding inventory of administration-related resources. Above all, the group defended nursing service administration against critics both inside and outside nursing, the former arguing, as they had traditionally done, that on-the-job administrative training was sufficient and the latter arguing that nursing administration duplicated programs already available in the College of Business and in the Graduate Program in Hospital and Health Administration.[34]

In 1987, the college formally reintroduced a nurse manager focus to the master's program, but it was the implementation of the doctoral program that provided the critical resources for the growth of nursing service administration at the master's level, helping to create a consolidated research focus in the area and also attracting both graduate students and faculty. By the 1990s, the college offered three options in nursing service administration at the master's level. The first of those was the Nurse Clinician/Manager track, a forty semester-hour program for students primarily interested in clinical specialization but seeking a secondary focus in nursing administration; the second was the Nurse Manager track, also a forty-semester hour program, for students desiring greater depth in the administration area; and the third was the Nurse Executive/MBA conducted jointly with the College of Business and initially funded by a grant from the Commonwealth Fund. In 1996, the college added a fourth option in nursing informatics.

The second focus of the doctoral program, gerontological nursing, also had a significant history at the College of Nursing, although less convoluted than was the case with nursing service administration. Since the undergraduate curriculum revision of the 1970s, nursing faculty had sought to integrate gerontological nursing content throughout the undergraduate program, in keeping with the increasing national attention to gerontological health care and Iowa's large and growing elderly population. In 1974, undergraduate teaching faculty began to conduct health screening clinics for ambulatory elderly in response to a need for clinical experience in health assessment for nursing students. Faculty conducted three to four clinics each semester in small towns, and students in their first semester of clinical coursework made physical assessments of an average of thirty to forty patients at each clinic. In the late 1970s, the College of Nursing also became actively involved in the university-wide initiatives in aging studies, and nursing faculty in 1982 approved and implemented a separate nursing elective, "Introduction to Gerontology." In addition, a resequencing of undergraduate courses in 1987 shifted the well-elderly screening clinics to the fourth semester of clinical coursework, affording students extended and intensified experience in the area.

The College of Nursing gradually added gerontological offerings to the graduate curriculum, developments linked to the demonstrated importance of gerontological issues in Iowa and to expanding faculty interest in gerontological research centered around the work of Toni Tripp-Reimer and Kathleen Buckwalter. In April 1988, the University Graduate Council approved the addition of a gerontological nursing track to the master's program. In fall 1993, the gerontological faculty conducted a survey of all community health agencies and longterm care facilities in Iowa and found heavy demand for gerontological nurse practitioners (GNP). Fifty-three community agencies and eighty-eight long term care facilities indicated a preference for hiring or contracting with a GNP within the next five years.; sixty-five of those agencies indicated that they would provide support for nurses in their agency to attend a GNP training program. In response to that survey, the gerontological nurse practitioner program began in fall 1994, and its first graduates completed their study in the summer of 1996.

Much as was the case with the graduate programs, the College of Nursing's continuing education offerings expanded significantly in the 1980s and 1990s. At the same time and in part because of state-mandated continuing education requirements, the assessment of continuing education needs in nursing became more formalized, involving input from the deans of the other health science colleges, from nursing staff of the University of Iowa Hospitals and Clinics, and from other sources around the state. The college's continuing education offerings included the continuation of some existing topical conferences and also the inauguration of several new conference series. The 1996-97 schedule, for example, besides a number of nursing seminars scheduled throughout the academic year, included the twenty-second annual school nurse conference, the eleventh annual traumatic brain conference, the ninth annual occupational health nursing conference, the twelfth annual gastroenterology nursing conference, the seventh annual longterm care conference, and the ninth annual clinical nursing conference. In addition, the College of Nursing, in conjunction with the Iowa City Veterans Affairs Medical Center and the University of Iowa Hospitals and

Clinics, maintained a technology laboratory open to students and all Iowa nurses for instruction in the appropriate use of current health care technologies, ranging from drugs to information systems to medical devices. As had always been the case, participant fees contributed the bulk of continuing education funding. In 1989-90, for example, fees accounted for ninety-four percent of the funding for thirty-seven programs that attracted more than 2,500 nurses. Meanwhile, extramural funding for continuing education varied widely from year to year, ranging from a low of just over $38,000 in 1982 to a high of more than $227,000 in 1987. In 1990, for the second time, the American Nurses Association Regional Commission on Accreditation awarded six years' accreditation to the College of Nursing for its continuing education program.

Administration, Faculty Development, and Research

Geraldene Felton assumed the deanship of the University of Iowa College of Nursing in 1981. Born in Norfolk, Virginia, and growing up in Philadelphia, Felton remembered her choice of a nursing career as a simple one. To be a nurse was, she said in a 1996 interview, the "only thing I ever wanted to be."[35] However, when Felton graduated from Philadelphia's Girls High School in the 1940s, career options were not so straightforward for young African-American women as that comment might suggest. A self-described "good student" in high school, Felton found that the University of Pennsylvania had filled its minority quota, and she enrolled instead in a diploma program at a Philadelphia hospital. Supported by the Cadet Nurse Corps in her last year of nursing school, Felton joined the US Army Nurse Corps upon graduation and, after orientation at Fort Sam Houston in San Antonio, Texas, and an initial assignment to a military hospital in Michigan, eventually was posted to a Mobile Army Surgical Hospital unit in Korea. The MASH units, as Felton remembered them, included a sizable female officer contingent and made up close-knit communities united around a common aim, remarkably free of the race and gender divisions so prevalent in American society at large in the late 1940s and early 1950s. Overall, the dean recollected, she had "never felt more like an American" than during her wartime field assignment.

After a yearlong tour in Korea, Felton moved to a staff nursing assignment in Japan and then to the nurse anesthetist program at Fitzsimmons Army Hospital in Denver, Colorado. Later taking reserve status, Felton enrolled at Wayne State University and received her BSN in 1960. School, she recalls, was "like eating peanuts," so enjoyable that she received her MSN, also from Wayne State University, two years later. Returning to active Army duty, Felton was back in school within a few years, this time at New York University, where she received her EdD in 1969 from the Department of Nursing Education. From there, she went to Hawaii where she organized a master's degree program in nursing at the University of Hawaii before a posting to Walter Reed Army Medical Center as deputy director of the Walter Reed Institute of Research, Department of Nursing, and as adjunct faculty member at the Georgetown University School of Nursing.

Felton resigned from the Nurse Corps in 1975, having, she felt, "outgrown" the Army and the sometimes frustrating constraints inherent in the military system. Ready for new challenges, Felton at first contemplated a less structured and perhaps more leisurely lifestyle as a research consultant, and, indeed, then and later, she served in a variety of consultant capacities to several institutions and agencies. However, she noted, too, the extraordinary number of vacant deanships in colleges of nursing and felt an obligation to make some larger contribution to the profession, which led in turn to the nursing deanship at Oakland University in Rochester, Michigan, where she oversaw the creation of a new baccalaureate nursing program, a program that she led for nearly six years.

Asked why, under the unhappy circumstances prevailing in 1981, she chose to accept the deanship at the University of Iowa College of Nursing, Felton responded that she did so "because of the challenge." For its part, the university's central administration, which appears to have given the new dean its unwavering support, chose Felton as much for her leadership experience and her nononsense approach to administration as for her lengthy resumé of research, publication, and professional offices. Confident in Felton's abilities and concerned for the future of nursing education at the university, administrators gave the new dean a relatively free hand in reshaping the college.

Felton set out immediately to reform the college's working environment. Her first step was to destroy the documentary record of the college's recent problems, a disconcerting decision to historians but an important symbolic act meant to focus attention on the future rather than the past. Felton insisted on orderly administrative procedures grounded in clear, written rules. In addition to administrative mechanics, the dean sought, in her words, to instill a "commitment to quality and excellence" in the College of Nursing,[36] a commitment grounded on the creation of a network of scientists and scholars linking the college to the university and to the larger world of nursing scholarship, all the while maintaining the excellence in teaching for which the college had been rightly noted since its creation. Given the college's limited resources, Felton focused her efforts on the development of promising younger faculty and on the recruitment of new faculty with solid research credentials, who could serve as role models for others. Realizing also that the college could not "do everything," Felton instituted a focused approach to research, concentrating attention and support in the two principal areas, nursing service administration and gerontological nursing, mentioned earlier.

In March 1982, the College of Nursing submitted to University of Iowa President James O. Freedman a five year strategic plan.[37] The nursing faculty, the report declared, must present the image of "an ethical, accountable, scholarly collective," with a keen appreciation of the content and goals of instruction and with an appreciation, too, that "research is an exciting and valuable professional activity." The image of academic idealism, the report warned, could not be sullied "without a catastrophic effect." The report then outlined several "shifts in priorities" set in place over the course of the previous year, including the implementation of a computer literacy program affecting both instruction and administration, the revision of faculty performance guidelines, and the strengthening of undergraduate, graduate, and continuing education efforts. For the future, the report recommended continued fine-tuning of undergraduate and graduate curricula, recruitment of "a faculty of quality, educational excellence, academic distinction and diversity," pursuit of extramural support for research and instruction, and closer integration of the college with the community of practicing nurses.

The new dean's firm goals and equally firm administrative style met with some resistance. In May 1983, just one month after settlement of the last of the court cases arising in 1979, press reports surfaced once again describing problems within the college, reports centered chiefly on charges of faculty harassment, violations of privacy and academic freedom, and copyright infringement. Significant though it was, this affair differed from the 1979 blowup in two key dimensions. First, it was far more limited in scope, involving grievances filed by a small number of faculty—"more than one but less [sic] than twelve," according to one press report and "one or two," according to the university administration.[38] Second, a good many faculty expressed frustration and embarrassment at a renewed public airing of dirty linen and, at a special faculty meeting, a sizable majority voiced their support for the current administration. At the same time, university administrators, most notably Vice President for Academic Affairs Richard Remington, charged that the local chapter of the American Association of University Professors exacerbated the situation through its "unbalanced investigation" of affairs in the college, and Remington decried claims by the AAUP chapter chair that matters in the College of Nursing had achieved "crisis proportions."[39]

The limited public record of those events began with May 1982 discussions surrounding the appointment of a new nursing faculty member at the rank of full professor with tenure.[40] Strongly recommended by the dean, approved by a vote of sixteen to zero among tenured professors and associate professors in the College of Nursing, and reflecting the urgent need to recruit qualified doctorally-prepared faculty, the appointment prompted objections from two faculty members who had abstained from the voting on the basis that the appointment had not received a "careful, thoughtful review" based upon "sound information."[41] The two then carried their concerns to a July meeting with university President Freedman centered on "the procedures and standards being used in appointments to the College of Nursing" and, more broadly, "the climate in the College."[42] Subsequently, conflict broadened to include grievances regarding teaching assignments, salary increments, the handling of grant money, and alleged misuse of intellectual property. Moreover, after extended but apparently inconclusive correspondence with various officers of the university administration, matters culminated in one faculty member filing suit in September 1984 against the dean, a former assistant dean, the university president, the vice president for academic affairs, and the State Board of Regents.[43]

An August 1983 informal report on the College of Nursing commissioned by Vice President Remington and submitted by Samuel C. Patterson, a professor of political science, provided an unusually blunt assessment of affairs in the college.[44] Assigned "to look into allegations which have been made, to recommend procedures to handle such complaints and allegations in the future, and to report findings from the inquiry to the Office of Academic Affairs," Patterson's direct and sometimes brutal review of the documentary and oral record led him to two broad conclusions. First, he noted that there were indeed significant problems "of policy and procedure" in the college, especially problems relating to the handling of intellectual property, privacy, and promotion and tenure decisions. "It behooves the Vice President for Academic Affairs and the College Dean," Patterson wrote, "to take necessary and effective steps to ameliorate the personnel problems involved here." Second and more important, Patterson returned again and again to what he at one point labeled the "long and tedious history" of "interpersonal problems" in the College of Nursing that he called "a distressing litany of incidents exhibiting considerable misanthropy, interpersonal distrust, lack of respect, petty behavior, bad judgment, infantile jangling, and, in general, an enormous waste of energies which ought to be channeled into productive scholarly activity." In tacit contrast to AAUP charges reported in the press, Patterson laid much of the blame on simple human failings which sometimes descended, he wrote, into an "incredible puerility in behavior."

In fact, the College of Nursing faculty and administration had taken significant steps to clarify many of the troublesome issues that had first surfaced in the 1970s and whose legacy had carried into the 1980s. In 1979, nursing faculty adopted new bylaws governing the College of Nursing faculty organization. The new bylaws defined two classes of members, voting members and voice only members, the former including instructors, assistant professors, associate professors, and full professors with primary appointments in the college. The new bylaws also established three councils—an academic council, a planning, development, and coordinating council, and a faculty welfare council, with the dean an *ex officio* member of each. In addition to the dean, an elected chair, five elected members, and two appointed members comprised the academic council, with responsibilities centered on the philosophy and objectives of academic programs, curriculum content and sequencing, and student affairs. Likewise, the dean, an elected chair, one tenured elected member, one non-tenured elected member, one elected member of instructor rank, and three elected at-large members constituted the faculty welfare council, its work focused on some especially sensitive areas, including recommendations regarding "guidelines, policies, and procedures related to faculty recruitment, selection, appointment, promotion and retention." Finally, the dean, an elected chair, four elected members, and the chairs of the academic council and faculty welfare council made up the planning, development, and coordinating council whose charge encompassed faculty development issues, promotion of the College of Nursing to external constituencies, and the scheduling of faculty organization meetings and the conduct of nominations and elections. Changes in the 1990s (Fig. 5.4) reduced the number of councils to two, a faculty council and an academic council, and added a dean's advisory group made up of the associate dean, three area chairs, the four office directors, the chairs of the academic and faculty councils, and the directors of nursing at the VA Hospital and the University of Iowa Hospitals and Clinics.

The college had also instituted more concrete promotion and tenure guidelines, specifying both academic credentials and expectations for research productivity. For instructors and lecturers, the new guidelines specified a minimum of a master's degree with an expressed commitment to research and an identified area of clinical interest. For assistant professors, the guidelines set the earned doctorate as the minimum credential, excluding appointments made prior to 1981, and required intramural or extramural support for a research product submitted to peer evaluation. For associate professors and full professors, requirements ratcheted upward accordingly. Appointment or promotion to the rank of associate professor hinged on the accomplishment of research that advanced the discipline, overall excellence in work, evidence of ongoing research productivity, and demonstrated ability to attract external research support, while appointment or promotion to the rank of professor required sustained scholarly activity and a combination of university, national, and international recognition for professional contributions.[45] By the early 1980s, then, the College of Nursing had, after much trial and tribulation, adopted essentially the same promotion and tenure requirements that applied elsewhere in the university.

Along with the promotion and tenure guidelines, the college administration, in consultation with the Faculty Welfare Council, instituted more detailed guidelines for faculty salary adjustments,

Fig. 5.4. College of Nursing Organizational Chart, 1995

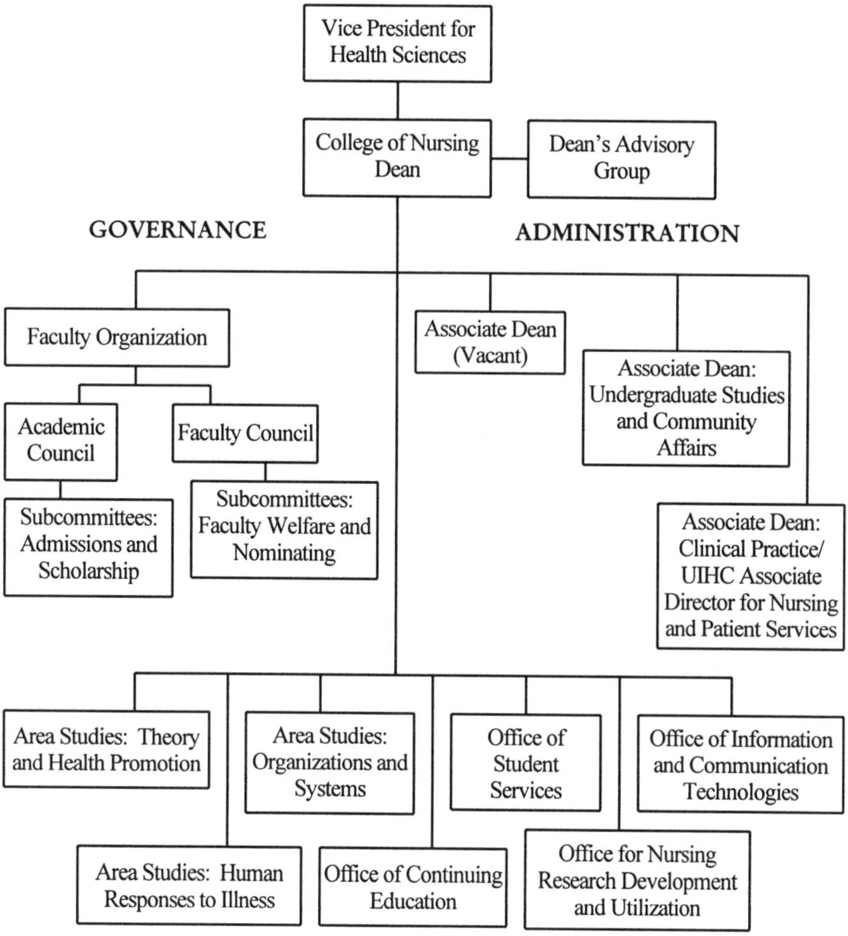

awarding salary increments on the basis of an overall performance score in teaching, service, and scholarship as determined by teaching peers, course coordinators, associate deans, and the dean. For faculty holding the doctorate, teaching counted for fifty percent of the total performance score, service for twenty percent, and scholarship for thirty percent. For faculty holding the master's degree, the respective percentages were sixty, twenty, and twenty. Finally, the College of Nursing, following the university's lead, also instituted formal evaluation procedures for administrators and the dean.

In addition, the college reorganized the teaching faculty in 1984 into "area studies groups." There were initially four areas—theory and methods, health promotion and maintenance, illness prevention and treatment, and organizations and systems. Later the number was reduced to three—theory and health promotion, human responses to illness, and organizations and systems. Aiming, in Dean Felton's words, to use faculty resources more "cost effectively" in the face of budgetary stringencies and to "better approximate the structure of nursing practices,"[46] the reorganization ended the longstanding distinction between graduate and undergraduate faculties and created a more supportive environment for junior faculty. Instituted in part at the suggestion of the university's central administration, the reorganization also shifted significant authority over hiring and teaching assignments, but not over budgetary matters, from the dean to senior faculty who served as area studies chairs. Finally, an Office of Continuing Education and an Office for Nursing Research Development and Utilization were also outgrowths of the 1984 reorganization.

Throughout the 1980s and into the 1990s, the college made significant improvements in the area of faculty development. In a 1982 self-study report to the National League for Nursing Board of Review for Baccalaureate and Higher Degree Programs, the college counted twenty faculty with doctoral degrees, either PhD or EdD. An additional ten faculty had completed doctoral coursework (ABD), and five more were involved in post-master's coursework. All told, thirty-five of seventy-nine total faculty, or 44.3 percent, in ranks from assistants-in-instruction—a category eliminated in 1987— to full professor either currently held or were actively pursing the doctoral degree. From 1985-86 to 1989-90, holders of the doctorate increased from 31.5 percent of total faculty numbers (28 of 89) to

49.4 percent, (39 of 79). More important and more striking was the college's ability to recruit doctorally prepared faculty at the assistant professor level, boosting the proportion of assistant professors with doctorates from eleven of twenty-two (50.0 percent) in 1985-86 to nineteen of twenty-six (73.1 percent) in 1989-90. In the latter year, twenty-eight of the thirty-nine doctorates among nursing faculty were awarded by the University of Iowa. Looking to the future, the college's 1989 strategic plan contained a pledge to "recruit, appoint, reward, and promote" faculty, including men and minorities, capable of earning "academic distinction."

By 1995-96, the college counted forty-three faculty with doctoral degrees out of a total faculty roster of seventy-two (59.7 percent). Thirty-five, or 81.4 percent, of those held doctoral degrees awarded by the University of Iowa. Among assistant professors, thirteen of nineteen (68.4 percent) held doctoral degrees, while eighteen of twenty associate professors did so. In the meantime, the college made modest progress toward ethnic and gender diversity within the faculty; in addition to one member in each of the African-American, Asian-Pacific Islander, and Native American categories, the faculty roster of 1995-96 included three males. By the mid-1990s, largely because of the heightened emphasis on research, the faculty had also undergone a *de facto* differentiation into a research-oriented, mostly tenure-track faculty group and a teaching-oriented, mostly non-tenure track faculty group whom the former, with obvious relief, often referred to as "worker bees." To further ensure faculty quality, the college in 1995 instituted "vitality" reviews every seven years for assistant and associate professors and every five years for full professors.

Faculty involvement in research and publication was one of the areas of greatest improvement in the 1980s and 1990s. In a 1985 article on the dean's role in the promotion of scholarship, Geraldene Felton noted that, in significant measure, "the excellence of our nursing college is defined by what we accomplish to advance knowledge," and the dean's role in that, as in other regards, was "essentially supportive and developmental."[47] However, Felton noted also that the dean's credibility in promoting research rested in large measure on her own research productivity. In a 1984 letter to university President James Freedman, Felton counseled that nursing research "must be defined broadly," and she referred to the definition formulated by the American Nurses Association Commission on Nursing Research (later, Cabinet on Nursing Research) which specified that "nursing research develops knowledge about health and the promotion of health over the full life span." Moreover, the ANA commission emphasized that nursing research was different from but complementary to "biomedical research...primarily concerned with causes and treatments of disease."[48]

An enlarged emphasis on research entailed a significant change in culture in the College of Nursing. One of the major issues in that regard was the apportionment of faculty time, which had traditionally been devoted overwhelmingly to teaching and related concerns. In October 1985, the College of Nursing's organizations and systems faculty held a debate on "working harder."[49] In general, faculty agreed that working harder, if it meant devoting more hours to the job, was not a feasible target. All seemed agreed, however, that "working smarter" was imperative if nursing faculty were to reconcile rising research expectations with increased educational demands, the latter of which would, if given free rein, absorb all available faculty time.

In 1980, the year prior to Geraldene Felton's arrival at the University of Iowa, the College of Nursing counted just under $10,000 in extramural research funding, a figure that rose to nearly $50,000 two years later. In 1984, extramural research funding jumped to $418,892, and through the remainder of the decade held in a range from $343,922 in 1986 to $615,047 in 1990. By the 1990s, nursing faculty were engaged in a variety of collaborative research projects with faculty from other colleges and departments, including anthropology, psychology, social work, medicine, and pharmacy, and the college's total research funding surpassed $1 million for the first time in 1993. The rapid rise in funded research paralleled a striking increase in grant submissions from an aggregate of $850,000 in 1983-84 to a high of more than $8 million in 1988-89. In both 1995 and 1996, total research funding exceeded $2.0 million. At the same time, faculty publications rose from forty in 1979 to 114 in 1990 and to 146 in 1994, while faculty presentations at national and international venues jumped from seventeen in 1980 to sixty-one in 1990 and to 101 in 1995.[50]

Behind the college's expanding research endeavor lay an increasingly sophisticated infrastructure of technology and programs.

Beginning in 1981, the college began a computerization program funded by a mix of federal grants, gifts, and university allocations. The college also instituted a program of summer developmental research fellowships for faculty in 1981, supplementing available university developmental programs. In addition, from 1984-85 to 1988-89, College of Nursing assistant and associate professors received more than $126,000 from National Institutes of Health Biomedical Research Support funds distributed by the university's vice president for educational development and research, a program superseded in the 1990s by a Central Investment Fund for Research Enhancement.

A growing roster of graduate student research assistants accompanied the increased focus on faculty research. The total of research assistant positions had risen from just seven in 1974-75 to nineteen already in 1980-81; by 1995-96, the college counted forty graduate research assistants. From the early 1970s to the 1990s, University of Iowa Graduate College allocations funded most research assistants, rising from $25,800 in 1980-81 to $66,150 in 1988-89 and held at just over $69,000 in 1995-96. Over time, however, the College of Nursing shouldered increasing responsibility for the funding of research assistants—thirty of the forty positions in 1995-96.

In 1984, as mentioned above, the college established an Office for Nursing Research Development and Utilization "to provide a structure and resource for faculty research and scholarship activities."[51] Early on, director Toni Tripp-Reimer and office staff focused much of their effort on procuring Division of Nursing postbaccalaureate training grants that supported several faculty in obtaining doctoral degrees. However, the office also began to nurture a research environment in the college, for example, conducting research-oriented seminars and encouraging travel to professional meetings as means to prepare faculty for research careers. In the late 1980s and 1990s, as the nursing faculty as a whole matured and especially as the college recruited more and more doctorally prepared junior faculty, the research office shifted more of its effort toward fostering research among younger faculty members, helping to plan longterm research programs, assisting in preparing grant applications, and holding mock peer-review sessions. All the while, the office provided varying levels of support for senior faculty, depending upon individual needs. In 1989, Dean Felton, Tripp-Reimer, and Sally Mathis, then Vice-President for Nursing Services at the University of Iowa Hospitals and Clinics, forged an agreement initiating a joint research office between the college and the UIHC Department of Nursing, with Kathleen Buckwalter as associate director. With the establishment of the doctoral program in the late 1980s, the Office of Research embraced broader programmatic goals, securing one five-year NIH institutional training grant for pre-doctoral students in 1990 (continued in 1996) and a second in 1995, making the college one of only two nursing schools in America to hold two such grants simultaneously.

Over time, much of the College of Nursing's research effort came to focus on two major initiatives. One of those was the Nursing Interventions Classification (NIC) project, aimed at developing a precise, standardized language to describe and catalog nursing interventions. The concept of a language of nursing was not new to the 1980s. Indeed, the University of Iowa College of Nursing curriculum committee had tried and failed in the late 1960s to compile a comprehensive list of nursing activities as a guide to curriculum design. In the 1980s, however, the concept of a taxonomy of nursing interventions emerged as a parallel problem to then ongoing discussion and work in nursing diagnoses, both areas—not coincidentally—of central importance in defining and justifying an autonomous nursing profession and in validating the work of nurses.

For a small core of University of Iowa faculty, the nursing interventions project grew directly out of their interest in nursing diagnoses and, specifically, their participation in the North American Nursing Diagnosis Association (NANDA). In 1982, the College of Nursing's Carolyn Crowell and Joanne McCloskey attended the Fifth National Conference of Nursing Diagnosis in St. Louis, an event that drew more than 160 educators and practitioners from across the United States and Canada. That 1982 conference, the expressed goal of which was "to identify diagnoses used in clinical practice in order to develop nursing's clinical science," focused on developing etiologies, defining characteristics of specific nursing diagnoses, and compiling a functional taxonomy.[52] By 1983, University of Iowa faculty had formed a "Nursing Diagnosis Interest Group" that embraced six subgroups assigned specific tasks or problems, one of which was "Developing Interventions for Specific Diagnoses."

Returning from a St. Louis NANDA conference in 1986, the University of Iowa group discussed creation of a taxonomy of nursing interventions to parallel the taxonomy of nursing diagnoses. Instigated by Joanne McCloskey and Gloria Bulechek, a small initial team of researchers from the College of Nursing and the University of Iowa Hospitals and Clinics held a series of meetings to explore the potential of the idea before beginning to develop a comprehensive classification of nursing interventions in 1987. Unlike the earlier work on nursing diagnoses, much of which was entirely new, the classification of nursing interventions drew upon on a rich collection of literature and experience in nursing, including existing practice activities and expectations as outlined in textbooks, nursing information systems, and the direct clinical experience of team members and survey respondents.

In 1990, the nursing interventions project won a three-year grant from the National Center for Nursing Research (now National Institute of Nursing Research), which supported an enlarged project team including a project assistant, research assistants, and consultants. By the mid-1990s, the Iowa Intervention Project team had attracted $1.7 million in funding, the bulk of that from the National Institute of Nursing Research. By the mid-1990s, too, the NIC project had spawned an impressive list of publications as well as a quarterly newsletter.[53] The results of phase one of the project—construction of a system of classification—appeared in 1992 under the title *Nursing Interventions Classification*, a compilation of 336 nursing interventions arranged alphabetically with bibliographies.[54] The results of phase two—construction of a taxonomy of interventions—appeared in 1996 as the second edition of *Nursing Interventions Classification*, a compilation of 433 numbered interventions organized in twenty-seven classes and six domains for convenience in clinical use and in computer data entry. In addition, the new taxonomy linked NIC interventions to NANDA nursing diagnoses.[55]

As work on nursing interventions progressed, faculty involvement widened and interests branched into related areas. In 1991, the original classification project gave rise to research into Nursing-Sensitive Outcomes Classification (NOC), headed by Meridean

Maas and Marion Johnson, a project that passed through similar stages of organization and development as had NIC. Aiming to provide a "comprehensive, standardized language and measurement for nursing-sensitive patient outcomes," the project's designers meant to link nursing interventions with specific patient outcomes. Eventually, a third component—the Nursing Diagnosis Extended Classification project, headed by Marsha Craft-Rosenberg and Connie Delaney and meant to update the NANDA classification system for nursing diagnoses—joined interventions and outcomes research. The combination of the three areas—diagnoses, interventions, and outcomes—promised to address the longstanding need for a reliable means to quantify the nature and worth of nursing practice. Eventually, too, work led by Delaney and Diane Gardner Huber on a nursing management minimum data set, modeled on the clinical minimum basic data set and designed to elaborate a set of nursing variables for routine collection at all health care institutions and agencies, grew out of the original NIC project.

Ultimately, the original work in nursing interventions classification came, in one way or another, to involve a majority of College of Nursing faculty. By the mid-1990s, classification research also drew increasing national attention, and several organizations, including the American Nurses Association, the Joint Commission on Accreditation for Health Care Organizations, and some health care agencies, approved NIC for a variety of uses. In addition, the International Council of Nurses integrated NIC into its International Classification for Nursing Practice (diagnosis and intervention), initial drafts of which were scheduled for circulation in mid-1997. In 1997, her decade of work on nursing interventions earned Joanne McCloskey the Sigma Theta Tau International Honor Society's Dorothy Garrigus Adams Award for Excellence in Fostering Professional Standards.

Those successes notwithstanding, continued dependence upon external funding in an era of federal budgetary cutbacks lent an uncertainty to the work, and participants sought a more permanent support structure. In late 1995, the State Board of Regents approved establishment of a Center for Nursing Classification Research in the college to house and support classification research and associated educational activities, the latter including Nursing Interventions, Outcomes, and Effectiveness predoctoral fellowships funded by the National Institute of Nursing Research. Simultaneously, the center's organizers created a fund-raising project to build a substantial endowment to ensure the center a permanent funding base.

The development of a research focus in gerontological nursing was in some respects similar to the case of nursing service administration. Most notably, gerontological research flourished initially on the efforts of a single faculty member, Toni Tripp-Reimer. At the outset, Tripp-Reimer, who holds a PhD in anthropology, approached gerontological research without specific prior training in the area; her interest in gerontological research flowed from her research into the influence of ethnic cultures in health care behaviors, a relationship most pronounced in elderly populations. In addition, the fact that Iowa's population had the third highest percentage of elderly over the age of sixty-five and the highest percentage of elderly over age eighty-five among the fifty states made gerontological research a good fit for the college and for the state.

Tripp-Reimer attracted the first College of Nursing research seed grants in gerontology during the late 1970s and early 1980s, with funds coming from the university-administered biomedical research fund, the American Nurses Foundation, and Sigma Theta Tau. In 1984, she received the first large federally funded grant in gerontological nursing research at the university, an award for the study of illness-related self-care responses among ethnic elderly. In subsequent years, Tripp-Reimer served three terms as chair of the university-wide Research Council, served continuously on the University Committee on Aging, served on the Executive Committee of the University Center on Aging, and chaired the external review committee of the University Aging Studies Program. At the same time, Tripp-Reimer earned a national reputation for her expertise in the combination of qualitative and quantitative research approaches and for mentoring other nurse scientists. From 1989 to 1992, she served on the NIH AIDS and Immunology Study Section and later on the NIH Nursing Research Study Section. She also served on the editorial boards of such journals as *The Gerontologist, Qualitative Health Research, Applied Nursing Research, Western Journal of Nursing Research*, and *Social Science and Medicine*.

At a slightly later date but in similar fashion, a doctoral focus in mental health and psychiatric nursing led Kathleen Buckwalter to gerontological research in Alzheimer's disease and related disorders as well as more general mental health concerns among the rural elderly. In 1983, Buckwalter received a three-year Geriatric Mental Health Academic Award, one of the first cohort of twelve fellows—eight psychiatrists and four psychiatric nurses—funded by the Mental Disorders of the Aging Research Branch of the National Institute of Mental Health. In the first year of her award, Buckwalter returned to full-time study in gerontology-related courses and earned a certificate in aging studies before devoting her second and third years to the development of graduate curricula and the selection of clinical research topics and sites throughout Iowa. Eventually, pilot studies of mental health issues at three sites led to larger externally funded projects.

By the mid-1990s, several nursing faculty were involved in major research and care programs dealing with gerontological issues. Meridean Maas, who joined the faculty after completion of her PhD in sociology and after many years' experience at the Iowa Veterans Home, became a key player in both nursing service administration and gerontological nursing, bringing to the college a combination of practical experience and skills in experimental design. In 1987, four college faculty—Tripp-Reimer, Buckwalter, Maas, and Rita Franz—formed a Gerontological Research Interest Group to critique gerontological nursing research proposals and manuscripts and to encourage research among junior faculty. With the advent of the nursing doctoral program and its concentration in gerontological nursing, the much-enlarged working group created a Gerontological Steering Committee to guide gerontological research and curricular development in the college. The Springer series of conferences in gerontological nursing initiated in 1992 was one product of the working group; a second was the development of the gerontological nurse practitioner program.

Alzheimer's disease also became a major focus of aging research in the college, including a National Caregivers Project led by Kathleen Buckwalter and directed at persons caring for victims of Alzheimer's and related disorders, a "Family Involvement in Care Study" led by Meridean Maas and Elizabeth Swanson and devoted to the study of interventions in Alzheimer's and other dementias, and a project funded by the National Institute on Aging targeting the dissemination of Alzheimer's-related information to rural health care practitioners. In addition, a university-wide strategic planning effort in 1989 led to establishment of the University of Iowa Center on Aging, with Donald Heistad of the College of Medicine as director and Buckwalter as co-director. In 1991, the center received an interdisciplinary training grant from the National Institute on Aging, which annually funded eight pre-doctoral and eight post-doctoral fellows. In 1995, Buckwalter became center director, with Heistad as co-director.

In the 1990s, the Office for Nursing Research and Development received a $1.7 million National Institutes of Health grant, most recently extended through 1999, to establish the Gerontological Nursing Interventions Research Center (GNIRC), with Tripp-Reimer as director and Buckwalter as co-director. Participating faculty's ongoing funded research in the field and demonstrated expertise in research training and research dissemination were principal factors in obtaining funding for the center, one of six focused research centers supported by the National Institute of Nursing Research, the only such center in the midwest region, and the only gerontological nursing research center in the nation. The center served a variety of research-related functions, including providing seed grants for research, conducting research training for faculty and graduate students, establishing collaborative links with faculty in the colleges of medicine, pharmacy, and liberal arts, and disseminating research findings to the scientific and practicing communities. The College of Nursing also sponsored four pre-doctoral and two post-doctoral fellows annually in a program entitled "Research Training in Gerontological Nursing," an effort funded by an Institutional National Research Service Award from the National Institute of Nursing Research.

College of Nursing faculty, including many of those involved in nursing service administration and gerontological nursing research, maintained research programs in other areas as well, including women's health issues, children's health, rural health concerns, management of pain in cancer patients, problems in nursing management and quality assurance in nursing practice, and the psychological and social ramifications of genetic testing. In addition, College of Nursing faculty collaborated on several research projects with staff of the University of Iowa Hospitals and Clinics Department of Nursing. Also, the dissemination of research findings to health care professionals and to patients and their families was, in the minds of most faculty, part and parcel of their research endeavors.

Through the 1980s and into the 1990s, increasing levels of College of Nursing faculty membership in professional organizations and honorary societies paralleled rising scholarly productivity. In 1988-89, 85.5 percent of nursing faculty were INA/ANA members; 19.7 percent were NLN members; 34.2 percent held memberships in the Midwest Nursing Research Society; 89.5 percent were Sigma Theta Tau members; 13.2 percent had been elected to membership in Sigma Xi, the honorary scientific research society; and 39.5 percent belonged to specialty organizations outside nursing. Moreover, at any one time in the late 1980s and early 1990s, at least five faculty participated as peer reviewers and as members of national research study sections. By 1997, the faculty included eleven Fellows of the American Academy of Nursing, including Geraldene Felton who was a 1973 charter fellow. Over the years, Felton's many professional offices included service as a member of the executive committee of the NLN Baccalaureate and Higher Degree Programs from 1983 to 1987, president-elect and president of the American Association of Colleges of Nursing from 1986 to 1990, first chair of the NIH Nursing Research Study Section from 1987 to 1991, and member of the National Advisory Council for the National Institute of Nursing Research from 1994 to 1998. After stepping down as dean of the college in January 1997, Felton became head of the National League for Nursing Accrediting Commission, the federally recognized accrediting agency for the nation's 1,655 nursing schools.

A few examples from a lengthening list of national and international nursing awards provide another measure of College of Nursing faculty development. In 1985, Myrtle Kitchell Aydelotte became an American Nurses Foundation Distinguished Scholar and was later named the first Sigma Theta Tau International Distinguished Fellow; in 1990, Joanne McCloskey joined the governing council of the American Academy of Nursing and in 1991 received the Midwest Nursing Research Society Distinguished Contribution to Research in the Midwest Award; in 1985, Toni Tripp-Reimer received the American Nurses Association Council on Cultural Diversity in Nursing Practice Award and in 1991 won the Elizabeth

McWilliam Miller Award for Excellence in Research from Sigma Theta Tau International; and, in 1985, Kathleen Buckwalter won the Region 2 Excellence in Research Award of Sigma Theta Tau and was elected to the Sigma Theta Tau International Research Committee in 1992. In the 1990s, both Buckwalter and McCloskey were selected as University of Iowa Foundation Distinguished Professors, and McCloskey and Tripp-Reimer received Iowa State Board of Regents Awards for Faculty Excellence.

By the 1990s, then, backed by rapidly expanding research programs and, to an increasing extent, by national reputations, College of Nursing faculty for the first time sat at the university table as the equals of faculty in other colleges and departments. Elizabeth Swanson's 1995 appointment as the university's associate vice president for health professions education, a position Swanson had held on an interim basis since May 1994, was a significant marker in that regard. In the wake of an administrative reorganization, Kathleen Buckwalter became the university's associate provost for health sciences in August 1997, with responsibility for academic programs in the health sciences and for advising the provost on the delivery of health care services.

Today's senior nursing faculty are acutely aware of the historical significance of the past decade's accomplishments for the college and for the nursing profession, noting that the successful faculty development efforts of the 1980s and 1990s marked the culmination of a struggle that began in 1949 and, against no small odds, extended through nearly four decades, interlaced at times with episodes of wrenching uncertainty and conflict. Moreover, senior faculty are aware, too, that, at least in most major respects, nurses' struggle for academic recognition at the University of Iowa College of Nursing embodied essential elements of the larger post-World War II history of nursing education in America.

Conclusion

With the convenience of hindsight, the history of nursing education at the University of Iowa lends itself to a simple, if somewhat arbitrary, four-part division, with due allowance for significant continuities from one period to another and, indeed, from the first period to the last. The first period, 1898-1949, extended from the turn-of-the-century opening of the University Hospital and its Nurse Training School—later the School of Nursing—to the establishment of the College of Nursing. The second period, 1949-1968, encompassed the critical formative years of the college, ending at a time when disparities between promotion and tenure practices in the College of Nursing and the rest of the university became acute. The third period, 1968-1990, was dominated by an occasionally acrimonious struggle to attain academic parity for the College of Nursing within the university. Finally, the fourth period, 1990 to the present, has been one of adaptation to environmental forces, most important the downsizing of government at both federal and state levels and the cost-driven reorganization of the health care system.

Early nursing schools like that conducted in the University of Iowa Hospitals were, for the most part, captives to the whims of hospital staff physicians and hospital administrators. The welfare of nursing students and an emerging nursing profession were, at best, secondary concerns, while the primary function of the hospital diploma school was to provide an inexpensive and dependable hospital workforce. Prior to the 1930s, when hospitals yet employed very few graduate nurses, the student nurse workforce was also a disposable one, cast for the most part into an uncertain future of private duty and public health nursing at the end of the three-year training program. Keeping in mind those inherent limitations, the University of Iowa School of Nursing was, by the 1930s, among the largest and best of its type, thanks to the exertions of a handful of dedicated nurses who became nurse-educators by necessity if not by training. Working within the confines of a male-dominated institutional setting, those leaders participated in the nationwide search to define and promulgate a professional identity for nurses and nursing, and they carved out a space in which young nurses learned professional ideals and essential leadership skills and in which nursing education began its slow integration into the university community.

The establishment of the University of Iowa College of Nursing in 1949 was part of a national trend toward baccalaureate education in nursing. While the founding of colleges of nursing constituted an essential first step toward a true nursing profession, one with command of its own educational and knowledge bases, the full realization of that goal was neither simple nor immediate. On the contrary, there remained a struggle for control over the nursing curriculum, perhaps best exemplified by the extended effort to extricate undergraduate nursing students from their hospital duties. There remained, too, a struggle for the resources to strengthen and extend nursing education at both undergraduate and graduate levels. Moreover, nursing's professional development hinged upon the much longer and more frustrating process of faculty development, the goal of which was the creation of a critical mass of appropriately trained nurse researchers and, in turn, a respectable body of peer-reviewed nursing research. Spurred by dedicated pioneers, nursing education made significant strides in several areas at the University of Iowa through the 1950s and 1960s, although faculty development clearly lagged well behind improvements in the quality of instructional programs. By the late 1960s, the gap between nursing faculty and their colleagues elsewhere in the university—measured in terms of academic credentials and research productivity—became a serious issue, prompting the university's central administration to grant the college the first of two exemptions from prevailing promotion and tenure guidelines.

In the years from 1968 to 1990, the College of Nursing came, however grudgingly at first, to face the issue of faculty development. When the college's initial five-year promotion and tenure exemption expired in 1973, the central administration, in the now famous "Vernon memo," extended the moratorium to 1980. In the meantime, however, nursing faculty as a whole made disappointingly little progress toward satisfying university promotion and tenure requirements. That was so for many reasons, including the extraordinary investment of time and energy in major revisions of both the undergraduate and graduate curricula, the lack of resources, both locally and nationally, to support faculty in obtaining doctoral degrees and to underwrite nursing research, the lack of a research culture and a deficiency of scholarly role models in the college, and, finally, increasing friction during much of the 1970s between the dean and a good part of the nursing faculty on a wide range of issues. Many observers, including some of the college's senior faculty, remain critical of the "Vernon memo" as well as Vice President May Brodbeck's initial 1979 decision to grant tenure at current rank to more than a score of nursing faculty, arguing that those expedients were, for the long term, a disservice to the college, calling into question the university administration's will to enforce its own regulations and, by implication, consigning the College of Nursing and its faculty to an inferior status within the university community.

Against that troubled backdrop, the 1980s brought what was perhaps an unexpectedly brisk turnaround in the fortunes of the College of Nursing. The foundations of that turnaround were many, not least the 1981 arrival of a new dean with an energetic agenda for the college, the recruitment of new faculty members with solid academic credentials and research potentials, and the concerted effort to instill a research culture in the college through various support mechanisms. By 1990, the college had emerged from its trials far stronger than ever before and no doubt stronger than most would have imagined during the uncertain times of the late 1970s. With its nationally recognized research programs and faculty, nursing had become a full-fledged academic discipline at the University of Iowa.

Events of the 1990s left faculty and administrators in the College of Nursing little time to celebrate their accomplishments, as the college has faced a new set of challenges posed by budgetary constraints and a fundamental restructuring of the health care system. In the name of cost containment, public and private third-party payers have implemented several variants of a basic managed care format in the 1990s, all of them centered on closely regulated access to health care services combined with greater utilization of clinic, outpatient, and home care services and fewer and shorter hospital stays. The managed care concept—in many respects a euphemism for managed access—threatened, for better or worse, the wholesale abandonment of much of what remained of the free-choice, fee-for-service principles that had long served as the foundations of American health care. It also threatened the tradition of cost-shifting upon which a good part of indigent care and health science education had rested in the post-World War II era.

While managed care came later to Iowa than to many other states, its effects were unmistakable by the mid-1990s; in 1996, after a decade of effort by a handful of the state's largest employers and strong endorsements from state commissions and agencies, more than half of Iowa's insured population was enrolled in managed care plans of one kind or another. In Des Moines, the state capital and the state's largest city, managed care plans covered nearly three-quarters of the insured population. The rapid shift toward managed care posed serious and immediate concerns for the nursing profession and especially for nursing education, both of which were, by tradition, heavily invested in hospital-based health care. For practicing nurses in Iowa as elsewhere, managed care often meant an aggressive downsizing of hospitals' professional nursing staffs and the increased utilization of nurse assistants, painful adjustments made worse by the routine exclusion of nurses from institutional planning. For the College of Nursing, Dean Geraldene Felton warned that changes in the health care environment necessitated "reforms in the kinds of practitioners we prepare, the skills and attitudes practitioners are taught, where health practitioners are trained, what services different health practitioners provide, and what research is most needed."[56] Under the circumstances, as one College of Nursing planning document phrased it, nurses must learn to "communicate, interpret, defend, and justify nursing practice to ourselves and others."[57]

Changes in nursing practice triggered an increased demand on educational resources at the College of Nursing, demand that outpaced the rate of growth of allocations from university funds in the 1990s. That shortfall forced the college to rely to an increasing—and increasingly worrisome—degree on other revenue sources, notably extramural grants and contracts, to underwrite research, instruction, and faculty development. From 1991-92 to 1995-96, university funds fell from 76.8 percent to 67.6 percent of the college's total funding base, leading, among other things, to a cut in full-time faculty slots from seventy-six in fall 1990 to sixty-eight in fall 1995, despite an increase in total undergraduate and graduate fall semester enrollments from 554 to 719. As a result, the college's fiscal year 1997 plan projected a cap on enrollment growth, setting goals of 350 basic BSN students, 60 RN-BSN students, 250 master's students, and 50 PhD students—a maximum enrollment of 710.[58]

Whatever the problems in adapting to a changing health care environment, nursing leaders at the University of Iowa and their colleagues across the nation also saw in the spread of managed care significant new opportunities for nurses' professional development. Nurses have long pressed claims for the efficacy of professional nursing care and have often touted nursing as "one of the best-kept secrets in health care," but their professional ambitions have foundered in part because of the lack of corroborating data and in part because of the lack of systemic pressures to entertain lower-cost alternatives to traditional hospital-centered and physician-controlled modes of health care delivery. The current combination of research into nursing diagnoses, interventions, and outcomes and the cost-conscious reconstruction of the health care market presents, in the eyes of some observers, including new College of Nursing Dean Melanie Dreher, constitute an unprecedented opportunity to bring nursing and the special talents of nurses into public view.

In response to changes in nursing education and practice, the University of Iowa College of Nursing had a faculty practice plan under active consideration by the mid-1990s. A faculty committee studied practice options, and the college sent representatives to the American Association of Colleges of Nursing Faculty Practice Conference in late winter 1996.[59] College of Nursing faculty already held adjunct appointments in the University of Iowa Hospitals and Clinics department of nursing, as they did also at various other local hospitals; however, nursing faculty and administrators saw a formal faculty practice plan as a way "to expand the potential roles that faculty members play" and "enhance the skills and contributions of faculty and strengthen the clinical experiences of students."[60] Grounded in part in the example of academic physicians whose mission, at least in theory, encompassed teaching, research, and direct patient service, the faculty practice concept would reintegrate nurse-educators in the clinical settings to some extent left behind in the move from diploma to baccalaureate programs a half century ago. Just as important, faculty practice would also afford academic nurses a means to define a space for nursing functions and within that space to address some of the salient issues affecting the profession at large, not least the stubborn problem of reimbursement for nursing services.

In May 1995, Geraldene Felton announced her intention to resign as dean of the College of Nursing, effective July 1, 1996. A nationwide search led to campus interviews of five candidates early in 1996 and to a June announcement of Melanie Creagan Dreher's appointment to the deanship, effective January 15, 1997, at which time Felton assumed the Kelting Chair in Nursing. Professor and dean of the University of Massachusetts School of Nursing since 1988 and also adjunct professor of anthropology, Dreher earned her BSN from Long Island University in 1967, a master's degree in anthropology from Columbia University Teachers College in 1974, and a doctorate in anthropology in 1977, also from Columbia University.   Dreher taught in the Division of Nursing, School of Health Sciences, at the University of Massachusetts from 1973 to 1976 and at the School of Public Health and School of Nursing at Columbia University from 1976 to 1983.   In 1984, she became dean and William R. Ryan Distinguished Professor in Transcultural Nursing Research at the University of Miami School of Nursing, positions she held until her departure for the University of Massachusetts in 1988.

During her career, Dreher was principal investigator on several community-based studies involving the health and development of women and children in Jamaica and, at the time of her appointment to the deanship at the University of Iowa, held a secondary appointment as professor of child health with the University of the West Indies Faculty of Medical Sciences.   Her research interests also encompassed cross-cultural studies of health care systems, the organization and financing of community health care, and the effects of substance abuse on health.   She was named a fellow of the Society for Applied Anthropology in 1987, a fellow of the American Academy of Nursing in 1988, Fogarty Senior International Fellow in 1993, and president-elect (1993-95) and president of Sigma Theta Tau International.   In addition, Dreher served on editorial review boards of journals in nursing, anthropology, and related fields.

Without question, the new dean assumed leadership of a college that was "complete in all its parts," possessed, by all accounts and by all measures, of caring and innovative faculty and staff, healthy research programs, a growing national reputation, and the enthusiastic support of thousands of alumni and friends who shared a commitment to the ideals of education, research, and service.   The support of alumni and friends, including their financial support, was essential in ensuring the college's viability over the years, and in 1995 the list of individual givers topped 1,400.   At the same time, the arrival of a new dean meant pervasive changes to the college, changes affecting administrative styles and policies as well as the college's broad range of educational and research programs.

Without question, too, the adaptation of nursing education to the demands of an evolving health care system presented the dean and the College of Nursing a stiff challenge; indeed, the nature and scope of nursing education were, for good reason, as intensely studied in the 1990s as at any time in the post-World War II era.[61] While observers differed over many key issues, including the fate of managed care and the prospect that physicians would reassert a significant measure of control over the provision of health care,[62] nurse educators sought nonetheless to accommodate their curricula to the likelihood of increasingly tight restrictions on hospital-based, high-technology health care, increased attention to preventive and ambulatory care, continued vertical and horizontal integration of the health care system, broader utilization of alternative delivery systems of whatever type, and a rapidly aging, multicultural population. More important, however, all hands agreed that the future of the University of Iowa College of Nursing, like its past, hinged most of all upon the unquestioned dedication of faculty and staff to their college, to their students, and to their profession.

Notes

1. See Arnold S. Relman, "The New Medical-Industrial Complex," *New England Journal of Medicine* 303 (1980), pp. 963-970.

2. Reporting on the effect of health care restructuring, particularly in hospitals, on the nursing profession and on the quality of care has been widespread; see, for example, Suzanne Gordon, "What Nurses Stand For," *The Atlantic Monthly* 279 (February 1997), pp. 80-82, 84-86,88; Laura Johannes, "On the Ward: Primary Nursing May Not Be Able to Survive the Push for Efficiency," *The Wall Street Journal* (Interactive Edition), October 23, 1997.

3. American Nurses Association press release, May 7, 1997.

4. See Ingeborg G. Mauksch, "Faculty Practice: A Professional Imperative," *Nurse Educator* 5 (May/June 1980), pp. 21-24.

5. Sara E. Barger and William C. Bridges, Jr., "An Assessment of Academic Nursing Centers," *Nurse Educator* 15 (March/April 1990), pp. 31-36. See also Barbara Murphy, ed., *Nursing Centers: The Time Is Now* (New York: National League for Nursing, 1995).

6. Geraldene Felton, "Preparation of Doctoral Students to Be Career-Minded Scientists and Scholars in Academia," p. 1, The University of Iowa College of Nursing Files.

7. Attributed to Ralph Nader in Starr, *The Social Transformation of American Medicine*, p. 400.

8. Iowa Hospital Association, *Iowa Hospitals: A Profile of Service, 1987*, p. 27.

9. American Hospital Association, *Hospital Statistics, 1992-93* (Chicago: American Hospital Association, 1992).

10. See Starr, *The Social Transformation of American Medicine*, pp. 396-398.

11. See *Marion Managed Care Digest, 1988* (Kansas City, MO: Marion Laboratories, Inc. 1988).

12. See Governor's Commission on Health Care Costs, "Final Report," 1982, pp. 9-10

13. Iowa Board of Nursing, Task Force on Statewide Planning for Nursing, *A Statewide Plan for Nursing*, 1988.

14. See, for example, "Whirlwind of Change Envelops University Hospitals," *The Gazette* (Cedar Rapids, Iowa), March 24, 1996.

15. Pew Health Professions Commission, "Critical Challenges: Revitalizing the Health Professions for the Twenty-First Century," November 16, 1995.

16. Institute of Medicine Division of Health Care Services, Committee on the Adequacy of Nurse Staffing in Hospitals and Nursing Homes, *Nursing Staff in Hospitals and Nursing Homes: Is It Adequate?* (Washington, DC: NRC, 1996).

17. Statistics are taken from "Advance Notes I" and "Advance Notes II" of the National Sample Survey of Registered Nurses, March 1996, Division of Nursing Worldwide Web site.

18. According to the Division of Nursing, federal funding under the Public Health Service Act for nurse practitioner and nurse-midwifery programs totaled more than $260 million from 1976 through 1996, with another $261 million invested in advanced nurse education—preparing nurse educators, public health nurses, and clinical nurse specialists—from 1975 through 1996.

19. See Loretta C. Ford, "Advanced Nursing Practice: Future of the Nurse Practitioner," in Linda H. Aiken and Clarie M. Fagin, eds., *Charting Nursing's Future: Agenda for the 1990s* (Philadelphia: J. B. Lippincott Company, 1992), pp. 287-299.

20. See *Iowa Code, 1997*, Chapter 147.107, "Drug Dispensing, Supplying, and Prescribing—Limitations."

21. See *Iowa Code, 1997*, Chapter 514C.11, "Services Provided by Licensed Physician Assistants and Licensed Advanced Registered Nurse Practitioners."

22. Evelyn Anderson, Patricia Roth, and Irene S. Palmer, "A National Survey of the Need for Doctorally Prepared Nurses in Academic Settings

and Health Service Agencies," *Journal of Professional Nursing* 1 (January/ February 1985), pp. 23-33.

23. "Males No Strangers to Nursing College," *The Daily Iowan*, March 30, 1982; "Clichés Don't Bother Nursing School Men," *The Daily Iowan*, December 13, 1984.

24. Peter T. Kilborn, "As Pay for Nurses Increases, So Does the Number of Men Entering the Field," *The New York Times*, November 29, 1992.

25. The University of Iowa College of Nursing, *Nursing News* (Spring 1982), p. 3.

26. See, for example, KF Langrock (Grandview College, Des Moines) to G Felton, May 11, 1983; JL Richards (Iowa Wesleyan University, Mount Pleasant) to G Felton, May 17, 1983; JV Stewart (University of Dubuque) to G Felton, June 2, 1983, Health, Box 6, JO Freedman Papers, 1982-83, The University of Iowa Archives.

27. College of Nursing, *Collegiate Review: Report of the Self-Study Committee, 1990*, College of Nursing Files.

28. A University of Iowa faculty member, Gloria Bulechek, was part of the National Center for Nursing Research ten-member expert panel on nursing informatics. The panel's March 1995 report, published under the title *Nursing Informatics: Enhancing Patient Care*, offered a detailed survey of the rapidly growing field as well as the panel's recommendations.

29. G Felton to JV Hinrichs, May 18, 1994, The University of Iowa College of Nursing Files.

30. The University of Iowa, *Parent Times* 40 (Fall 1996), p. 5.

31. The American Nurses Association's American Nurses Credentialing Center (ANCC) offered certification exams in more than two dozen specialty areas by the mid-1990s.

32. See Mary E. Duffy, "Innovation as a Survival Strategy," in *Patterns in Nursing: Strategic Planning for Nursing Education* (New York: National League for Nursing, 1987), pp. 53-56. By the 1990s, there were just two such nursing doctorate programs in operation, but nurse educators appeared more and more concerned over the adequacy of associate degree, diploma, and baccalaureate programs alike.

33. William L. Holzemer, Laura Hart, and M. Patricia Donahue, "Nursing Doctoral Education in Iowa: A Feasibility Study," The University of Iowa College of Nursing Files.

34. See, for example, Joanne Comi McCloskey, Diane Gardner, Marion Johnson, and Meridean Maas, "What Is the Study of Nursing Service Administration?" *Journal of Professional Nursing* 4 (March-April 1988), pp. 92-98; see, also, "The Iowa Model: A Proposed Model for Nursing Administration," *Nursing Economic$* 9 (July/August 1991), pp. 255-262.

35. Geraldene Felton interview with the authors, June 20, 1996.

36. Geraldene Felton to College of Nursing Faculty and Staff, March 6, 1981, The University of Iowa College of Nursing Files.

37. The University of Iowa College of Nursing, "Long Range Planning, 1982-87," March 1982, Box 6, 1981-82, JO Freedman Papers, The University of Iowa Archives.

38. "UI Nursing College Dispute Opens Old Wounds," *The Daily Iowan*, May 9, 1983; "Nursing Professors Vow Fight for Change," *Iowa City Press-Citizen*, May 9, 1983.

39. "Teachers, Administrators Trade Charges at U of I Nursing College," *The Register* (Des Moines), May 8, 1983; see also, Faculty Organization Minutes, May 6, 1983, Box 6, Health, 1982-83, JO Freedman Papers, The University of Iowa Archives.

40. See G Felton to K Moll, May 27, 1982, Health, Box 6, 1981-82, JO Freedman Papers, The University of Iowa Archives.

41. RJ McKeighen and BS Thomas to G Felton, June 3, 1982, Health, Box 6, 1981-82, JO Freedman Papers, The University of Iowa Archives.

42. R McKeighen and BS Thomas to G Felton, July 19, 1982, and R McKeighen and BS Thomas to JO Freedman, July 19, 1982, Box 6, 1981-82, JO Freedman Papers, The University of Iowa Archives.

43. *Barbara Thomas* v. *Geraldene Felton, et al.*, US District Court for the Southern District of Iowa, Davenport Division, No. 84-109-D-1.

44. Samuel C. Patterson, "Problems in the College of Nursing: A Report," August 1983, Box 6, JO Freedman Papers, 1983-84, The University of Iowa Archives.

45. "Collegiate Policies for Faculty Appointments, Evaluations and Promotions," Fall 1981, The University of Iowa College of Nursing Files.

46. Dean Geraldene Felton, quoted in "UI Nursing Faculty to Reorganize," *The Daily Iowan*, June 28, 1984.

47. Geraldene Felton, "The Deanship and the Promotion of Scholarship in Nursing," *Journal of Professional Nursing* 1 (January-February 1985), pp. 8, 65.

48. From G Felton to JO Freedman, May 15, 1984, "Recent Academic Achievements," Box 6, JO Freedman Papers, 1983-84, The University of Iowa Archives.

49. College of Nursing, *little f.y.i.*, January 31, 1986.

50. The University of Iowa College of Nursing, "Research and Scholarly Productivity, 1995"; College of Nursing Self-Study Committee, *NLN Self-Study Report, 1990*, Vol. I—Narrative.

51. College of Nursing Self-Study Committee, *National League for Nursing Self-Study, 1990*, Vol. II—Exhibits, p. 222.

52. The University of Iowa College of Nursing, *little f.y.i.*, April 23, 1982.

53. The University of Iowa College of Nursing Worldwide Web site contains a wealth of information regarding the NIC and the Center for Nurs-

ing Classification, including a bibliography of publications stemming from the research effort. The authors are also indebted to Joanne McCloskey for her personal recollections of the genesis and development of the classification project.

54. Joanne C. McCloskey and Gloria M. Bulechek, eds., *Nursing Interventions Classification* (St. Louis, MO: Mosby—Year Book, Inc., 1992).

55. Iowa Intervention Project, *Nursing Interventions Classification* (St. Louis, MO: Mosby—Year Book, Inc., 1996).

56. G Felton to JV Hinrichs, May 18, 1994, The University of Iowa College of Nursing Files.

57. The University of Iowa College of Nursing, *FY 1997 Process for Budget and Operating Plan*, p. 62.

58. *Ibid.*, p. 65.

59. *Ibid.*, p. 63.

60. The University of Iowa College of Nursing, *Strategic Plan, July 1995* (Revised October 1995), p. 7.

61. For an excellent overview of the current state of nursing education, its strengths and weaknesses, and recommendations for future development, see Myrtle Kitchell Aydelotte, "Nursing Education: Shaping the Future," *Charting Nursing's Future*, pp. 462-484.

62. On the fate of managed care, for example, see Eli Ginzberg and Miriam Ostow, "Managed Care A Look Back and a Look Ahead," *New England Journal of Medicine* 336 (April 3, 1997), 1018-1020; on the prospects of a resurgence of physician control, for example, see Robert Kuttner, "Physician-Operated Networks and the New Antitrust Guidelines," *New England Journal of Medicine* 336 (January 30, 1997), pp. 386-391.

Appendix A: Presidents of the University of Iowa and Directors of Nursing Education

Presidents of the University of Iowa

1855-1859	Amos Dean
1859-1862	Silas Totten
1862-1867	Oliver Spencer
1867-1868	Nathan Leonard (Acting)
1868-1870	James Black
1870-1871	Nathan Leonard (Acting)
1871-1877	George Thacher
1877-1878	Christian Slagle (Acting)
1878-1887	Josiah Pickard
1887-1898	Charles Schaeffer
1898-1899	Amos Currier (Acting)
1899-1911	George MacLean
1911-1914	John Bowman
1914-1916	Thomas Macbride
1916-1934	Walter Jessup
1934-1940	Eugene Gilmore
1940	Chester Phillips (Acting)
1940-1964	Virgil Hancher
1964-1969	Howard Bowen
1969-1981	Willard Boyd
1987-1988	Richard Remington (Acting)
1988-1995	Hunter Rawlings III
1995-	Mary Sue Coleman

Directors of Nursing Education

1897-1900	Jennie S. Cottell
1900-1901	Florence E. Brown
1901-1903	Susan G. Parrish
1903-1904	Antonia Epeneter
1904-1906	Bertha Wilkinson
1906-1907	Helen Balcom
1907-1912	Mary E. Nesbit
1912-1916	Josephine Creelman
1925-1926	Lois B. Corder (Acting)
1926-1928	Mae MacArthur
1928-1947	Lois B. Corder
1948-1949	Lola I. Lindsey
1949	Myrtle E. Kitchell

Appendix B: Deans of the University of Iowa College of Nursing

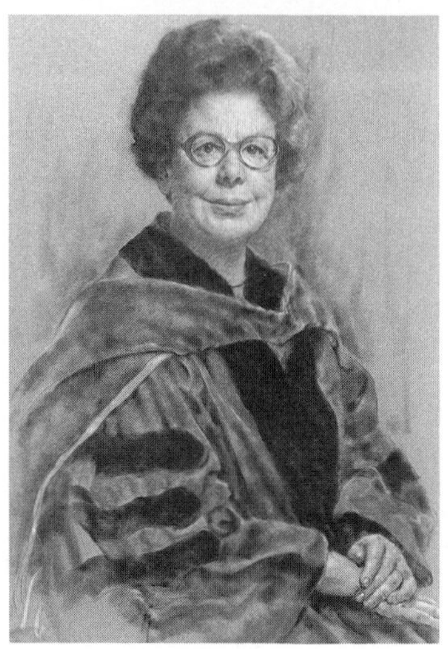

Dean Myrtle Kitchell Aydelotte
1949-1957
(College of Nursing Collection)

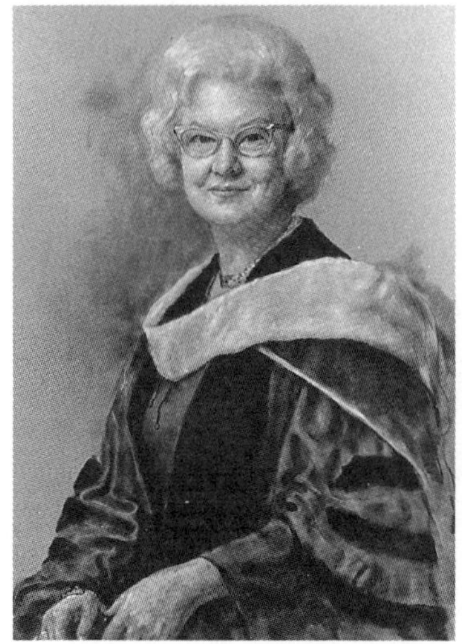

Dean Mary Kelly Mullane
1959-1962
(College of Nursing Collection)

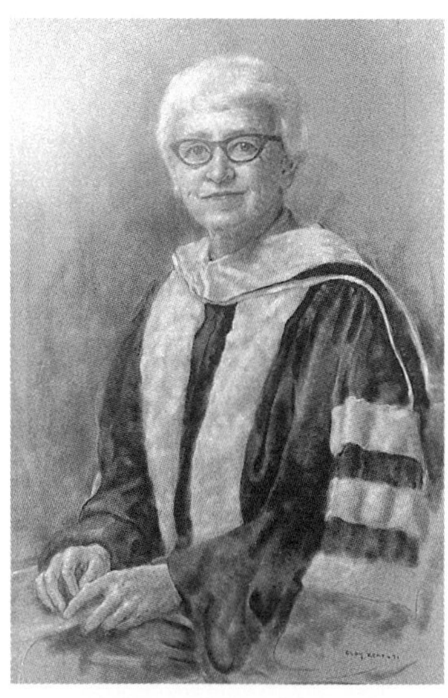

Dean Laura Corbin Dustan
1964-1972
(College of Nursing Collection)

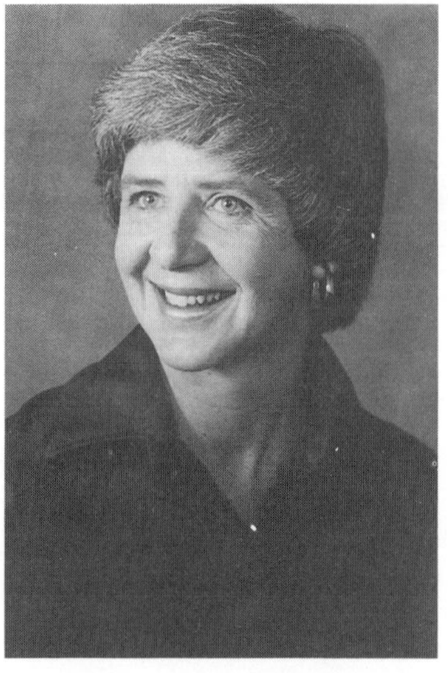

Dean Evelyn R. Barritt
1972-1979
(Courtesy of Evelyn Barritt)

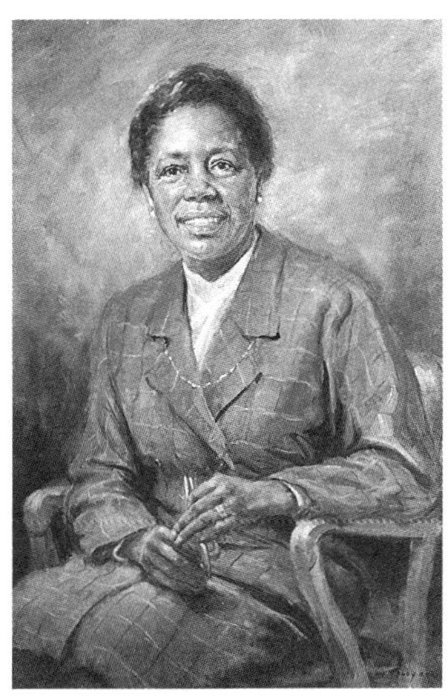

Dean Geraldene Felton
1981-1997
(College of Nursing Collection)

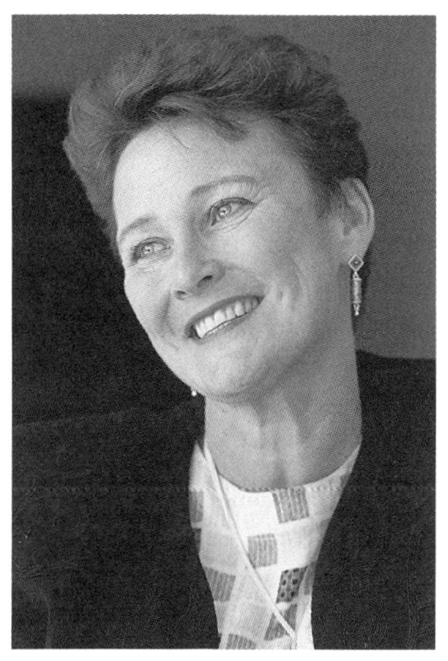

Dean Melanie Dreher
1997-
(University Relations News Services)

Interim Deans of the College of Nursing

1957-1959   Etta H. Rasmussen
1962-1964   Etta H. Rasmussen, Florence Sherbon, Marjorie Lyford
1971-1972   Etta H. Rasmussen
1979-1981   Sue R. Rosner

Appendix C: The College of Nursing Pin

Etta Rasmussen

The University of Iowa College of Nursing pin bears similarities—across time and culture—to the distinctive decorations and symbols worn by members of other groups sharing common backgrounds, achievements, and purposes. In Europe, for example, the system of heraldry stretches to the middle ages; in America, there is a long history of badges or pins associated with membership in lodges, clubs, fraternities, high school classes, and the like. It appears that the first nursing school pin was given to graduates of the Bellevue Hospital School of Nursing in 1880.[1]

In his history of the University of Iowa Department of Internal Medicine, Walter L. Bierring ascribed the turn-of-the-century Nurse Training School pin to a committee of three medical faculty: Lawrence Littig (Internal Medicine), Elbert W. Rockwood (Chemistry), and Bierring (Pathology and Bacteriology).[2] Although Bierring did not assign a specific date to the pin, Littig resigned in 1903, thus the pin presumably originated prior to that date. Also, a 1906 report of the university's Board of Regents noted that, in addition to monthly stipends, nursing students would receive "the pin."

The nursing pin is made up of three icons, each significant in its own right: the circle, the cross, and the laurel wreath. The circle symbolizes the cycle of life; the laurel symbolizes triumph and virtue; and the cross sysmbolizes compassion and understanding. Until 1964 the cross was in two colors, red for valor and gold for purity. Originally, the letters UHTS (University Hospital Training School) appeared on the arms of the cross, and the word IOWA appeared in the center of the cross. In 1952, alumnæ and student groups authorized change in the lettering from UHTS to SUCN, the latter for State University College of Nursing. Since 1965, when "State" was dropped from the university's name, the words UNIVERSITY OF IOWA COLLEGE OF NURSING appear in gold lettering on a black circular field around the cross. Also in 1965, when the manufacturer encountered increasing difficulty in producing a true color for the red, the pin was redesigned, preserving the cross and the surrounding laurel wreath and black field but with the red and gold motif changed to black and gold (the university colors).

Throughout its history, the distinctive School of Nursing/College of Nursing pin—samples of which are depicted below and on the facing page—has symbolized graduates' pride in the high standards of the nursing program.

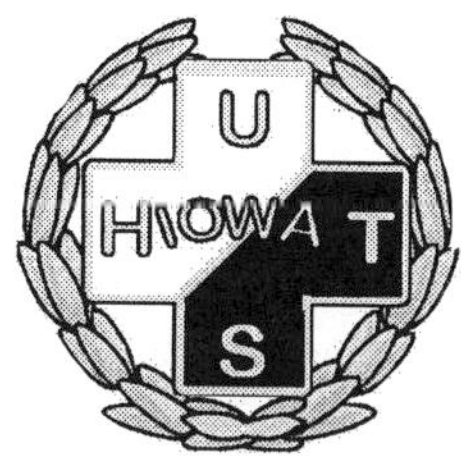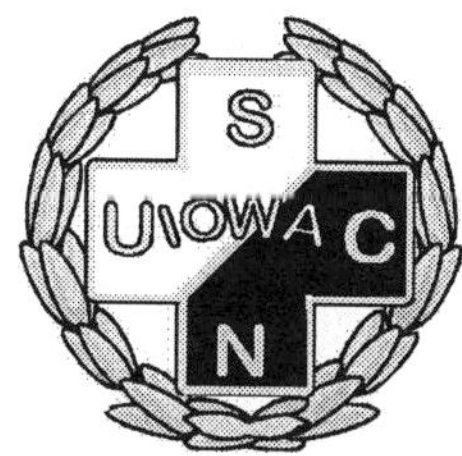

The pin on the left depicts the style prior to 1953; the one on the right was the style from 1953 to 1964. Both were 2 centimeters in diameter, with lettering, laurel wreath, and field outlines in gold, the upper left field of the cross in yellow enamel, and the lower right field of the cross in dark red enamel.

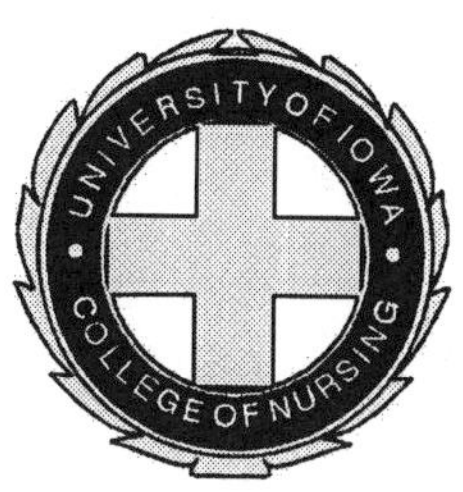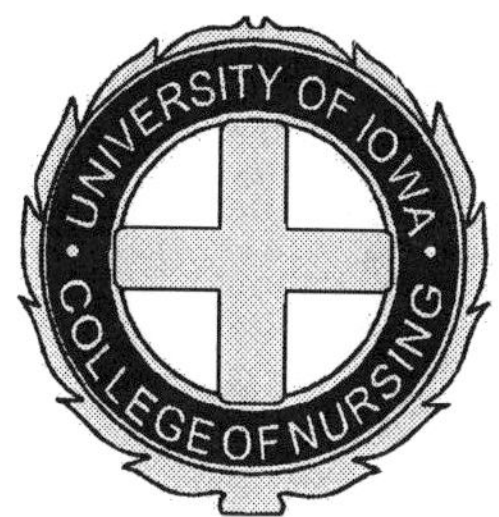

The pin on the left, used from 1965 to 1977, was 2.4 centimeters in diameter and slightly convex; the one on the right, used from 1977 to 1982, was 2.7 centimeters in diameter and flat. In both cases, the lettering, laurel wreath, and cross were gold, with black circular fields.

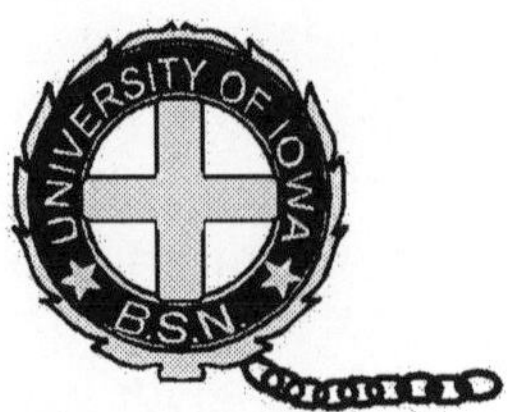

The pin above, used from 1982 to the present, is 1.6 centimeters in diameter, with lettering, laurel wreath, and cross in gold, and the circular field in black. A lightweight four-centimeter chain may attach the pin to an associate degree or diploma pin.

Notes

1. Further information on nursing school pins may be found in Lorraine J. Carbary's article in *RN* 34 (December 1971).
2. See Bierring, *A History of the Department of Internal Medicine, State University of Iowa College of Medicine, 1870-1958* (Iowa City, IA: State University of Iowa, 1958).

Index